The Spark Solution

THE
Spark
Solution

A Complete Two-Week Diet Program
to Fast-Track Weight Loss and Total Body Health

BECKY HAND, R.D., M.Ed.,
and
STEPFANIE ROMINE,
editorial director at SparkPeople.com

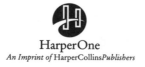

HarperOne
An Imprint of HarperCollins*Publishers*

HarperOne

This book is written as a source of information only. The information contained in this book should by no means be considered a substitute for the advice of a qualified medical professional, who should always be consulted before beginning any new diet, exercise, or other health program.

Grateful acknowledgment is given to the following photographers for the use of their work in this publication: color photo insert: Catherine Murray; pp. 247–51: Elliot Giles; p. 316: Catherine Murray; pp. 361–62: Malinda Hartong; p. 363: Arthur Cohen; p. 364: Jeffrey Hosier Photography

THE SPARK SOLUTION: *A Complete Two-Week Diet Program to Fast-Track Weight Loss and Total Body Health.* Copyright © 2013 by SparkPeople, Inc. All rights reserved. Printed in the United States of America. No part of this book may be used or reproduced in any manner whatsoever without written permission except in the case of brief quotations embodied in critical articles and reviews. For information address HarperCollins Publishers, 10 East 53rd Street, New York, NY 10022.

HarperCollins books may be purchased for educational, business, or sales promotional use. For information please e-mail the Special Markets Department at SPsales@harpercollins.com.

HarperCollins website: http://www.harpercollins.com

HarperCollins®, 📖®, and HarperOne™ are trademarks of HarperCollins Publishers.

FIRST EDITION

Designed by Terry McGrath

Library of Congress Cataloging-in-Publication Data
Hand, Becky.
The spark solution : a complete two-week diet program to fast-track weight loss and total body health / Becky Hand, R.D., M.Ed., and Stepfanie Romine, editorial director at SparkPeople.com. — First edition.
    pages cm
ISBN 978–0–06–222828–4
1. Reducing diets. I. Romine, Stepfanie. II. Title.
RM222.2.H2273 2013
613.2′5—dc23   2012046664

13 14 15 16 17 RRD(H) 10 9 8 7 6 5 4 3 2 1

To everyone who wants to finally take control of their lives and reach their biggest goals, the healthy way

Contents

Introduction

Chris "SparkGuy" Downie,
founder and CEO of SparkPeople.com

Meet Erin. She's thirty and lives in Florida. Happily engaged and recently promoted at work, she loves her life. She wakes up feeling great, rarely stops moving throughout her waking hours, and goes to sleep each night with a smile on her face. Life isn't perfect, but every day feels better than the last, she says.

Erin is so committed to this life that it's hard for her to remember what it was like before, when she weighed almost twice what she does now. When she had little energy to stay awake after work and all she wanted to do on her days off was sleep. When she was in excruciating pain from even the smallest physical efforts and walking around the block seemed like torture. When she looked in the mirror and didn't recognize the woman she'd become and didn't know how to change her life.

She wanted to marry the love of her life, raise babies together, and do all the fun things she could only watch from afar. When she moved to Florida from New York, she was excited about the year-round sun, access to the beach, and all the theme parks and outdoor festivals. But most of the time, she stayed inside or came home early because she was tired and in pain. Life was passing her by, and she felt helpless. Looking back now on the day she decided to change everything, it feels like a dream—a nightmare—but she's grateful for it. Looking back, the worst day of her life was also among the best, because it was the first day of the rest of her life.

The harness was stuck. No matter what she did, Erin couldn't fasten the safety belt around her middle. She held her breath, sucked in her stomach,

and tried wiggling in her seat. Her fiancé, JT, then tried, but to no avail. People were laughing and pointing, and the line was backing up. The roller-coaster operator came over to see what was wrong.

It was the day after Erin's longtime boyfriend had proposed to her, and they were at a Florida theme park to celebrate. The joy that hadn't left her face since he got down on one knee was replaced by fear and panic. Finally, it clasped.

Her humiliation turned to relief and then terror as the ride began. Was the harness secure? Would it hold her weight, or would she plummet to her death on what should have been a day of celebration? The ride lasted a mere three minutes, but every moment felt like an eternity. She held her breath, gripped her fiancé's hand, and prayed for it to be over. It soon was, and her giddiness returned, until they picked up the photos taken on the ride. Her stomach dropped as she looked at the woman in the photo. She knew she had gained weight, but really? That was what she looked like?

I look like a pillow stuffed into a wastebasket, she thought. Right then and there, she knew something had to change. She and JT wanted to start a family, but Erin asked herself, *How can I take care of kids if I can't take care of myself?*

After years of trying maple-syrup cleanses, all-meat fad diets, and every diet pill in the pharmacy, she was ready to lose the weight for good. No more quick fixes or searches for an instant cure.

This is it, she told herself. *It has to be the right way. Nothing ever worked before because I didn't do it the right way.*

"How to live a healthy life," she typed into her browser; she was not going to look into diets. SparkPeople.com popped up in her search results and she joined immediately. She got started on her new life and never looked back.

"I started slow, didn't change all my habits at once," she said. Instead of downing two liters of cola—up to 878 calories a day—she drank water. She added one new, healthy habit at a time, adding more new ones when the existing ones felt easy. This new way of living wasn't about restriction, as she had feared. It was about *freedom.* She could make all the healthy choices she wanted, with real results. She was excited about this new life.

Six months after finding SparkPeople, Erin had lost several pants sizes, had broken her after-work fast-food habit, and felt more confident than

ever. She had shattered her initial goals and was well on her way to reaching more. She was motivated, and she was committed. But not *that* day. That day, she was terrified. She and JT had returned to their favorite amusement park, and she was about to ride the roller coaster where she nearly got stuck the day after their engagement. Her palms sweated and she struggled to catch her breath. She panicked as doubts flooded her mind: *What if I still can't fit? What if I still need help getting in? What if people laugh?*

JT held her hand and looked her in the eyes. "I'm so proud of you," he said. She squeezed her eyes shut and reached for the buckle. *Click!* It snapped, without effort. Erin exhaled and looked at JT. "Told you so," he said.

Those next three minutes were the best of her life. With the man she loved next to her, the one who'd been by her side no matter what size she was, she was now literally flying high without a care in the world. She was full of energy and felt like she could do anything. She laughed, thinking how a roller-coaster ride represented the journey that had brought her full circle in just six months.

When Erin saw the photos, she began to cry. There was a woman who fit comfortably into the seat. There was a woman who was happy. There was a woman who had succeeded. "I realized how my effort had resulted in this wonderful moment," she said. "I am prouder of myself than I ever have been before. Prouder than the day I graduated high school. Prouder than the day I got my college degree. Prouder than the day I got a promotion. And why? Because I always knew I could do those things. But losing the weight? That was something I never thought I could do. But I did do it. And that feeling of accomplishment—more than just how I look—boosts my self-esteem more than I ever could have imagined."

You know how we all say "someday, I'll . . . ," and for many of us "someday" is code for "never"? Erin was one of those people, but with her new, healthy lifestyle, she is actually taking on those "someday" goals one at a time, with energy left over for everything else life brings her way.

Almost five years later, Erin is 117 pounds lighter. She is at a healthy weight for the first time since childhood, and she's at the weight she's been trying to reach since age fourteen. Erin was promoted at work to a position that has her on her feet all day. She spends her weekends with JT, exploring Florida, not sitting on the couch. She has energy to do what she needs

to do to stay healthy, such as exercise, and lives her life to the fullest. When she has a rough day or her enthusiasm wanes, to boost her motivation she thinks back to those two roller-coaster rides. For Erin, this new life is fun!

Erin used to think of weight loss as being on or off the diet bandwagon. Now, she uses an analogy that's common among SparkPeople members: losing weight is a journey, not a destination. And with the Spark Solution, you can get started quickly and on the right path, which keeps your motivation levels high.

Erin likes to visualize the journey as a trail through the most scenic countryside she can imagine. To get to a healthy weight, she walked a while, ran sometimes, and encountered hills and even a few plateaus. This road will always be there, and you can move at your own pace. Even "if you stop to smell the roses, have a picnic, or rest," she says, you won't be left behind or suddenly find that your path has disappeared.

Those first two weeks, Erin said, were crucial to her success. Though Erin started with small steps, she saw big changes in her energy levels, motivation, and metabolism. She discovered a new way to think about weight loss, which made all the difference in her overall success. And she learned how to avoid the event that most likely leads to failure with weight loss: giving up. She didn't give up when she ate a cookie, because she knew it wouldn't negate the days of healthy choices she had made. (She can now eat a cookie without guilt.) She didn't quit when walking around the block left her out of breath. (She's training to run her first 5K race.) And she didn't turn back. She was building momentum even in her first days on the plan, and she knew she would lose the weight this time. She's now comfortably maintaining her goal weight.

Healthy living is about living! "I realized how *good* it felt," Erin says. Two weeks from now, you'll say the same thing.

Welcome to the Spark Solution, the complete two-week diet program to jump-start weight loss and total body health. Whether you want to lose 10 pounds, 50 pounds, or 100 pounds, this book is going to change how you think about weight loss. It will set you up for a lifetime of healthy living by helping change the way you think about weight loss and setting goals that will lead to long-term success.

At SparkPeople, we believe that how you lose weight matters, and how you *start* to lose weight has a huge impact on your short- and long-term

success. We surveyed our most successful "losers" to prove it. We learned what those successful people did in their first two weeks and, more important, what those who failed did in *their* first two weeks. We documented what to do and what not to do and built that into this program. Starting out with a proven easy-to-use program and building no-fail tactics into your first two weeks puts you at a great advantage for success. We will help you reach your goals, and you'll have fun while doing it. These next two weeks matter. These next two weeks will change your life.

Over the next fourteen days, you'll follow the Spark Solution plan, developed by the experts at SparkPeople.com, one of the largest healthy-living and weight-loss destinations on the web, and based on the substantiated success of our members who have lost weight and kept it off. This program is bolstered by two groundbreaking surveys. The first reached out to thousands of members to find out what worked and what didn't. The results were clear: Those who failed did so within the first two weeks, and we know what they did wrong. Those who succeeded were motivated from day one and even more motivated after two weeks on the program, thanks to the goals we helped them set. We'll share what we learned from both groups.

From there, we asked a smaller, more elite group of successful members to tell us what helped them. It's these members, like Erin, who share their stories and tips throughout this book. Like all of you, these members wanted to lose weight. Like many of you, they had tried to lose weight and quit, repeatedly. But when they came to SparkPeople, something changed. Something clicked. They built momentum, changed their mind-set about weight loss, and boosted their metabolism through simple swaps and healthy habits. Rather than giving up on their goals, they stayed motivated until they reached them—and then set more. Now we get to share their stories and the secrets to their success with you. They failed before ultimately achieving success, and now you get to glean the wisdom they acquired from those setbacks.

If you've had misstarts, if you've tried to diet but gave up, if you've lost weight and gained it back, finally there's a way to get a fresh start without wasting time and energy. If you're starting this journey for the first time, it will be the *only* time; for you, with the Spark Solution, there will be no *next* time.

Like Erin, our members have tried everything. Those soup diets didn't work. Skipping meals or restricting food during the day worked for a while, but their motivation quickly waned. They ended up right where they started, with no idea how to get excited to try again—until that last time, with SparkPeople. Their "experiments" with weight loss were over for good. They found the Holy Grail: sustainable weight-loss success.

Guessing and testing was fun in elementary school science class, but it's tedious when you're an adult trying to get yourself on the right track. You're busy. You don't have time for weight-loss tactics that don't work. We know that. These next two weeks are designed to jump-start your weight loss. Our plan provides you with everything you need: three meals a day plus two snacks, and a workout plan that can be catered to your lifestyle. The Spark Solution focuses on three overlapping areas:

1. *The "Metabolic Makeover"* is the crux of our meals and workouts. Our plan uses the best of what works to optimize your metabolism, giving you both the know-how and the drive to get started on the right track toward lasting change. We structured our plan to boost your metabolism every step of the way, from the frequency and amount you're eating to the types of workouts you're doing. Even the ingredients in our meals are part of your metabolic makeover and will help you optimize your body's potential without giving up foods you enjoy or going hungry. Many people start trying to lose weight by skipping meals, eating too few calories to sustain daily activities, and other actions that actually slow or interfere with their metabolism. To be successful, your body's metabolic processes—your ability to burn calories—needs to function optimally, to work with you not against you, as you begin your weight-loss plan.

2. *The "Mind-Set Makeover"* helps you look at healthy eating and exercise as a means to live life to the fullest, gain energy, and boost confidence. Beyond your body, we also tackle what many dieters report to be their number one hurdle: the mind. We build on the results you'll see as you experience the metabolism makeover. We interpret the latest scientific research on weight loss and goal setting into simple actions that will help you reconsider how you think about healthy living. We focus on the positive, with tips from our members and experts, plus provide stats about what we've learned from those who've succeeded.

3. Finally, "Motivation and Momentum" focuses on building motivation and joins the other parts of the program in helping you build a strong foundation for your journey to better health and weight loss. On Day 1 of the plan, you press the reset button on your diet history and your battles with food. The past doesn't count anymore. You make one healthy decision, which leads to another healthy decision and another and . . . you get the picture. Your program builds on previous days to create a tightly woven safety net. You will not fail or grind to a halt. We won't let you. You won't let you. Gone is the vicious cycle of dieting and guilt. In its place is a virtuous cycle of healthy living. Better nutrition begets easier and more frequent exercise, and vice versa, which boosts metabolism. The better you feel, the more motivated you are to keep reaching toward your goals, and the more you keep going, the better and more motivated you feel.

Throughout the book, we offer simple yet effective mind-set and motivation makeovers as ways to build even more momentum in these first two weeks, which will make healthy living easier and more enjoyable. This combination of metabolism, mind-set, and motivation is sure to spark you forward toward lasting weight loss and a healthy, energized life.

What Can Happen in Two Weeks?

Plenty. In two weeks you can . . .

  reduce your cravings, especially those for sugary and processed carbs;

  start to stabilize your blood sugar;

  positively affect your cholesterol levels;

  succeed at the first small steps you take, so your confidence grows;

  increase your momentum and motivation day by day;

  lose at least 4 to 6 pounds of body fat, not water weight;

  create a deficit of at least 14,000 calories;

Six Reasons You're Not Losing Weight Already

So many people try and fail when it comes to weight loss. What are they—and you—doing wrong? It's not a matter of willpower or not trying hard enough. You may be approaching weight loss in the wrong way. Do any of these scenarios sound familiar?

1. You use exercise as an excuse to eat more. You're eating back all the calories you burn, not creating any calorie deficit.

2. You're not eating as healthfully as you think you are. You need to know exactly what you're eating—and how much—to really see the scale budge.

3. You never change your exercise routine, walking the same three-mile loop four times a week or taking the same weight-lifting class every week. All exercise burns calories, but to achieve the results you want, you need to balance calorie-burning cardio with muscle-building strength training, and change it up.

4. You're inconsistent, adhering to a rigid program for a few days, then—overwhelmed by cravings and run down from all the activity—you lose motivation and steadily revert to old habits. Or, to cope with what's going on inside your head, you down an entire bag of chips or box of cookies as a stress reliever, then you give up entirely. This cycle of feast or famine wreaks havoc on your metabolism and your motivation. Balance is key to sustainable weight loss.

5. You're relying on exercise alone to lose weight. Diet and exercise are like soap and water—beneficial on their own, but to really achieve results you must have both.

6. You're relying on unhealthy diet tactics for a quick fix. You skip meals, exclude entire food groups, or use diet pills to lose weight. Losing weight shouldn't compromise your health or well-being. For you to stick with it, weight loss has to be healthy and energizing, not exhausting.

Are you guilty of any of the above weight-loss tactics? That might be why you're not losing weight, and that's exactly why you need the Spark Solution.

get fourteen chances to wake up and make today the best, healthiest day of your life; and

gain a new, positive outlook on life, one with the belief that you can finally reach your goals.

After two weeks of eating this way, you might notice that your hunger is under control, you no longer need that third cup of coffee in the morning, or you're actually eating—and enjoying—your vegetables!

After two weeks of exercising, you might find that you're huffing and puffing less or you can add another mile to your walk or another ten minutes on the elliptical. You will have more energy than you've had in some time.

Plus, with the Spark Solution's metabolic makeovers to boost your body's efficiency, our mind-set makeovers to change how you think about healthy living, and our Spark Solution recipes and workouts, you may also . . .

notice clearer skin and healthier nails,

have more energy for the activities you enjoy most,

start to feel satisfied rather than stuffed after meals,

feel better about yourself in ways you never thought possible, and

realize that this healthy living isn't so bad. In fact, it makes you feel great. And it's actually something you can live with for life.

All of that sounds good, right? We agree. But we also have to warn you that everyone is different—your results might be either more dramatic or subtle at first. Be patient. Remember that lasting weight loss comes slowly and steadily. There is a big difference between how you put on the weight and how you'll take it off with this program. Unlike with most programs, which make you suffer before you see results, with our two-week jump start, you'll start to feel great right away, and you'll be much more likely to hit your ideal weight-loss goal over time, and stay there.

Imagine for a moment that all you needed to do was swallow a pill or make a wish and all your excess weight would be gone. What would

keep you from gaining the weight back? How would you deal with the underlying issues that caused your weight gain in the first place? Whether it's post-baby weight, the result of an injury, a side effect of an emotional wound, or day-to-day stress, those extra pounds provide wisdom as we shed them. We posed that same question to members in a precursor to our secrets-of-success survey and found that 75 percent of those who reached their goals would not wish away the weight or take a pill, while the ones who gave up were almost exactly the opposite: 72 percent wanted to take the easy way out.

With the Spark Solution, you don't need a magic pill. In just the first fourteen days, you'll gain the knowledge, confidence, and encouragement to keep going. You'll have achieved goals, with more on the horizon. You'll have both long-term and short-term plans. You'll know what to do when times get tough, when you're confronted by office candy jars or birthday cupcakes or diet saboteurs.

You'll look in the mirror and say to yourself, *This is not the only two weeks. This is the first two weeks of the rest of my life.*

Creating the Spark Solution

Based on more than ten years of experience working with more than fourteen million members and tens of thousands of people who have been successful at losing weight and documenting the foods and actions that got them there, the Spark Solution starts you on the path to long-term healthy living, or gets you back on the path if you've tried losing weight in the past. Our members track their food and their workouts, and we can see what works and what doesn't every day. Each month members add another twenty million entries to our database, which now numbers in the hundreds of millions. We packed in the best of what we know really works for weight loss and healthy living, along with the latest science and research on metabolism and motivation, to create the Spark Solution 14-Day Plan.

The SparkPeople community and program have been praised in studies at prestigious medical schools, and *Good Housekeeping* magazine called us "the online program that works." Though our plan comes to life through

the stories of those who've lost weight successfully, it's firmly rooted in science and backed by more than a decade of data.

This fourteen-day plan is specifically arranged to start you off on the right foot, from the time you wake up on Day 1. Each simple step, each well-timed meal, each boost of confidence from a small goal achieved will combine with what came before and build, over these two weeks, to gain momentum, boost metabolism, increase energy, and form a mind-set for success. Both what you do and how you think are critical in those first days and can mean the difference between quickly falling off the bandwagon or long-term success.

Advice from Those Who've Been Where You Are

Before those surveys, we knew we had a plan that worked, but we hadn't formally documented from a wide number of people who had successfully used our plan which aspects helped them the most. The number one take-away: Those who succeeded in the first two weeks didn't set out to change their entire lives, but attribute their ultimate success in reaching long-term weight-loss goals to the motivation they were able to sustain throughout those first fourteen days. The ones who failed lacked the motivation to keep going, even for just two weeks.

We're creating a new paradigm of weight loss: Be ready to change from Day 1, but you don't have to change your whole life all at once. Be committed to a healthy lifestyle versus a short-term diet, but you need only be prepared to take it one step and one goal at a time, at the pace that's right for you.

The Spark Solution does three things differently. First, we remove the pitfalls commonly associated with weight loss by creating a plan that wants you to succeed once and for all. We don't want return customers. We don't want you to "go on a diet . . . again." We want to help you reach your goals and be the healthiest you can be, starting now.

Second, we help you press the reset button. There's no place for self-loathing or negative thoughts about your body or your potential. Your inner skeptic is silenced, and your inner believer is awakened. Starting now, you will believe in yourself, because you can and you will do this.

And knowing that makes all the difference in your long-term potential for success. We hear over and over from our members who tell each other, "If I can do it, anyone can do it!" Accepting a new mind-set about weight loss will allow you to slowly build back your confidence until nothing can stop you, with your health and in other areas of life.

Third, we created our program to help you feel real results in just two weeks. You will feel better. You will lose weight. You will notice changes in your mind-set and your metabolism. You will feel satisfied, and you will feel energized. Your life will change. You'll have the energy to get off the couch and play with your kids, to wake up in the morning and start the day with a positive outlook, to be there for your partner, your friends, your coworkers and still have energy left for you.

Ours is a program based on *yes*. Yes to believing in yourself, not using self-loathing as a way to fuel weight loss. Yes to setting goals that you can reach, not challenging yourself to impossible weight-loss feats that end in failure. Yes to eating food that nourishes you and fuels your life, not restricting yourself so you end up overeating later. Yes even to enjoying dessert in right-size portions, not banishing certain foods from your life forever.

You're here because you want to change, just like those members we surveyed. What sets them apart from those who failed? They're ready to commit. They're in this. They know it will be a process, that little steps add up to big change. They take it one step at a time, and before long, they believe in themselves 100 percent. They finally let go of the old mentality that held them back.

Regardless of the kinds of changes they made, those weight-loss winners stuck with their changes and added more. Those members have banished the word *try* from their vocabulary and dived straight into the program with us. The hard part was short-lived, and any doubt was soon replaced with motivation; it's part of the mind-set makeover.

"It is not easy to change habits, but I just decided I was going to start with the things I needed to change the most—give up soda, exercise more, and monitor my calories—without making excuses," says Elizabeth, age thirty-two, of Virginia, who lost well over 100 pounds. "I just did it, and I saw results."

Those who succeed take weight loss seriously from the get-go, because they know what it's like to fail on fad diets, to waste money on gadgets that make lofty promises, and to feel unhappy in their own skin.

"The first two weeks of my new lifestyle were all about proving to myself that I could do it, that I could change and break old habits," says thirty-three-year-old Lisa. And change she did. Lisa lost more than 5 pounds in those first two weeks, and more than 90 pounds overall.

"I love my new life, and I have surprised myself in so many ways," Lisa wrote on SparkPeople.com. "I love how my body feels when I take care of it by putting good things in it. I don't get sick as often. I love to be active, and every day I delight in the little things that I used to be unable to do—like not have to worry about needing a seat-belt extender on an airplane!" A working mom, Lisa had been overweight since childhood and was morbidly obese when she started with SparkPeople. Today she's running half marathons while her two young daughters cheer her on. She sticks with SparkPeople because it works not only to lose the weight but also to keep it off.

For the first time, we surveyed the hundred or so people whose weight-loss stories we use to inspire others and spread the word about SparkPeople. They've been on the covers of national magazines, seen on morning TV news shows, and featured in books, blogs, and on our website. This all-star team lost more than 9,590 pounds combined, and most have kept the weight off. Every single one of them follows a healthy lifestyle rather than a diet, and it was that desire to be healthier that motivated them to lose the weight. Even better, they lost an average of 4.4 pounds in the first two weeks, and 43 percent lost more than 5 pounds in those first two weeks. A whopping 95 percent credit the first two weeks for setting the stage for their long-term success. Their responses were so strong and their results so impressive that we integrated them into this program, which combines nutrition and fitness plans from our experts with real-life tips, tricks, and stories from our most successful members.

With such impressive results, I bet you're wondering what kind of torturous exercise and restrictive diet (yum, more bean sprouts!) we have planned. You'll be elated to hear that you won't go hungry, and you won't be sweating for hours in the gym over the next two weeks. You don't need a gym membership (most work out at home or outdoors), and you'll be eating food that's delicious, nutritious, and comforting.

Here, we've juxtaposed what the successful group did during the first two weeks against what those who gave up did instead:

The Questions	The Success Stories	The Quitters
Were they dieting or following a healthy lifestyle?	Zero percent thought of themselves as "on a diet"	34 percent thought of themselves as "on a diet"
How much weight did they lose in two weeks?	70 percent lost 4 pounds or more	44 percent lost less than a pound
Did they think they got off to a good start?	Yes	No
Did they consider certain foods to be "bad" and off-limits?	No	Yes
On Day 1, how high was their motivation?	63 percent felt they were very motivated	29 percent felt they were very motivated
By Day 14, how motivated were they?	73 percent remained very motivated	78 percent were neutral or unmotivated
How many tried to build momentum during those first two weeks?	Almost half built momentum	Only 15 percent tried
How many built a strong foundation?	More than half built a strong foundation of healthy habits	Again, only 15 percent
How many ate breakfast?	44 percent ate a healthy, filling breakfast	Only 19 percent ate any breakfast—mostly a small one, with no concern for healthiness
How many ate more protein?	35 percent	21 percent
How many drank more water?	89 percent	65 percent
How many slept more?	18 percent	15 percent
How many ate three meals a day?	28 percent	11 percent
How many ate more fiber?	29 percent	23 percent
How many ate more fruits and veggies?	73 percent	48 percent
How many ate more whole grains?	40 percent	18 percent
How many ate more low-fat dairy?	12 percent	3 percent
How many practiced portion control?	67 percent	24 percent

What's more important than this comparison is what the success stories *didn't* do: 80 percent didn't spend hours in the gym—they worked out for less time than those who failed; 78 percent didn't quit when they ate a cookie or had a second helping—they believed in eating everything in moderation; 100 percent didn't give up when their motivation waned—they took a long-term view. In the end, their top motivators entailed laying a strong foundation of healthy habits, feeling better about themselves, and feeling healthier. They all say they're still following a healthy lifestyle program today.

As you can see, getting healthy—and staying healthy—begins with three steps: change your diet, start working out, and take the small steps that lead you to believe you can do it. Just changing what you eat doesn't work, because it's only part of the plan. You also need to change your mind-set about weight loss and get moving. During those first two weeks, 72 percent of our success stories changed their diets *and* started exercising.

"I began to walk every day on my lunch break," says Tammy, who lost 37 pounds and has kept the weight off since 2008. You don't need to start out working out every day, but with your increases in energy, you probably will want to. Tammy also made simple food swaps, which made a big difference over time. "I replaced processed foods with whole foods, such as fruits, vegetables, and whole grains. These steps gave me the ability to increase my healthy habits over time rather than saying I was on a diet. I wanted this to be a long-term change in how I looked at food and exercise. Most of all, I've learned an awful lot about myself: what motivates me, what I want out of life, what I need to do to get there."

It doesn't matter what you do, but you need to move most days. Most of our success stories exercise an average of 4.6 days each week, often in the morning so a busy day is no excuse to miss a workout (more than half work out in the morning). Does going from no exercise to daily exercise sound overwhelming? Don't worry. You can start from where you are to build your program. And you can start with a simple walk, or break up your workouts into shorter segments.

Remember Erin? She "hated" exercise and started with walking just a few minutes twice a week. Over the course of her 117-pound weight loss, she added in power walking, light jogging, swimming, step aerobics,

strength training, elliptical training, cardio DVDs, and yoga. She focused on what she really enjoyed, a list that kept expanding as she improved her fitness levels.

From our surveys we also learned that these individuals with amazing success stories don't rely only on the scale to measure progress; they notice how their clothes fit, how they feel, how much energy they have, and how many inches they've shed. One of Erin's early goals was to fit into a size 20 (now she's a size 8), and she rewarded herself not only for losing pounds but also for dropping pants sizes.

By Day 14, these winners believed in the path they were on, and that small steps would take them all the way to their ultimate goal. For the first time in a long time, they had hope, and they knew that the Spark Solution would help them get to where they wanted to be. They believed they could do it.

If they can do it, why can't you?

"I've realized the only way to do this is to change my lifestyle and to make healthy habits permanent," says Erin. She reached her goal over three years ago, and she's continuing to get stronger and healthier by setting new goals. Slow and steady is the way to build a sustainable weight-loss plan.

Even Erin's "permanent" healthy habits started with those first two weeks, so now let's learn how this book can help you achieve success the way she did.

How to Use
the Spark Solution

Our experts, led by our dietitian Becky Hand and editorial director Stephanie Romine, teamed up to write this book and guide you through the next two weeks. The workouts were designed by Nicole Nichols, a certified personal trainer and group fitness instructor who's also the editor-in-chief of SparkPeople.com. Our healthy cooking expert, Chef Meg Galvin, created the recipes.

The book is divided into four parts. In Part 1, you'll learn how fourteen days can change your life. Rather than bombard you with all you'll ever need to know about healthy eating and exercise, we focus on what you need to know right now.

From there, we dive into the fourteen-day plan in Part 2. We tell you what you'll need to get started; aside from a trip to the supermarket to stock up on some healthy foods (nothing too weird or expensive), you don't need much. Read through each day's plan ahead of time, and find a few minutes to prep your meals either after dinner the night before or in the morning. We offer time-saving tips with each recipe along with shortcuts to "Make Tomorrow Easier," which tell you what you can do ahead of time. (If you're really short on time, use the suggestions in "The Spark Swaps Assembly Line" in the "Food for Life" section of Part 4.) Each day you'll see comparisons of the Standard American Diet (SAD) and the Spark Solution's Spark Swaps meals and snacks. We show you the effect that our style of eating will have on your weight loss, not only each time you sit down at the table but also cumulative throughout the days, weeks, and beyond. We explain why we swapped certain ingredients,

offer shortcuts in the kitchen, and share tips for personalizing your meals while sticking to the plan. You'll also follow our workout plan, and each day we tell you exactly what to do. On strength-training days, you'll follow the plan as written; on days you do cardio exercise, you get to choose the activity, while we tell you how long and how hard to work out. (If you want inspiration, check out the "Menu of Workouts" in the appendixes.)

We know life happens, so we offer "Fit It In" tips to help you stick to your healthy habits when you're short on time. If you want to do more, we tell you how to do that as well. You'll also set two manageable goals each day, with the intent of making over both your metabolism and your mind-set as you follow the plan, plus a quick visualization exercise, which will help you keep your eye on the prize. The recipes and exercises we reference throughout your fourteen-day plan can be found in Part 3. You'll also find your entire two-week "Spark Solution Fitness Plan" in Part 3.

After two weeks, you'll head into Part 4, "What Comes Next." We aren't leaving you high and dry after your fourteen days are up. We give you more freedom but offer plans for Week 3 and Week 4, then fill you in on what you'll need to know to keep going. You'll learn how to distinguish between true hunger and cravings, with a list of ten reasons we eat when we're not hungry. We tell you why rewards are important, and you'll find out how to avoid and overcome plateaus. (They happened to even the most successful members, with surprising results.)

"Motivation and Momentum" is perhaps one of the most important chapters of the book. It covers motivation, and the lack thereof, which many of us battle. You'll learn from Dean Anderson, our resident behavioral psychologist, how to keep your spirits high and avoid quitting when the urge arises. In "Food for Life," we will break down nutrition into bite-size chunks, with a focus on sustainable weight loss. You'll also learn how to navigate your way through the kitchen, even if you hate to cook, and how to save time and still eat right by boosting the nutrition of convenience foods. In "Fit to Live," we dive a little deeper into the basics of exercise. You'll learn how to change your plan as your fitness level increases and how to avoid wasting time doing exercises that don't work, with more Spark Swaps to help you get fit in less time.

That's it. Are you ready to get started? The next fourteen days will fast-track your weight loss and change your life!

The 14-Day Jump Start

The Magic of Two Weeks

Quite simply, dieting and weight loss come down to calories in versus calories out. But as with most things in life, it's not that simple. A calorie is the unit used to measure the energy value of food, and 3,500 of them equal a pound of body fat. Burn 3,500 calories and you'll lose a pound. Consume 3,500 more than you expend and you'll gain a pound.

Think of an old-fashioned scale. On one side are calories in, from everything you eat and drink. On the other are calories out, those that you burn by exercise, daily activity (showering, doing the dishes, working in the garden), and the body's activities that keep you alive (breathing, pumping blood, and digesting food, among them).

So, if all you have to do to shed a pound of body fat is burn 3,500 calories, why is losing weight so difficult?

We don't live in a vacuum, and in today's society we're surrounded by calories, which makes resisting food (and the calories therein) that much more difficult. Food isn't just in the obvious places, like our homes, the supermarket, and restaurants, but almost every public place too: movie theaters, gas stations, the kids' sporting events, and every store you enter. Social functions, such as book clubs, PTA meetings, and church groups, revolve around food, even when food isn't central to the activity. Keeping track of all those calories—especially bites, sips, and tastes—and resisting food at times when you're not really hungry can be difficult, to say the least. We'll delve more into that when we talk about motivation.

Plus, while the body is meant to move, the laws of physics still apply: an object in motion will stay in motion, and an object at rest will stay at rest. We like to sit, and our lives accommodate that habit. We sit in our cars, at our desks, and on our couches. And it feels good—until it doesn't.

Getting yourself moving is the hard part. Keeping yourself moving is slightly easier. First comes motivation, then comes momentum. And over the next two weeks, you'll develop both.

Why Two Weeks?

Think of all you know about the "old" way of dieting, from personal experience or hearing from others who have been on the diet roller coaster a few times. The same experiences come up time and again:

"I went off my diet this weekend. I'll have to 'start my diet' again on Monday."

"I started to lose weight, but I totally blew it over vacation and gained it all back. I give up. I'll never lose weight."

"I started a diet and was doing well, but after a few days I got stressed out and ended up eating a pint of ice cream, so I quit."

"I was feeling good until I got on the scale. All that effort and the scale barely moved. I quit."

What's the common thread? These sentiments come directly from people who attempted dieting with the old quick-fix view, which ended in a "quick ditch." These people quit within the first two weeks.

With the Spark Solution, this isn't a diet in the old definition: restrictive, temporary, and punitive. When we say "diet," we mean a habitual pattern of eating, what to eat for a lifetime of optimal health. The first two weeks are the beginning of a lifetime of healthy eating and exercise.

Our members reported astonishing results in the first two weeks, and those results became the Spark Solution program we use throughout this book. Two weeks—fourteen days—is the proven amount of time necessary to begin a life change, according to the results that we saw among our most successful members. Two weeks is long enough to feel results, but not so long as to feel intimidating.

Regardless of how much weight they lost, our members overwhelmingly reported that they felt successful after two weeks. That feeling of motivation, that growing confidence, was key to building the momentum they needed to reach their next goals and take the option of quitting off the table.

Plus, two weeks is ample time for your body to begin repairing itself both mentally and physically. Almost 40 percent of our members cited

health as an area where they wanted to see improvement, and all of them reported that they started to feel and see changes. Cravings subside, especially for sugary and processed carbs, as your body starts to thrive on your new diet full of lean proteins, smart carbs, and plenty of fruits and vegetables. Thanks to your new way of eating, you may see your blood sugar stabilize. And these changes start to positively affect your cholesterol levels. Without a steady stream of sugar and fat, your body is able to settle down and return to "normal."

Two weeks is enough time to establish new habits, set some goals, and see real results. You might not see everything that's happening, but you'll feel them inside and out. All you have to do is get started and stick with it.

People who fail tend to do so in these first two weeks. The chart in the introduction showed how they fell short. Once you make it through the initial fourteen days without quitting, with as much or more motivation than when you started, you're more likely to reach your goals. Our surveys found that those who succeeded in losing weight were much more likely to do so if they had done the "right" things in the first two weeks. And, more important, those who failed lost motivation because they didn't do those things.

Finally, starting with a new mind-set and hitting the reset button on your weight-loss approach allows you the completely limitless opportunity of choosing the path that works this time and reaching goals you may have never thought possible. Your mind will be focused through daily reminders, goals, and visualizations, which set you up for success. Giving up thoughts of a quick fix will ultimately lead you to a *real* fix, where your actions and thoughts create a healthy approach to living. Weight loss will result, but so will many more things: goals will be reached, energy levels will increase, and you'll enjoy a happier life. Changing your body starts with changing your mind.

More About the Metabolic Makeover

For a moment, think of your body like a car (your dream car—something hot, flashy, and fast; no clunky jalopy or boring sedan). Your body, like your car, needs some TLC. You have to get regular tune-ups, avoid running out of gas, and change the oil and fluids regularly, right? If you have a lead

foot, are prone to slamming on the brakes, or drive erratically on a regular basis, your car will be fine for the short-term, but overall its performance will suffer.

Your body is the same. If you're a couch potato, if you skimp on sleep, or if you overeat regularly (or, alternately, skip meals), you'll be fine, for a while. Eventually, you'll start to feel sluggish, you'll gain weight, and you might even end up broken down on the side of the road, metaphorically speaking.

Take care of your body with adequate sleep, nutrient-rich food (with occasional treats), and regular exercise, and your body will return the favor. You'll feel better and perform better in your daily life.

All the positive and negative things you do to your body affect your metabolism, which is like the body's engine. Metabolism refers to the rate at which your body operates. For our purposes, we're focused specifically on how your body burns calories rather than storing them as body fat. If your body doesn't know when your next meal is coming, due to a pattern of fasting for weight loss, or if it doesn't get enough fuel on a regular basis, it can bring weight loss to a standstill. You can become tired, sluggish, and fatigued, and you'll lack the energy for your workouts, even your basic daily activities. That's why most women should eat no fewer than 1,200 calories a day and men, no fewer than 1,500.

If you consistently give your body far more calories than it needs, it can't keep up and has no choice but to store it as fat. If you rarely exercise or spend most of your time sitting, your body grows accustomed to a lethargic lifestyle and will lower your basal metabolic rate (the number of calories you need just to get through your basic daily activities, like breathing and digestion).

While other factors, such as changing hormone levels during menopause, low thyroid conditions, and polycystic ovarian syndrome, can also affect your metabolism, you can still see results from small tweaks in your diet and activity level with our plan.

Two things are guaranteed: you will move more and you will eat less than the average American. The Standard American Diet consists of 2,700 calories a day, according to the USDA, and as of 2011, three in ten Americans reportedly didn't exercise at all, according to a Gallup poll.

The good news is that even small steps make a big difference. And notice that we didn't say you'd be eating less often. You'll eat three meals

plus two snacks daily. How you exercise is up to you. Find activities you enjoy, that suit your lifestyle and your abilities. We'll get into the specifics in the next chapter.

The Eight Habits of Super Successful Dieters

The following eight habits, in no particular order of importance, will be the most powerful you can adopt. They are the essential and proven truths that will lead to sustained weight loss and health. They helped our successful members keep their motivation levels high throughout the first two weeks and beyond.

1. *Stay motivated, no matter what.* What separated the successful members from those who gave up was all in their heads: motivation. On Day 1, they were motivated and ready to commit to this journey. By Day 14, they were just as motivated, or even more so. They didn't all find motivation in the same ways. Some focused on becoming healthier parents, while others wanted a better body; some made it a point to share their goals with everyone, while others wanted to wait until they saw the scale budge before telling their loved ones; and some were spurred by a life-threatening diagnosis, while others decided to get healthy because their pants were too tight. They, like you, had their own reasons to lose weight. The ones who didn't lose sight of their goals, remembered the reasons they set out to do this in the first place, and celebrated every accomplishment along the way—those were the ones who succeeded. That's why we've built so much motivation into the Spark Solution.

2. *Write it down.* Whether you use SparkPeople.com to track your food and workouts (find out more about signing up for a free account to complement this book on page 364) or you jot down everything in a notebook, keeping a log of your calories in and calories out is imperative to success. In fact, a 2008 study published in the *American Journal of Preventive Medicine* found that you can lose twice the weight just by keeping a food diary. It's easy to forget what crosses your lips, especially things like grocery store cheese samples, swigs of your husband's beer, or tastes while cooking dinner. Writing them down reminds you that all calories—

not just those eaten at mealtime or while sitting down at a table—count. Many of us think we're eating within an acceptable calorie range, only to discover later that those nibbles and tastes here and there are breaking the calorie bank. Seeing your calorie intake in front of you will also help you stay motivated.

3. *Eat what you want, but in right-size portions.* Measuring food is a dieter's best-kept secret, and it's a key part of keeping a food diary. Buy a set or two of measuring cups and spoons. Measure everything you eat or drink. While your eyes can deceive you about portion sizes, these tools don't lie. It will be a real eye-opener. Measuring food prevents supersizing and returns you to right-sizing. Reading labels is piggybacked on this tip, and it's a small step that yields big results. A 2012 survey by the Centers for Disease Control and Prevention found that women who read nutrition labels weigh on average about 8 pounds less than those who don't. For the average American woman, who weighs in at 165 pounds, those 8 pounds represent about 5 percent of her body weight.

4. *No forbidden fruit, so to speak.* No food is off-limits. If you want an ice cream sundae, go for it. You can keep going to your weekly happy hour with the office too. Have that glass of wine. At your neighbor's potluck, dig in with fervor when she presents you with her homemade lemon meringue pie.

According to a 2007 study of female dieters in the journal *Appetite*, restricting or banning certain foods (such as chocolate, the access to which was restricted in the study) leads to increased desire in the form of cravings. Those cravings can in turn result in uncontrolled binges. Such an attitude toward food can also bring about feelings of guilt, anxiety, and depression.

There's one caveat: to lose or maintain your weight, you can have it all, just not all at once and not all the time. And you have to watch your portions. As long as you know how much you're eating and you're meeting your nutritional goals for the day, you can include any food as an occasional treat.

5. *Balance your calorie account.* Think of your calorie budget as you do your household budget. You have 1,500 calories in your account to spend each day. Yes, you can have the slice of lemon meringue pie for 300 calo-

ries, leaving you 1,200 calories to spend that day. Once you withdraw all 1,500 calories, you have no more to spend. You can't borrow from yesterday or tomorrow except on special occasions, and you shouldn't get in the habit of banking calories for a giant splurge or binge. (Also, in a study published in the *Journal of Nutrition,* researchers found that people who ate 70 percent of their calories throughout the day lost more weight than those who ate 70 percent of their calories at night.)

6. *Don't burn out.* One of the biggest mistakes people make is adopting the weekend warrior approach to exercise. After months or years of not moving much, you hit the gym and try to work out as much, as hard, and as long as you can. Quickly you lose steam, sidelined by soreness, fatigue, or—worse— injury. Start with shorter workouts and you'll be able to exercise more frequently, building endurance and strength without burning out. A recent Danish study, published in the *American Journal of Physiology,* found that exercising thirty minutes a day had the same effect on weight loss as exercising sixty minutes a day. Researchers suggested that the results can be explained by the fact that with shorter workouts you are more likely to have energy left over for other activities that day and in the days following a workout. (Consistent, long exercise sessions may also lead you to eat more, so that's another reason we vary the duration and intensity of your workouts.)

If you're overwhelmed by exercise, start by counting steps using a pedometer. Aim for more steps every day, with the ultimate goal of at least 10,000 per day.

7. *It's about healthy eating* and *exercise, not healthy eating* or *exercise.* Exercise and healthy eating are equally important parts of the weight-loss equation, and a 2005 study in the *International Journal of Obesity* bolstered that argument. A study of overweight and obese adults found that the most effective way to lose weight and keep it off for a year or more is to combine a healthy diet with exercise. We agree.

Start working out without changing your diet, and your hard work will go unnoticed. Change your diet without working out, and you might see results for a while, but you'll soon hit a dreaded plateau. You can only reduce your calorie intake a certain amount before your body rebels and becomes exhausted, but by adding exercise or changing up your routine, you'll continue to achieve success. With our plan, you'll make manageable

changes to both your meals and your moves, which will leave you with plenty of energy and enthusiasm to keep living this way.

8. *You can't go it alone.* Even if you're the only person in your circle of friends, your family, or your office who is trying to lose weight and become healthier, you're not alone. Lack of support has long been identified as a major hurdle for those trying to lose weight. A study of 438 overweight adults enrolled in a diabetes-prevention program found that those who had support from family or friends reported significantly better results than those who did not have a support system. As time passed, those with support continued to see progress, according to a 2012 study in the journal *Clinical Medicine and Research*.

If you don't have someone at home to whom you can turn, online programs like SparkPeople work too. A 2007 study published in the *American Journal of Medicine* found that you can trust what you read on the Spark-People message boards and recommended that healthcare professionals direct their patients to the site.

Share your goals with your loved ones and seek out others who are also on this journey—at the gym, in a support group, or online—and you'll find that your hardest days become a little easier. There's no reason to keep your goals a secret, so when you're ready, tell people. Write those goals on a whiteboard in the kitchen, post them on your Facebook timeline, or tell your best friend the next time you have a night out. Early on, identify those people in your life who are going to cheer you on through thick and thin. Positive people will boost your confidence and self-esteem with support and encouragement when the going gets rough.

These eight habits will launch you toward success and keep you motivated. As you've probably discovered, they all contain a running theme: balance. Balance is critical.

This is perhaps most clearly seen when it comes time to step on a scale. The problem with weighing in is that most of us give the scale too much power. If daily weigh-ins motivate you, keep it up but stick to the following guidelines. And if stepping on a scale stresses you out, weigh yourself once or twice a week, not daily. A scale is only one tool for measuring weight-loss success. Sure, we all want to see the numbers go down quickly and frequently, but losing a pound means you've had to create a deficit

of 3,500 calories, and that won't happen overnight. If you step on a scale daily, you're likely to see fluctuations. There are plenty of reasons: you're nearing the start of your menstrual cycle, if you're a woman; you just ate; you haven't gone to the bathroom yet; you ate a lot of salty food; or you just worked out and sweated a lot. It's normal for your body weight to fluctuate up to 5 pounds per day, so create a routine for your weigh-in to offset those variances. For best results, weigh yourself at the same time of day, in the same place, on the same scale, wearing approximately the same amount of clothes. Starting with Week 1, set up a weigh-in routine and stick with it. Don't let the scale control you, and remember that weight is just one measure of success. (You'll learn more about body measurements at the beginning of the 14-Day Plan.)

Balance is important at every meal too, both in the plan we laid out for you and those you'll choose for yourself after the first two weeks are up. We want you to be able to have your cake and eat it too. That's why we believe in either-or, rather than all-or-nothing. This means you have choices to make each time you sit down to a meal. Do you want a glass of wine with dinner or chocolate mousse for dessert? A few chips with salsa before your meal or an extra tortilla with your fajitas? Sour cream on your baked potato or butter? When you're counting calories, every calorie counts, but that doesn't mean you have to deprive yourself. It just means you have to decide what matters most to you at this meal.

"But I want it now" is the Veruca Salt school of thought. Do you remember the spoiled rich girl from *Charlie and the Chocolate Factory*? She wanted it all right now, and look where that got her—right down the chute with the golden egg. As you weigh your options, take a look at what's on the menu at home or at a restaurant and decide what matters most to you.

As a study of balanced eating, let's imagine you're grabbing dinner at a popular fast-casual Mexican restaurant before a movie. The line is long, your belly is grumbling, and the choices are numerous and coming at you fast. Burrito or bowl? If you get the burrito, you can probably skip the rice since you have carbs covered. If you skip the tortilla and get the bowl (good choice, as those plate-size wraps can have more than 300 calories each), go for the rice, brown if they have it. Next up are the proteins: meat or beans? Chicken, steak, or pork? Lean protein is important, so you choose the chicken because you can see it's white meat, which you know is lower

in fat. Now come the toppings. Choose your salsas and load on all the veggies you like.

Finally, the good stuff, the extras: guacamole, cheese, and sour cream. Though a good source of calcium, cheese isn't adding much to the meal here. Will you really taste it with all those other ingredients? Likely not. Get it if you want, but then skip the other two. That leaves the guacamole and sour cream. Are you craving the cool creaminess of sour cream? Or do you prefer the richness of the cilantro-laced guacamole? Put them together and their flavors will compete. Choose one and enjoy every bite of your balanced meal. You've just made a whole series of healthy decisions, and you have a dinner that will fill your belly without wrecking your entire day.

Our plan sets you up for success by giving you options and putting you in control. Help us help you by setting realistic goals that will balance your desire to improve your health with your need to keep living your life. Don't set yourself up for failure with a goal that's unattainable. Balance is critical here as well. Unrealistic weight-loss goals can have a negative impact on the success of your weight loss and weight maintenance, as reported in 2003 in the *Journal of Consulting and Clinical Psychology*. You didn't gain the weight overnight, and you won't lose it overnight either. You can't lose 20 pounds before your high school reunion in two weeks, but you can lose it in a couple of months, just in time for summer. If you have 100 pounds to lose, you could reach goal weight by this time next year.

Scale goals aside, be realistic with your workout goals too. Avoid definites (always and never). Instead of "never eat chocolate," aim for "eat one square of my favorite dark chocolate on days I work out." Restrictions simply don't work, but balance does. When you give yourself the freedom of flexibility, failure is no longer an option. We simply balance out any indulgences or missteps along the way. Had a huge birthday dinner with friends last night? Balance it out by eating your daily intake of calories and taking an extra twenty minutes of exercise. While in a perfect world each day and each meal would be perfectly balanced, you can also aim to create balance from day to day. Balance equals success.

The Spark Solution
Metabolic Makeover

Tina wanted to feel better about herself. She wanted her clothes to fit better. She wanted more energy. And she really wanted sexy knees, a flat stomach, and toned upper arms. She wasn't going to give up so easily. She started tracking her food, and she took the first steps toward what would ultimately be a 90-pound weight loss. Strong and steady was her motto, and she was motivated. Each decision to wake up and exercise, every time she resisted the urge to overindulge her sweet tooth, it solidified her resolve. Rather than relying on sheer willpower, she had this foundation, a history of good decisions, behind her.

"Learn that saying no to yourself is actually how you say yes to a healthy lifestyle," she said. "This is the life I always wanted, and every good choice I make is the reason why I deserve it."

Tina, now thirty-two, never gave up, because she knew that "each day there are moments of motivation to encourage us." Her drive to succeed was no longer about willpower but about resiliency. She knew that even if she slipped up (and she did—everyone does, to varying degrees), she knew she had multiple chances and strategies to make healthy decisions. Her momentum built. She couldn't stop.

"As my weight-loss goals inch closer and closer," she wrote on her blog, "I often look back on the series of milestones and self-discoveries marking my journey. They're brief, trivial moments and thoughts, but they have brightened my day and helped me advance my weight-loss attempts little by little."

By the end of her first year, Tina got the sexy knees, flat stomach, and toned upper arms she wanted, plus a boost in confidence and the ability to love herself again. She entered a modeling contest sponsored by her favorite clothing store and felt brave enough to ask others to vote for her. "I am ultimately beyond satisfied with the body and the spirit that I now own. I have my flaws, and I have learned to deal with them or accept them. What a difference this year has made to my life, my health, and my happiness," she said. "As I celebrate today, I look forward to continuing this journey into the coming years, because my tomorrow is now."

Momentum, Not Magic

It's Day 5 of your new diet. You worked super hard all week: tons of salads, plenty of workouts, and no "bad" food. You were determined to reach goal weight by sundown on Friday, just in time for your big weekend plans.

The time is here. You step on the scale, eyes closed, heart hopeful. And then you see it. The number on the scale. You lost . . . half a pound. Half a pound? Half a pound! After all this work?

You feel defeated and frustrated, discouraged by the constant struggle to lose weight. You're tired, drained of all energy, thanks to the hour you put in on the treadmill with no recovery snack. You're frazzled and sore from head to toe. "Why is this so hard?" you yell at no one in particular. "Why can't someone just tell me what to do to lose this weight once and for all?" Then you stomp off to excavate the pint of chocolate chip cookie dough ice cream buried deep in the freezer.

We've all been there—even Tina. But she didn't give up and neither should you.

"You can't think of it as a diet," says Harvey, who lost 63 pounds. "If you think of this as a diet, you may lose weight but it's going to come back. It's a *lifestyle change,* knowing what you are putting in your body and how it makes you feel. You have to be in the right frame of mind for it to stick."

While there's an app for almost everything in our instant-gratification society, there's no shortcut to weight loss. And since we're surrounded by massive portions of highly processed foods loaded with fat, sugar, and salt and simultaneously bombarded by ads for cleanses, diet pills, and supplement scams, it's no wonder that losing weight is so hard.

Enter the Spark Solution. Our Spark Swaps meals aim to nourish your body, repair your sluggish metabolism, and optimize your energy while fighting off intense food cravings and insatiable hunger. You'll shed body fat and have more energy. You'll learn which foods are dragging you down, as well as those that truly fuel your engine. You'll figure out how to more efficiently use your time at the gym, as well as other fitness tricks to keep your body working long after the workout ends. Finally, you'll develop other daily habits that can burn more calories and ward off hunger.

Let's start with the food.

Healthy Eating: How, What, and When to Eat to Spark Up Your Metabolic Furnace

SparkPeople has only about forty employees, which is pretty incredible considering we operate six websites and write books. This fact matters because we pride ourselves on our efficiency and effectiveness. We know time is precious—ours and yours. Rather than share everything we know about nutrition right here, right now, we focus on what you need during the first two weeks. Throughout those fourteen days, we'll give you a day-by-day guide filled with proven tips, simple and healthy recipes created by our chef, and all the confidence you'll need to succeed. Then we offer a more in-depth look at nutrition in Part 4, which looks ahead to Week 3, Week 4, and the rest of your life.

Let's live in the moment and talk about the first two weeks. Each day, you'll eat three meals and two snacks for a total of about 1,500 calories, give or take 50 calories. (Don't forget to write them down or track them online, but you also have a detailed meal plan in Part 2.)

Your daily meal plan is divided as follows:

Breakfast: 325 calories

Lunch: 375 calories

Dinner: 400 calories

Two Snacks: 100 calories each

Dairy: two servings as part of a meal or as a snack, 100 additional
　　calories each

TOTAL = 1,500 calories

No Crash Diet

The thinking goes that if you cut calories and lose weight, you can cut
even more calories and lose even more weight faster. You now know the
reality is different. Cut your calories too much and weight loss sputters
and soon grinds to a halt, because you've exhausted your body, putting
the brakes on your metabolism and your ability to perform daily activities
with vim and vigor.

That's why the Spark Solution plan centers on eating 1,500 calories a
day. (See page 35 for more information on adding or cutting calories to
the plan based on your activity level and build or body type.) Your total
daily calories should be low enough for weight loss yet high enough to
nourish and satiate you. Our plan is designed to create healthy, steady
weight loss while giving you the energy to work out and get through your
busy day. You'll have the energy to take the stairs instead of the escalator
at the mall. You'll have the drive and focus to take on that extra project at
work. You'll get excited about playing ball with your kids, and you won't
be dragging at the end of the day. With the Spark Solution, you will truly
be a calorie-burning, fat-busting, high-performing machine.

Those who follow a structured eating plan—with predetermined meals
and snacks, plus a grocery list—are more likely to lose weight than those
who wing it, according to the results of a six-month study published in
the journal of the International Association for the Study of Obesity. We
want you to be as prepared as possible, so you'll use our meal plans for
the first two weeks (although in Week 3 and Week 4 you'll get the chance
to create your own if you so desire).

Most people can and will lose weight using our plan as written, losing
2 pounds or more a week; however, some of you might need to modify
the plan to suit your lifestyle and body type. If you fit into one of the following categories, please adjust your meal plan accordingly. We've
accounted for these exceptions:

If you . . .	Why do you need to modify?	What do you need to do?
are a woman who is 5'2" or shorter	Your smaller stature means you need fewer calories. Due to your size, you likely weigh less to begin with, which means each pound represents a higher percentage of your body weight compared with someone taller.	Consume about 1,200 to 1,300 calories daily. You can either decrease the portion sizes of your meals or cut out one snack daily. Each day, you'll need 3 servings of vegetables, 2 servings of fruit, 5 servings of grains or starchy vegetables, 2 servings of proteins, 2 servings of dairy, and 1 serving of fat. Rather than losing up to 2 pounds a week, an appropriate weight-loss goal is up to 1 pound.
are a woman age 50 or older, premenopausal, or have gone through menopause	As you age, your metabolism slows, so you need fewer calories.	
have a condition that affects metabolism, such as low thyroid function, polycystic ovarian syndrome, or an endocrine disorder	Having a medical condition that slows your metabolism reduces your calorie needs.	
are over 6 feet tall	Your height means your body requires more calories than someone shorter.	Add 100 to 200 calories each day (for a total of 1,600 to 1,700 calories) by adding extra servings of vegetables, fruit, whole grains or starchy vegetables, protein, or fat. You can add another snack or an extra half serving of your main dish at lunch or dinner.
have a highly strenuous, physically demanding job	You're more active than the average person, which means your body will require additional calories each day.	

If at any time during the plan you find yourself losing weight more quickly than you expected, or if after a week or so you are losing weight more slowly than expected, you can further adjust your plan to suit your lifestyle and your body's needs.

We constructed our meals with some key concepts in mind to either boost metabolism or leave you looking and feeling better. These concepts are simple enough to fit into even the busiest days, yet they yield tremendous results with both your weight loss and well-being. Like other healthy habits, they'll soon become second nature. And this is the goal. Say goodbye to restrictive diets and hello to your ideal weight and healthy lifestyle.

"Making these changes to my lifestyle helped me feel much more in control of my life," said Amber, 62 pounds lost. "I now know that I can reach any goal I set my mind to."

Burn, Baby, Burn

Fiber-filled whole grains, legumes, fruits, and vegetables require the body to "burn hotter" as it digests these foods and converts them into energy, a process called thermogenesis. Research published in 2011 in the journal *Food and Nutrition Research* found that whole, unprocessed foods actually increase the calories you burn and can boost your metabolism. The findings indicated that meals containing processed foods decrease thermogenesis by about 50 percent. This means that if you eat unprocessed foods, you'll burn twice as many calories. That's why our recipes and meal ideas, though designed to be fairly quick and easy, focus on "real" food.

> *"Eating more protein, fruits, and veggies while reducing sugar has helped a great deal with weight loss. Getting rid of the junk to eat more whole foods makes a big difference."*
>
> —*Denise, 87 pounds lost*

Load Up on Fruits and Veggies

Fruits and veggies are packed with water, dense in nutrients, and comparably light on calories, and all but a couple are virtually fat-free. They are key to satiety and keeping the body burning. They also contain a wide variety of disease-fighting phytochemicals that will help your body look and feel its best. We use fruits and veggies to fill the plate without filling your waistline.

Fruits and veggies have health benefits that reach far beyond weight loss. The Academy of Nutrition and Dietetics (formerly the American Dietetic Association) recommends eating two and a half cups of vegetables and two cups of fruit per day, which adds up to about half your plate at

every meal. It is well-evidenced that eating fruits and vegetables can protect against a number of diseases and conditions, including heart disease, hypertension, diabetes, cancer, chronic obstructive pulmonary disease (COPD), diverticular disease, and cataract formation.

According to a 2005 study in the *American Journal of Clinical Nutrition,* eating more fruits and veggies, specifically those rich in the carotenoids beta-cryptoxanthin and zeaxanthin can help you cut your arthritis risk. To boost the anti-inflammatory, protective benefits of those carotenoids— which are the yellow, orange, and red pigments found in plants—eat oranges, papaya, tangerines, kale, collard greens, spinach, Swiss chard, mustard greens, red pepper, okra, and Romaine lettuce.

If you're trying to quit smoking, a 2012 study in the journal *Nicotine and Tobacco Research* found that what goes on your plate can have an effect on your success. Those who ate the most fruits and vegetables were more likely to have fought the urge to smoke after one month, compared with those who didn't eat their veggies. As it turns out, fruits and veggies make cigarettes taste worse, which can help people quit.

If you are searching for the fountain of youth, look toward the salad bar rather than the beauty bar. People who eat the most vegetables have rosier complexions, according to a 2012 study presented in the online journal *PLOS ONE.*

Rather than focusing on the complex nutrition behind antioxidants, we encourage you to eat a variety of colors of fruits and vegetables each day. Each color corresponds to a different set of antioxidants, each with a unique set of health benefits. We don't want you to think that any one veggie is better than another; eat them all!

> *"Eating more veggies and fruit was one of the key components of my weight loss. Eating vegetables and learning how to make them taste delicious helped me from feeling deprived and hungry. I had no idea how filling and yummy veggies could be! Fruit became so sweet and yummy to me too. I still eat tons of fruits and veggies because they are so tasty, filling and healthy. I mean really, what's better than a sweet, juicy peach?"*
>
> *—Elicia, 92 pounds lost*

Pump Up the Protein

Protein is a triple threat when it comes to weight loss. Not only does it help maintain your muscle mass as you lose body fat, but as you incorporate more exercise into your daily routine, protein will help you build more muscle tissue and recover from your workouts. Plus, protein is your insurance policy against a growling belly and hunger-induced cravings, as reported in 2004 in the *Journal of Nutrition*. That's because, compared with carbs or fat, protein makes you feel fuller longer. We included plenty in every recipe (and at least 60 grams a day), so you won't feel hunger when your next meal or snack is still hours away.

> *"I definitely eat more protein now than I ever have. I have always been a carb addict. I find myself trying to consciously make more effort to eat higher protein meals, and I find that I feel fuller longer and feel satisfied with a smaller tasting of the carbs."*
>
> —*Christy, 95 pounds lost*

Three Meals, Two Snacks

Eat too often and your body never learns to deal with reasonable hunger levels. Go too long between meals and your energy level and blood sugar drop and your metabolism suffers. Research published in the *American Journal of Clinical Nutrition* in 2005 found that skipping meals and having irregular mealtimes can cause you to overeat and burn fewer calories throughout the day. By evenly spacing your meals throughout the day and placing your two snacks at your hungriest times in the day (for most of us, that's mid-afternoon and after dinner), hunger is under control and the body is kept energized. This keeps blood-sugar levels steady and prevents hunger-induced binges. A 2004 study in the *Journal of the American College of Nutrition* found that planning to have an evening snack can reduce the urge to binge or excessively graze after dinner.

*"I would snack all day long before, or skip
meals. I now eat regular meals."*

—Yvonne, 150 pounds lost

Breakfast Served Daily

One of the most common diet downfalls is skipping a morning meal, either because you're not hungry or you want to bank calories for later in the day. Bad idea. Having breakfast within the first two hours after you wake up provides your body and brain with the energy needed to function. Eating breakfast wards off hunger later in the day and lessens afternoon binge eating. Plus, those who eat breakfast tend to eat fewer calories overall, as reported in the *Journal of the American College of Nutrition* in 2003.

A regular morning meal can also help prevent hunger-related stomachaches, headaches, and fatigue. Breakfast does just that: it breaks the fast your body endured while you slept and kick-starts your metabolism and your day. Ours are easy and tasty. You'll eat meals like Fruity French Toast, Spicy Tomato-Egg Muffins, and Slim Sausage Gravy with Better "Buttermilk" Biscuits, plus quick-fix dishes like sweet and nutty oatmeal, whole-grain toast with tasty toppings, and scrambled eggs, including milk and fruit.

*"Before SparkPeople, I would eat all day. I wouldn't eat
breakfast but I would make up for it by eating a morning
snack, lunch, an afternoon snack, a large dinner, and a
huge pre-bed meal, which consisted of a big bag of chips."*

—Amber, 62 pounds lost

Choose Carbs Carefully

Despite decades of diets telling us otherwise, carbs are not the enemy. You need them. They are brain food, after all. But sodas and other sugary beverages, baked goods, and any foods made with highly processed

white flours and refined sugar are often just a waste of calories. These highly refined, nutrient-void foods send a surge of sugar into your bloodstream, leading to sugar highs and crashes and requiring massive amounts of insulin for recovery. This increases your risk of packing on the pounds, particularly the belly fat. This surge of energy has no staying power, which means you'll likely end up needing more food sooner than expected, and the more you eat them, the more you crave them. Our plan contains fewer carbs than the Standard American Diet (45 to 65 percent of your daily calories on our Spark Solution plan come from carbs), and we focus on whole grains and other smart carbs, such as fruits,

The Whole Story Behind Whole Grains

Not all whole grains are actually whole, but food labels and the companies who wrote those labels would like you to believe otherwise. Manufacturers play tricks on consumers by labeling items with useless terms like "cracked wheat," "stone-ground grains," or "seven-grain goodness." These terms essentially mean nothing; they're still processed grains.

Consider these two scenarios:

- *You pick up a loaf of bread that's golden brown and topped with a crunchy coating of nuts and seeds. Though it looks wholesome (another meaningless word on packages) and nutritious, this bread was made with enriched, refined, white varieties of wheat flour (often labeled just WHEAT FLOUR). It has added coloring to make it look brown like true whole-grain bread, and the seeds and other accoutrements on the crust trick you into thinking it's better for you. In reality, this loaf of supermarket bread is just refined white bread with a clever disguise.*

- *You see the words "whole grain" on your morning cereal box. You examine the nutrition facts and ingredients lists. The first item listed is whole-wheat flour. But you see additional ingredients, including several varieties of sweeteners. If all those ingredients were combined, sugar would be the number one ingredient; since they're not, this cereal seems more nutritious than it really is. In some "whole-grain" cereals—and*

vegetables, beans, and low-fat dairy, whenever possible. These carbs are a double whammy: they provide key nutrients and important fiber. You'll load up on smart carbs like sweet potatoes, brown rice, beans, and even fruits and veggies, plus whole-grain breads, pasta, and tortillas. These smart carbs are an ideal fuel for your body and brain, and they provide the key nutrients and fiber to protect against disease and promote a healthy body weight. That's why quinoa or brown rice, for example, are better choices than white rice or a slice of white bread. That's also why potatoes—even the white ones with the skin on—are on our list of smart carbs.

crackers, cookies, and the like—most of the calories come from sugar, not any grains. You might also notice that whole-wheat flour is listed first, with several other enriched or refined flours listed after it. Again, this means your cereal, crackers, or bread isn't whole grain.

To ensure you're getting real whole-grain products, look for the 100% WHOLE GRAIN stamp from the nonprofit Whole Grains Council. This label means the food contains only whole grains and no refined grains, with a minimum of 16 grams of whole grains per serving. (Don't try to do the math because it gets confusing, but 16 grams is considered a full serving of whole grains.)

That stamp is a good first step to weed out hidden refined grains, but you should still read the ingredient list and the nutrition facts label to also weed out excess sugar and salt. If there is no stamp on the label (not all companies use the stamp), look for the word "whole" in front of any type of grain, seed, or grain product: whole-wheat flour, whole-rye flour, whole-corn meal, or whole oats. This is telling you that the whole grain was truly used in making the bread, cereal, or pasta. If you only see "wheat flour," "corn meal," etc., you are not getting true whole grains.

An easy way to ensure you're getting whole grains is to eat them whole. Seek out some that may be new to you, such as amaranth, brown rice, buckwheat, bulgur, farro, millet, quinoa, wheat berries, and wild rice. Eating grains whole is also cheaper than buying them in crackers, bread, or other forms.

There's another kind of carb that helps keep hunger at bay: resistant starch. While commonly classified as fiber, resistant starch is a carbohydrate that doesn't digest in the small intestines the way other carbs do. Instead, it moves to the large intestines, where it ferments and is used as fuel for probiotics, the healthy bacteria in your gut that benefit your body. Resistant starch comes in four forms, three of which are naturally derived from foods like legumes, under-ripe bananas, raw potatoes, and cooked-and-cooled potatoes and grain products. The fourth is added to foods and does little to curb hunger, according to studies, but the other three boost weight loss and help curb hunger. So, if you either don't have access to a microwave or prefer to eat your leftovers cold, you're actually doing your body a favor.

> *"I switched out all white foods to whole grains and whole foods. This controlled my hunger. I felt fuller longer and more satisfied. I was hesitant at first to try this, but in time learned to enjoy this habit."*
>
> —*Roxanne, 75 pounds lost*

Fill Up with Fiber

Fiber is a dieter's best friend. It can't be digested, so it just passes right through you. It adds no calories to your day, and it helps prevent constipation, which can be common when losing weight. Let's be frank: eating fiber makes for perfect poop. Because fiber—what your grandma called "roughage"—adds bulk to your food. It also wards off hunger and fills up your belly, because it takes longer to pass through your system.

You'll stay full and satisfied, and you'll be regular, thanks to 25 grams or more of fiber found in our daily meal plan, which uses fiber in its natural form: whole grains, fruits, veggies, and beans. We avoided foods with "added processed fiber," as they will not help you eat less and keep weight off in the same way. A 2011 study in the journal *Appetite* found that adding fiber to a liquid, for example, does little to squelch hunger, compared with eating naturally fiber-rich oatmeal. And a 2012 study reported in the *Journal of the Academy of Nutrition and Dietetics* found that this added fiber

(think fiber in yogurt or other foods that wouldn't naturally contain any or much of it) not only has little effect on satiety, but can also cause stomach upset, gas, and bloating.

> *"I made a goal to eat more fiber because I know eating fiber will fill me up faster than non-fiber foods, which when combined with drinking more water equals eating fewer calories. Eating fewer calories means losing weight."*
>
> —Diane, 80 pounds lost

Savvy About Sweets

If we banned all desserts from the program, we know most people would throw down the book and quit before they even started. No food is inherently "bad," so we believe that as long as you're eating sweet treats in the right portions and staying within your calorie range, you can eat dessert daily. We control the portions to avoid blood-sugar spikes and crashes. Plus, removing the forbidden nature of sweets can help many people avoid bingeing on them, as reported in the journal *Appetite* in 2007. Our sweets integrate healthy ingredients whenever possible, such as fruit, whole-grain flours, and flavored yogurts, in addition to the ice cream and chocolate you crave.

> *"I always have a low-calorie dessert because I enjoy it, and allowing myself to have a sensible treat keeps me from bingeing."*
>
> —Melissa, 100 pounds lost

The Calcium Connection

Aside from keeping bones strong and healthy, which is especially important to women as they age, calcium and vitamin D may help fight the

battle of the bulge. Preliminary research published in the journal *Obesity Reviews* in 2012 suggests that the pair helps burn body fat too. Therefore, we include two servings of fat-free or low-fat milk or yogurt daily. And for all you cheese lovers, there's plenty in our recipes. Thanks to the protein found in dairy, you can meet your nutrient needs, maximize your metabolism, and ward off hunger.

Not a milk drinker? You can achieve the same nutritional benefits from nondairy milks and yogurts fortified with calcium and vitamin D.

> *"I have found that when I really try to get in my calcium, I make better snack choices. By doing this I can stay in my calorie range and not have a flux in my blood sugar."*
>
> *—Anne, 126 pounds lost*

Sleep Soundly

Skimping on sleep can seriously impact your weight and overall health, as reported in the journal *Obesity Reviews* in 2009. Chronic sleep deprivation has been linked to increased risk of diabetes and heart problems, and it can also send your "hunger hormones" into overdrive, leading to an increased appetite and more food cravings, especially for those quick carbs you're trying to avoid. Adults require at least seven hours of good sleep per night, which gives your body the time needed to repair cells, recover from workouts, and perform all the other vital, behind-the-scenes functions necessary to keep you healthy and happy. Track your sleep habits and, if needed, add an extra fifteen to thirty minutes a night each week until you've reached the ideal amount for you.

Regular workouts and eating less sugar can improve sleep quality, so just following our program can have an impact on your shut-eye. If you don't think you have time to sleep, consider cutting back on your down time. According to a 2006 study in the journal *Obesity Reviews,* replacing just one hour of inactivity—such as time spent watching TV or surfing the Internet—with sleep "is likely to result in a substantial reduction in calorie intake."

*"Getting enough sleep is an ongoing challenge
for me, but I've found when I'm more consistently
getting a good night's sleep, it helps with
my weight and my energy levels."*

—*Denise, 57 pounds lost*

Keep the Fat

Fat also satiates, so it's another way to ward off hunger. While you won't find any deep-fried dishes or greasy sauces in the Spark Solution menu, you will feel satisfied with the healthy fats included in our meals and snacks. Diets that are too low in fat have some telling signs: dry skin, dull hair, and brittle nails among them. Your body also needs fat to make your bathroom visits more comfortable, due to its lubricating qualities, and to process some vitamins. The fats the Spark Solution relies on are mostly of the heart-healthy variety, and they help keep other areas of the body running smoothly too. In the kitchen, fat is necessary to create texture and flavor in foods. Foods too low in fat take on the texture of cardboard and lack that comforting "mouth feel." Our plan includes enough fat to satisfy while still meeting the American Heart Association Nutrition Committee's recommendations for a heart-healthy diet and the 2005 recommendations from the Centers for Disease Control and Prevention.

"I try and stick to healthier fats, but I'm not afraid of fat."

—*Amber, 99 pounds lost*

Exercise: How to Keep Your Metabolic Furnace Sparked

It's six in the morning on a Thursday. Your alarm just went off—you've been getting up early every day this week to exercise. Monday, you started off strong by power walking and jogging four miles. Tuesday, you felt great, so you ramped it up with an hour-long indoor cycling class, which

promised to burn a thousand calories. By yesterday, you were tired and didn't want to go to the gym, so you did a full-body strength workout DVD at home. Today you plan to spend ninety minutes on the elliptical to make up for the burrito you scarfed down last night that was the size of your head.

You roll out of bed, stumble into the bathroom, and stare at yourself in the mirror. Dark shadows circle both eyes. Your whole body aches. You want nothing more than to go back to bed. And that's exactly what you do, hoping the extra hour of sleep will make you feel human again.

Isn't exercise supposed to give you energy? Then why do you feel like you were hit by a truck? And how are you supposed to lose weight when working out makes you so hungry you want to eat everything in sight?

While it's true that you can always burn more calories with extra exercise, your body has its limits. And when you're just starting out, less is more. Too much exercise too soon can lead to exhaustion, overtraining, and even injury.

"When starting, don't overdo it, or you risk making yourself so sore you don't want to work out anymore," warns Bobi, who lost 70 pounds. "Take it slow and in time you can challenge yourself to reach greater fitness goals after you have laid a solid base."

Crystal, who ultimately lost 71 pounds, fell into that trap of too much too soon. "I began exercising daily," she said. "Most days I did at least thirty minutes to an hour of exercise. I didn't know not to exercise the same body part two days in a row, like the legs, so I think I may have gone overboard at first, but eventually I got into a good routine. I had much more energy. Exercise makes me feel so much better all around."

Our workout plan is designed for optimal results and jump-starting new habits, but it is designed for real people with real lives. This approach is proven, and we're excited to share it with you. We focus on efficient, effective exercise that does more in less time and with little or no equipment. You won't spend hours working out because the goal here is sustainability. You want to break the old patterns of ups and downs, binges and busts. You can't be expected to adhere to restrictive diets, so why should you be expected to work out like a machine seven days a week? There's a real danger in setting up unrealistic goals and pushing beyond physical limits. Just as with the meal plan, our Spark Solution workouts are

suitable for beginners, but those who have been exercising regularly can modify them to suit their needs.

Our plan, designed by Coach Nicole, consists of a combination of cardio, strength training, and flexibility with bonus points for any activity that gets you out of bed and off the couch, even if it doesn't require you to lace up your sneakers.

Each week you'll alternate cardio and strength training for six days, then take one full rest day. You'll start with twenty to thirty minutes of cardio, working up to thirty to forty-five minutes during Week 2. Strength training will take twenty to forty-five minutes. After each workout, you'll spend a couple of minutes stretching, and you'll look for ways to make each day more active than the last.

Coach Nicole will explain exercise in more detail in "Fit to Live" (page 327), but for now remember this:

Type of Exercise	What It Does	Why It Matters	How Often You'll Do It
Cardio	Gets your heart pumping and keeps it that way for at least 10 consecutive minutes	Burns fat Strengthens your heart and lungs	Three days a week Week 1: 20 to 30 minutes Week 2: 30 to 45 minutes
Strength training	Exercises performed against resistance from a machine, a weight, or even your own body	Builds muscles Strengthens bones, tendons, and ligaments	Three days a week
Flexibility (stretching)	Exercises to lengthen your muscles and develop or maintain range of motion	Reduces injuries Improves coordination Enhances your posture	A few minutes after every cardio and strength session

Her plan combines all three to boost your metabolism during your workout—and long after the sweat dries. Here's how:

Don't Skimp on Strength

The more muscle you have, the more calories you'll burn, which is why it's so important to incorporate strength training into your workout routine when you're losing weight. Unlike body fat, muscles burn calories even when they're at rest, which is how strength training also boosts your

metabolism. You don't have to get ripped or lift heavy weights. Even light to moderate strength training can preserve or increase bone density, which is especially important for women, and if you lose a great deal of weight, it can tighten your skin and reduce flab.

Without consistent strength training, muscle size and strength decline with age. An inactive person loses half a pound of muscle every year after age twenty. After age sixty, this rate of loss doubles. But muscle loss is not inevitable. With regular strength training, muscle mass can be preserved throughout your life, and any muscle lost can be rebuilt.

> *"Adding strength training has been a new change for me. I have found that it challenges me in a different way, and I love the way my muscles look and feel after training. I wish I had started this sooner!"*
>
> —*Christy, 95 pounds lost*

Take It Easy and Work Hard

We are creatures of habit, but our metabolism gets lazy when we do the same exercises day after day. This plan alternates steady-state cardio, in which you exercise at the same pace or intensity for the duration of your workout, with intervals, in which you alternate short bursts of faster or higher intensity efforts with periods of easier, slower exercise. This keeps your body on its toes and revs up your metabolism. Stick exclusively with steady-state cardio all the time (walking three miles every day, four times a week, for example), and that workout will no longer challenge your body. It won't require as many calories to recover from the effort, and you'll soon plateau with your weight loss. We make small changes in the time or intensity of your cardio workouts to keep you and your body focused on your goal. Think of your workouts as playtime for adults, and because we constantly change up the workouts, you'll never get bored of the "game."

> *"I've been doing intervals for a while, and believe me, it works. No more boring cardio. This really gets you moving, and anyone can do it. Do just enough so you feel it, [but] not so much that you feel like giving up."*
>
> —*Lala, 37 pounds lost*

Cheat On Your Cardio

Running, walking, cycling, salsa dancing, power yoga—they're all great calorie burners. No matter which type of cardio you choose, you should alternate it with other activities at least once a week. Cross-training adds variety to your workouts, prevents boredom, and—you guessed it—keeps your metabolism working efficiently.

> *"I've added lots of variety to my routine, which helps keep me from getting bored and helps to keep me fit. So now rather than just walking and doing circuit training videos I have added running, yoga, hiking, Pilates, kickboxing, and many other things to my repertoire."*
>
> —Elicia, 92 pounds lost

Off the Couch and Out of Bed

Even if you are someone who can exercise one hour every day without experiencing burnout or injury, twenty-three hours remain. How are you spending them? Each day we ask you to estimate and track the number of minutes you spend on your feet or doing something other than sleeping, eating, or sitting. Grocery shopping (pushing a full cart, walking around the store, and hauling bags to and from the car) counts. So, do the trips you make to the copier, the water cooler, and the restroom a few times a day. And the ten minutes you spent having a tickle war with your toddler—that counts too. You will burn thousands of extra calories over time, and it keeps your metabolism from hibernating between workouts. By setting a goal for these NEAT minutes each day—what is referred to as non-exercise activity thermogenesis—you'll find ways to get moving, which will not only burn calories and boost metabolism but also give you more energy and motivation to keep moving.

> *"The improvements I made in my routine, habits, and health have allowed me to live a more active lifestyle. Not just going to the gym, but in general we do more as a family. We go hiking together, we spend the day at the zoo walking around, we go to the park and play games, walk around the neighborhood, spend days*

at theme parks, etc. These are all things that were a
challenge to me before I changed my ways. Thanks to
a lot of smaller changes, I can now say I lead a healthy
lifestyle, and it's a much happier life than the one I knew
before. Life looks a lot better away from the couch."

—*Stacey, 97 pounds lost*

The Awesome Side Effects of Regular Exercise

- Your metabolism speeds up, thanks to added muscle.
- Your body adjusts to the stress of exercise, and you feel rejuvenated.
- Your immune system improves, helping prevent illness.
- Your strength and endurance improve, making exercise (and daily tasks) easier.
- Your mood and energy level stabilize.
- You sleep better at night.
- You look and feel better.
- Your motivation to keep going increases.

Let's Get Started

THE SPARK SOLUTION 14-DAY PLAN

The First Two Weeks of the Rest of Your Life

Today's the day you start the program and begin making the changes that will stick with you the rest of your life. It's *all* going to change, but what you'll notice is how simple the Spark Solution is to use each day. You're not changing everything overnight. Why? Because that is exactly what went wrong the last time you dieted—and the time before that. Anyone of us who has attempted at least one diet knows that the change-everything approach does not work. That's why the Spark Solution is different. Each day and each week we'll set goals, and every goal will build upon the next, creating a cycle of motivation.

How you start your weight-loss program has a huge impact on success, both short-term and long-term. This fourteen-day plan features the formula that has worked for tens of thousands of SparkPeople members who have each lost from 10 to 150 pounds or more.

As we discussed, the plan is easy. We cut calories through simple swaps with the Standard American Diet (aptly given the acronym SAD) and create a plan that fills you up while slimming you down. Our Spark Swaps meals focus on not just cutting calories but loading up the plate with foods that nourish your body, give you energy, and keep your metabolism revved up. This 1,500-calorie-per-day plan helps you lose weight while fighting cravings and warding off hunger, as well as preventing huge blood-sugar spikes and crashes.

To put the meals in perspective, we compare our Spark Swaps to a similar SAD meal and show you the impact that making these changes can have on your diet. We show you not only the calorie difference between the two meals, but we also explain why we made the changes to the meals, reinforcing the core principles of the Spark Solution diet in a practical, real-life way.

Since diet and exercise go hand in hand, we also give you a daily workout. You choose the type of activity that's right for you, and we tell you how long and how hard to work out to achieve the best results and optimize the time you spend exercising. And at the beginning and end of each day you'll get a healthy dose of motivation, to give you the support you need throughout the program, plus a quick survey, to help you monitor your progress beyond the scale.

You can start any day of the week, but most people find it easiest to start on a Monday, with some prep work on Sunday. No matter when you start, you'll want to find an hour to grocery shop and schedule your workouts. (In the appendixes, you'll find detailed shopping lists for Week 1 and Week 2, along with a customizable shopping template.)

Keep in mind that the number on your scale isn't going to budge immediately. It takes time (and a deficit of 3,500 calories) to lose a pound. We know you want to see results instantly, so you'll see how each meal, each workout, and each decision affects your overall success. Trust that each positive thing you do to get closer to your goal is creating change within your body, which will eventually turn into results. You will feel healthier, stronger, and simply better almost right away, which in turn will motivate you to keep going. Then the weight will start to come off and stay off for good.

Before You Begin: Weighing In and Measurements

As you now know, not feeling pressure to weigh yourself daily is one of the "Eight Habits of Super Successful Dieters," but you'll need to weigh yourself before beginning the program so you know how much weight you've lost each week.

Top Tips for Stress-Free Weigh-Ins

Wear as little as possible.

Weigh yourself at the same time of day.

Weigh in at the same place and on the same scale.

Record the number in a journal or on SparkPeople.com.

Even when the scale is barely moving, your body can be changing in other ways, such as in the amount of body fat or muscle mass. Your clothes might be looser after one week, and you might even have lost some inches. We recommend taking measurements every month or so after the first two weeks.

On SparkPeople, we encourage our members to write about their goals and their progress, either in a private journal or on a blog where others can offer support and motivation. We encourage you to do the same. Though it's not imperative, we recommend taking a few minutes to write about the daily insider tips and mind-set and metabolic makeovers, along with the challenges and highlights of your day. Your journal will soon become another tool to build your momentum and keep you motivated.

A Day in the Life

Did you know that the average American consumes 2,700 calories a day? Many of us eat much more—up to 4,000 calories! Every day, we'll compare a day's worth of SAD fare to our Spark Swaps meals, then calculate the

How to Take Measurements

Body measurements can be a useful way to track your progress. Many times you'll see a loss of inches even if the scale isn't moving. To ensure accuracy, measure in exactly the same place and under the same conditions each time. Here are some instructions and tips to help you. When you're done measuring, you can track your measurements on SparkPeople to see how your body changes over time.

Bust: Place the measuring tape across your nipples and measure around the largest part of your chest. Be sure to keep the tape parallel to the floor.

Chest: Place the measuring tape just under your breasts or pectoral muscles, and measure around the torso while keeping the tape parallel to the floor.

Waist: Place the measuring tape about a half inch above your belly button (at the narrowest part of your waist) to measure around your torso. When measuring your waist, exhale and measure before inhaling again.

Hips: Place the measuring tape across the widest part of your hips and buttocks, and measure all the way around while keeping the tape parallel to the floor.

difference in calories consumed and burned to show you how you create a calorie deficit during the week. This diet in our Spark Solution plan is based on 1,500 calories, with three meals and two snacks, including a sweet treat.

Throughout the fourteen-day plan, we offer "Spark It Up" tips to take your program up a notch, plus "Make It Work" solutions to bust through excuses and help you find time to exercise on even your busiest days.

Let's get started.

Week 1

Your fridge is stocked with healthy food and quick meal ingredients. A water bottle is full and by your side. Your motivation is at an all-time high. You're ready for this.

Planning is key. First-timers, make sure you have enough time to prep your healthy breakfast before work, pack your lunch the night before, and set a reminder on your phone so you won't skip your walk. If you're a pro and already have a fitness plan in place, stick with it, but use our workout suggestions as a way to boost your calorie burn or increase your exercise frequency, intensity, or duration.

Note: Most of our meals include fruits and vegetables on the side. This is a place in the plan where you have some leeway. Choose fresh, frozen, or canned (drained and rinsed) fruits and vegetables, depending on your budget and your preferences. And, if we've suggested a vegetable or fruit you dislike or can't find in your supermarket, you can swap in another one (e.g., cantaloupe for honeydew, or broccoli for asparagus).

DAY 1

INSIDER TIP

Slow and Steady Works

"I told myself that I would change two habits every week; not as a diet, but as permanent lifestyle changes so that they weren't temporary. I compounded the effect by continuing to add two new healthy habits every week."

—Solomon, 139 pounds lost

MIND-SET MAKEOVER

Starting now, on Day 1, you're done with regrets. When you go to sleep tonight, think about everything you did right, not what you should have

done better. Focus on the positive—eating five servings of fruits and vegetables, walking during your lunch break, or finishing everything on your to-do list. Tomorrow is another chance to make more healthy decisions. Focus on that instead.

METABOLIC MAKEOVER

Start your day by drinking one cup (eight ounces) of water. Chances are you go to the bathroom first thing in the morning and your hydration levels are at the lowest level they'll be all day. Drinking water in the morning energizes the body, replenishes the fluids your body has gotten rid of, and helps you maintain your hunger levels. (Thirst can often be mistaken for hunger.)

BREAKFAST

SAD		Spark Swaps		Calories Saved
2 eggs 3 slices bacon 2 slices white toast with 2 pats butter 1 cup orange juice Coffee with 2 tablespoons half-and-half	736 calories	Bacon-Swiss Scramble (page 150) with spinach 1 slice whole-grain toast with 1 teaspoon unsalted butter 1 small orange Coffee with 2 tablespoons skim milk	320 calories	416

Bacon Overload. Think of bacon as you would a seasoning or condiment. Don't count it, or any cured meat, as a main source of protein.

OJ Is Okay but Oranges Are Better. Juice lacks the fiber that the whole fruit provides. Fiber equals feeling full equals bye-bye, hunger!

A Tale of Two Quiches. Bacony, cheesy quiche lorraine and spinach-filled quiche florentine inspired this breakfast makeover. First, we ditched the fat-laden crust made with white flour and served whole-wheat toast on

the side. Next, we used low-fat Swiss cheese, cut the bacon down to one slice, and used one whole egg and one egg white to cut cholesterol. The result? An entire breakfast for fewer calories and less fat than a slice of quiche. Don't like spinach? Swap mushrooms, onions, or tomatoes.

Making Bacon. Though we include bacon in this meal plan, there's no way you will make it through a pound of bacon before it spoils. We recommend dividing the pound in half, wrapping one half in two layers of plastic wrap and freezing it for later use. Lay out the slices of the other half pound on a rimmed baking sheet. Preheat the oven to 375°F, then bake for 15 minutes. Drain on paper towels and store in single-serve portions in the fridge or freezer.

LUNCH

SAD		Spark Swaps		Calories Saved
12-inch ham and cheese sub with mayonnaise 1-ounce bag of chips Soda	1,131 calories	Turkey and cheese sandwich on whole-grain bread with light Dijon mayonnaise, lettuce, and tomato 1 ounce unsalted pretzels Flavored water	334 calories	797

No Recipe Needed. We want you to get comfortable making your own meals, so there's no recipe for this simple sandwich. Stick to your serving sizes (3 ounces meat, 2 slices bread, and as many veggies as you can pile on) and keep condiments in check.

Lighten Up. Light mayonnaise has 40 calories less than regular mayonnaise but all the creaminess you crave. Boost its flavor by mixing it with salsa, hot sauce, mustard, pesto, or jam.

Smart Move. If your office orders boxed lunches, immediately give away the cookies and chips to save up to 600 calories.

Sayonara, Soda. Nix one 12-ounce soda from your diet a day and that'll amount to 18.6 pounds lost a year. Swap a 20-ounce soda for water, and you'll drop 31 pounds.

SNACK

SAD		Spark Swaps		Calories Saved
Cookie from the office cafeteria	410 calories	1 cup celery sticks (2 ribs) with 1½ tablespoons natural unsalted peanut butter	162 calories	248

Craving That Cookie? Split it with a friend to lessen the sugar crash later on and save calories. Skip your other snack.

Sneaky Swap. We know, we know. Celery is not a swap for a cookie, especially if you're craving sweet. The celery will give your mouth plenty of time to chew, which should satisfy any urge to eat out of boredom. And the natural peanut butter offers healthy fats and protein, which will keep you satisfied all afternoon. Sprinkle on some cinnamon to sweeten your snack.

DINNER

SAD		Spark Swaps		Calories Saved
1 serving boxed "helper" meal	460 calories	One-Dish Dinner: Southwestern Chicken and Rice (page 203) 1 cup diced pineapple 1 cup skim milk	457 calories	3

Lose the Box. Boxed meals save time but not much else. We checked out the nutrition label on a "whole-grain" variety of a popular helper meal.

The second ingredient was sugar! That's not going to help one bit. Thankfully, you can ditch the box and create a tasty, economical one-skillet meal in just twenty minutes.

While the calories are close, ours provides a well-rounded meal that is low in fat, sugar, and salt. This is a great example of how important it is to look at more than just calories when choosing food.

SNACK

SAD		Spark Swaps		Calories Saved
1 cup chocolate ice cream	285 calories	1 banana with 1 cup low-fat chocolate milk (1 cup skim milk with 2 tablespoons light chocolate syrup)	184 calories	101

Instant Milkshake. Combine the banana and the low-fat chocolate milk in a blender with a few ice cubes for a cool after-dinner treat.

Screaming for Ice Cream? Serve it in a teacup not a salad or cereal bowl. Your serving will seem more satisfying.

SAD Total	Spark Swaps Total	Deficit
3,022 calories	1,457 calories	1,565 calories!

DAILY TOTALS

Calories: 1,457	Sodium: 2,071 mg*	Fiber: 26 g
Fat: 35 g	Carbs: 205 g	Protein: 100 g

*Even though lunch today is higher in sodium, when paired with other low-sodium meals, you'll still stay within your limits for the day. Further cut salt by using rotisserie turkey rather than deli meat.

Fitness That Fits

CARDIO: 20 MINUTES

Choose any activity and accumulate minutes in two 10-minute chunks or all at once. Work "somewhat hard" (8 out of 10) so you are slightly breathless the entire time. Need help deciding what to do? Check out the appendix for a list of workouts, and see the chart on page 245 for more information on how hard you should work.

Our Pick: elliptical machine (250 calories burned)

FLEXIBILITY

Spend 5 to 10 minutes stretching all major muscle groups after your workout.

NEAT: 30 MINUTES

Daily Deficit: 1,815 calories
Week-to-Date Deficit: 1,815 calories

SPARK IT UP: MULTITASK

Walk after dinner while talking to your friend on the phone. Twenty more minutes amounts to 112 more calories burned.

MAKE IT WORK: WORK OUT WHILE YOU WATCH

Have a meeting and need to skip your workout? Tonight do jumping jacks during commercial breaks while you watch TV.

Make Tomorrow Easier

Grill, bake, or poach 2 pounds of boneless, skinless chicken breasts and store them in single-serve portions in the fridge. You'll need a pound (which will yield 12 ounces of cooked chicken) for tomorrow night's dinner. Use the rest for lunches throughout the week.

You can also prep the Quick Chicken Enchiladas (page 206) tonight (or even in the morning) and bake them tomorrow night.

Daily Reflection

HOW DID YOU FEEL TODAY?	Poor		OK		Excellent
	1	2	3	4	5
I made healthy food choices based on the Spark Swaps meal plan.					
I was physically active, following the Fitness That Fits workouts.					
I felt motivated to stick with the Spark Solution program.					
I am ready to take on tomorrow and all that it has in store for me.					

What were the highlights of your day? What were the challenges? How can you use today's highs and lows to make tomorrow better and easier?

DAY 2

INSIDER TIP

It Really Does Add Up

"It's the little things I add in that have given me a more active lifestyle. Walking briskly around the store when I do my shopping, walking my dogs, parking farther away from the store, taking the stairs, cleaning house more vigorously by doing things like faster vacuuming or dusting. They may seem small, but the calories burned add up."

—Amanda, 54 pounds lost

MIND-SET MAKEOVER

Envision yourself doing something at your goal weight that you can't do at your current weight, whether it's fitting into an airplane seat, riding a

roller coaster, or walking up a flight of stairs without feeling winded. How does it make you feel to see yourself actually doing it without pain or discomfort? Use that feeling to help you reach your goals today.

MOTIVATION MAKEOVER

Put a picture of your motivation on your phone or within sight on your desk. Do you want to get healthy for your kids? Look hot at your high school reunion? Hike the Grand Canyon? Whatever your motivation, keep it physically in sight so you don't figuratively lose sight of the prize.

BREAKFAST

SAD		Spark Swaps		Calories Saved
2 cups fruity cereal 8 ounces 2 percent milk	322 calories	½ cup old-fashioned oats 2 packed teaspoons brown sugar 1 cup blueberries 3 tablespoons chopped or sliced almonds ½ cup skim milk	405 calories	(83)

Perfect Oatmeal. Bring 1 cup water to a boil in a heavy saucepan. Then reduce the heat to medium, stir in the oats, and simmer uncovered until thick, about 3 to 4 minutes. Transfer to a bowl and top with the brown sugar, blueberries, almonds, and milk (or serve on the side).

Comfort Food. There's something so comforting about cereal. It harks back to childhood: the Saturday morning routine of filling the bowl, hoping the toy would fall into your bowl, pouring in the milk, and trying not to spill it as you carry it to the TV to watch cartoons.

Those sugary cereals of yore were such a treat, and for good reason. A bowlful has more than 7 teaspoons of added sugar. That's sure to leave a bad taste in your mouth.

Cereal is one of the most common foods we mismeasure. A serving is ¾ to 1 cup, depending on the cereal, but most bowls will easily fit at least twice that. And how easy is it to go back for seconds?

Oatmeal is just as comforting, but it's a whole grain packed with fiber and protein. Your belly won't be growling for seconds after this breakfast.

You'll note that today's breakfast has more calories than the SAD version; that's because we're focusing on keeping you full until lunchtime.

Did You Know? One of the reasons processed foods taste so sweet is that food manufacturers add salt as well as sugar to balance the flavor. One serving of cereal has 360 milligrams of sodium.

Take a Pause. Each time you sit down to eat a meal or snack today, pause before taking a bite. Forget about taste for a moment and consider your other senses. Breathe deeply and smell your food (without picking up your plate). Take a close look at the colors and textures. Then take a bite. Chew carefully and slowly, considering the rest of your senses as you eat: taste, of course, but also the sound and feel of the food. Eating with all your senses truly helps you appreciate your food.

LUNCH

SAD		Spark Swaps		Calories Saved
Tuna salad on whole-grain bread from a bistro	840 calories	Curried Tuna Salad Sandwich (page 176) 1 cup cucumber slices and baby carrots 2 tablespoons light ranch dressing for dipping ½ cup cubed honeydew melon	359 calories	481

Tuna, Take Two. Tuna salad somehow made itself into a health food. A scoop atop a lettuce leaf alongside butter crackers was the de rigueur diet plate for years. While tuna packed in water is a lean protein, tuna salad is usually

smothered in gobs of mayonnaise, with a few bits of celery thrown in for crunch. Even at a fast-casual bistro, tuna salad remains a fat bomb that gets most of its flavor from mayonnaise.

We gave this lean lunchtime staple an exotic twist. A bit of curry powder makes it more interesting, some dried cranberries add unexpected sweetness, and cucumber offers much-needed texture. A mix of olive-oil mayonnaise and fat-free plain Greek yogurt keeps the salad creamy yet low in fat.

Swapping a tablespoon of mayonnaise for plain Greek yogurt saves 79 calories and 10 grams of fat. That's a pound a year with just 1 tablespoon less mayonnaise!

Skip the Sandwich. Nix the pita and dip your veggies into the tuna salad or serve the tuna salad over lettuce.

SNACK

SAD		Spark Swaps		Calories Saved
Fast-food strawberry banana smoothie	440 calories	Just-as-fast real-food smoothie: purée 4 ounces light strawberry yogurt with half a banana and 1 cup fresh or frozen strawberries until smooth	173 calories	267

The reason commercial smoothies taste so good is that they're often sweetened, sometimes with actual sugar and sometimes with apple juice, which is very high in sugar.

Them Bananas. Want a thick, creamy—and sweet—smoothie at home? Let bananas ripen, then peel and slice them. Freeze them in a ziplock bag and add to smoothies as needed. The bananas thicken your smoothie and keep it cool without diluting any flavor the way ice can.

Desktop Dining. Make your smoothie the night before and store it in the freezer in a sealable plastic cup. It should thaw by snack time.

DINNER

SAD		Spark Swaps		Calories Saved
Chicken enchiladas	854 calories	Quick Chicken Enchiladas (page 206)	504 calories	350
		1 cup skim milk		
		½ cup fruit cocktail packed in water or juice		

Lost in Translation. The word "enchilada" comes from a Spanish verb that means "to add chili pepper," but based on what we see on most restaurant menus, that's been interpreted as "to add cheese—as much as possible." Ours keeps the cheese but puts it on top so you can taste every gooey bite. The sauce is packed with veggies, and we fill ours with lean chicken (though you could swap extra-lean ground beef) and white beans along with a flavorful salsa.

Mind Your Manners. This dish doesn't require a knife, but go ahead and use one anyway. Using a knife *and* fork when you eat slows you down, allowing your brain more time to tell your body when it has had enough.

SNACK

SAD		Spark Swaps		Calories Saved
1 ounce potato chips	152 calories	12 almonds	82 calories	70

Chew On This. There are plenty of reasons we eat. In the afternoon, we often snack out of boredom or stress. If you're craving something crunchy, choose almonds instead of chips. You'll save on salt and get a boost of calcium, protein, and fiber.

Easy as it is to toss a handful of nuts in your mouth, slow down. Eat your almonds one at a time, chewing well and pausing between each one. Nuts are a dense food, but they're small in size so it's easy to overeat if you're not being mindful.

SAD Total	Spark Swaps Total	Deficit
2,608 calories	1,523 calories	1,085 calories

DAILY TOTALS

Calories: 1,523	Sodium: 1,644 mg	Fiber: 32 g
Fat: 34 g	Carbs: 228 g	Protein: 95 g

Fitness That Fits

STRENGTH TRAINING: TWO SETS OF TEN REPS
Perform the exercises in the Spark Swaps Strength Workout (page 247) in the order listed, moving quickly from one exercise to the next for one set, then repeat for a second set. For exercises performed on one side at a time, perform all reps (repetitions) on each side before switching. Then move on to the next exercise.

Calories Burned: 72

FLEXIBILITY
Spend 5 to 10 minutes stretching all major muscle groups after your strength training.

NEAT: 45 MINUTES
Daily Deficit: 1,157 calories
Week-to-Date Deficit: 2,972 calories

SPARK IT UP: JUST ONE MORE
Add an extra set to tonight's workout and, time permitting, do 10 minutes of cardio to warm up and cool down.

MAKE IT WORK: PICK UP SOME HELP
Use rotisserie chicken and fresh salsa from the grocery store to speed up dinner even more.

Daily Reflection

HOW DID YOU FEEL TODAY?	Poor		OK		Excellent
	1	2	3	4	5
I made healthy food choices based on the Spark Swaps meal plan.					
I was physically active, following the Fitness That Fits workouts.					
I felt motivated to stick with the Spark Solution program.					
I am ready to take on tomorrow and all that it has in store for me.					

What were the highlights of your day? What were the challenges? How can you use today's highs and lows to make tomorrow better and easier?

Habits of Fit People

Don't Make Exercise Excuses

The excuse people most often make for not exercising is a lack of time, but the truth is, we're all busy. You can complain about it. You can theorize that everyone else must have it easier than you do. However, let's be honest: we all have commitments and obligations; we just choose to prioritize them differently.

One of my favorite Nike ads says, "Someone busier than you is running right now." Take a moment to let that resonate. I like to think about this phrase from time to time as motivation. No matter how busy I feel I am each day—and I am definitely busy—I know there are people who do much more than me each day and still maintain a healthy lifestyle. That thought inspires me to stay committed to exercise, even on days when I swear I don't have time to work out.

If you still feel too busy to work out, you do have some options:

Break up your workout into smaller chunks throughout the day, such as ten minutes in the morning, at lunch, and after dinner—three ten-minute workouts benefit you just as much as one thirty-minute workout.

Try a shorter workout. On my busiest days I sometimes only have time to exercise for ten or twenty minutes, but I still get out there and give it all I've got rather than let that all-or-nothing mentality convince me that I might as well do nothing.

Turn off the tube. If you have time to watch TV, you have time to exercise. Try watching your favorite shows while you exercise, if you don't want to cut back on your screen time. The publication Preventing Chronic Disease *from the National Center for Chronic Disease Prevention and Health Promotion found that watching more than two hours of TV a day was associated with a higher weight-to-height ratio, along with higher rates of obesity and overeating.*

Life is always going to be busy, stressful, and difficult, but we must learn to weave workouts and other healthy habits into our lives. It might take some reprioritizing. It might mean saying no to others or asking for help. But it can be done. All the fit people in the world can attest to that.

—Nicole Nichols

DAY 3

INSIDER TIP

These Things Take Time

"Don't expect everything immediately. Celebrate little steps because many little steps cover a great distance."

—Amy, 82 pounds lost

MIND-SET MAKEOVER

We settle into ruts and get comfortable with our habits because breaking them and stepping away from what we know can be scary. Start small. Try something new—a new running route, a different brand of yogurt, a blue pen instead of black—anything to make today feel different from yesterday. How does it feel to try something new, no matter how small?

METABOLIC MAKEOVER

Eat away from the computer or TV all day long. Though we recommend that you always eat at a table, free from distractions, we know that in today's busy world that's not always possible. Try it for just one day. Notice any difference in your hunger levels or your enjoyment of the food you're eating.

BREAKFAST

SAD		Spark Swaps		Calories Saved
Frozen spinach-feta wrap	260 calories Plus, 25 percent more sodium and half the protein	Spinach-Feta Breakfast Wrap (page 168) 1 cup watermelon cubes	313 calories	(53)

The Bigger Picture. Here's where our swaps get tricky. If you look only at calories, you might think our meal was the wrong choice. Step back and see the big picture. The grab-and-go option from your favorite coffeehouse has more sodium and half the protein as ours. Plus, we add watermelon for a well-rounded meal.

Stretch It Out. Strong ingredients like feta cheese impart tons of flavor, even in small amounts. Two tablespoons of feta stands out more than an equal amount of a mild cheese like mozzarella.

LUNCH

SAD		Spark Swaps		Calories Saved
Chicken Caesar salad	560 calories	Lighter Chicken Caesar Salad (page 182)	456 calories	104
		½ cup grape or cherry tomatoes		
		16 seedless grapes		
		1 carton (6 ounces) light Key lime pie yogurt (or another flavor)		

Hail, Caesar. Caesar salads are a lunchtime standby, from corner delis to white-tablecloth restaurants, but they're not exactly light. The dressing is loaded with salt and fat, plus cheese is often in the dressing as well as sprinkled on top. Aside from the lettuce, there's no other vegetable—just fried croutons.

Choose Your Yogurt. Whether you choose regular or Greek yogurt is up to you. We like light yogurt. It tastes like a treat, but it's nutritious too.

SNACK

SAD		Spark Swaps		Calories Saved
Cheese crackers from a vending machine	190 calories	Avocado Toast:	159 calories	31
		1 slice whole-wheat bread, toasted		
		¼ avocado, mashed		
		Black pepper to taste		

Go Beyond Guac. Not all fats are created equal, as you've learned. Cheese crackers are full of saturated fat, salt, and preservatives without the calcium and protein found in real cheese.

Avocados are a source of heart-healthy unsaturated fat and boast fiber too. Avocado Toast stretches this fruit beyond the usual guacamole and gives you the same contrast of creamy and crunchy as the crackers, without the sodium overload.

To make this super snack, toast a slice of whole-wheat bread. Top it with the mashed avocado. Sprinkle it with black pepper, smoked paprika, or lime juice, cut it into wedges, and eat immediately.

DINNER

SAD		Spark Swaps		Calories Saved
Homemade cheeseburger (made with 80 percent lean ground beef) and frozen french fries with loads of ketchup	922 calories	Inside-Out Burgers (page 199) Baked Garlic-Herb Fries (page 217) 1 cup skim milk	480 calories	442

Better Burgers. Who doesn't like a game of hide-and-seek? The usual burger-and-fries dinner is hiding loads of fat. Seek out ours instead, which has secrets of its own. Extra-lean beef can be dry, so we stuff it with onion and herbs for a juicy, tasty burger.

Fixed-Up Fries. On its own, the potato is somewhat bland, which is why we love to load up our fries with salt and ketchup. You can achieve that same crunchiness by baking potato wedges at a high temperature. We took them up a notch with garlic and herbs. Without loads of oil adding excess calories, you'll have room to dip.

Dip Do-Over. Ketchup is a panacea for bad food. Consider skipping the red stuff (or at least choosing a low-sodium, no-added-sugar version) and dipping your fries into something more creative (with fewer calories). Try mustard, salsa, plain Greek yogurt mixed with herbs, or . . . nothing at all!

SNACK

SAD		Spark Swaps		Calories Saved
Blueberry cobbler (homemade)	290 calories	Berry Cobbler Cup (page 230)	138 calories	152

Dieting White Lie. If it's made with fruit, you can eat as much as you want. This fallacy applies especially to desserts, it seems. Traditional cobbler drenches low-calorie berries in sugar, then smothers them in a buttery crust with white flour and more sugar. Tasty but certainly not light.

Our version takes mere minutes (in the microwave), and it's portion controlled so you won't be tempted to serve yourself too much or reach for seconds. Still sweet, it allows the natural flavor of the berries to shine.

SAD Total	Spark Swaps Total	Deficit
2,222 calories	1,546 calories	676 calories

DAILY TOTALS

Calories: 1,546	Sodium: 1,941 mg	Fiber: 28 g
Fat: 34 g	Carbs: 207 g	Protein: 112 g

Fitness That Fits

CARDIO INTERVALS: 30 MINUTES

Choose any form of cardio and alternate between high intensity and low intensity using this guide: 1 minute of "all out" (9 out of 10) followed by 3 minutes of "moderate" (6 out of 10). Repeat this sequence of intervals 6 times (24 total minutes). Warm up before and cool down after for 3 minutes each.

Our Pick: running at a 10-minute-mile pace, with intervals of running at a 9-minute-mile pace (390 calories burned)

FLEXIBILITY
Spend 5 to 10 minutes stretching all major muscle groups after your
workout.

NEAT: 30 MINUTES
Daily Deficit: 1,066 calories
Week-to-Date Deficit: 4,038 calories

SPARK IT UP: BOOST THE BURN
Do an extra set of intervals to burn 25 percent more calories.

MAKE IT WORK: BREAK IT UP
Break your cardio intervals into three 10-minute sessions. Do one set in
the morning, one at lunch, and one while making dinner.

Make Tomorrow Easier

Mix up the Breakfast Cookies (page 152) while the burgers and fries are
cooking, then bake them after dinner.

Daily Reflection

HOW DID YOU FEEL TODAY?	Poor		OK		Excellent
	1	2	3	4	5
I made healthy food choices based on the Spark Swaps meal plan.					
I was physically active, following the Fitness That Fits workouts.					
I felt motivated to stick with the Spark Solution program.					
I am ready to take on tomorrow and all that it has in store for me.					

What were the highlights of your day? What were the challenges? How
can you use today's highs and lows to make tomorrow better and easier?

DAY 4

INSIDER TIP

Fake It Until You Feel It

"Dress the part. Act the part. Suck it up. That was my first mantra. Dress the part of who you want to be that day: put on your workout clothes. Act the part: be active. Suck it up: if people or situations get to you, suck it up and let it out later during a good workout or vent with a friend."

—Beth, 235 pounds lost

MIND-SET MAKEOVER

Today, think about getting up and exercising first thing in the morning instead of sleeping in. (And maybe do it, if your schedule permits.) How does it feel to start your day on a healthy note? How can you put that extra time in the morning to good use? When the urge to oversleep, skip a workout, or avoid some other healthy-living task arises, ask yourself this question: What would I do instead? Stepfanie uses this tactic when she's tempted to skip Spinning or running after a long day of work. The answers—not much, take a nap, watch TV, etc.—sound pretty lame when she says them out loud, so nine times out of ten, she ends up working out as planned.

METABOLIC MAKEOVER

Sitting is bad for your health, but if you work a desk job, it's hard to avoid it. Set a timer on your phone or write a reminder on your calendar. Get up every hour, even if it's just to stand up and stretch your legs. Walk to the kitchen to refill your water bottle, print something so you have an excuse to get up from your desk, or close your office door and hold plank position for thirty seconds (see page 251 for details). You won't regret moving, but you'll regret not moving at the end of the day when you're stiff and tired.

BREAKFAST

SAD		Spark Swaps		Calories Saved
Gas station breakfast:	731 calories	1 Breakfast Cookie (page 152)	419 calories	312
1 cinnamon frosted toaster pastry		1 medium apple		
1 12-ounce bottle chocolate milk		1 cup skim milk		

Rough but Ready. We all have those mornings. The dry cleaning needs to be dropped off. The kids missed the bus. Everyone overslept. The gas gauge is on empty. Turn around a stressful morning with a healthy breakfast. Prep a batch of these cookies once a week and keep them on hand (or stash some in the freezer) for crazy days. Grab one, along with an apple and a container of milk, and breakfast is ready—fast.

Double Take. Toaster pastries come two to a package, but a serving is one pastry. Deceiving, isn't it? Even the kind made with whole grains and "real fruit" doesn't constitute a healthy breakfast or count as a serving of either whole grains or fruit. Add the full-fat chocolate milk and you have a heavy breakfast that will send your blood sugar soaring, then leave you famished long before lunchtime.

Skim Milk Skeptics. We know that switching from 2 percent or whole milk to skim (fat-free) can be a bit of a challenge at first. If your distaste for skim is preventing you from getting your daily dairy, 1 percent is an acceptable swap. The difference in fat is small, but it does add a nice richness. Once you're used to 1 percent, consider mixing half skim and half 1 percent and eventually make the switch.

LUNCH

SAD		Spark Swaps		Calories Saved
Sweet-and-sour chicken with white rice	1,435 calories	Sweet Orange-Miso Chicken and Veggies (page 189) with ½ cup cooked brown rice 1 cup skim milk	444 calories	991

Food Court Failure. With the abundance of bright veggies and steamed rice, Chinese food appears to be a good choice. It must certainly be lower in calories than the fried chicken sandwich and fries, right? Wrong. A crispy chicken sandwich with mayonnaise and fries has almost 1,100 calories, and a full take-out container of the mall standby sweet-and-sour chicken has even more. The chicken is usually deep-fried dark meat, the veggies cooked in oil, and the rice served in large portions.

Stock Up on Sauces. Keep a batch of the miso and other favorite sauces on hand for quick lunches throughout the week. If you're really pressed for time, choose a low-sodium, light-on-the-sugar bottled sauce that you can add to veggies, lean chicken or beef, and brown rice.

SNACK

SAD		Spark Swaps		Calories Saved
1 ounce nacho-flavored tortilla chips	150 calories	1 ounce baked tortilla chips 1 ounce (2 tablespoons) hummus	133 calories	17

Crunch Time. When it comes to snacking, we often crave a texture or taste rather than something specific. When crunchy is what you crave, more than likely a banana won't satisfy you. You want chips. But which ones?

The nacho-flavored chips have little if any real cheese but plenty of things you can't pronounce and salt. Lots of salt. Swap them for baked tortilla chips (low-sodium or unsalted, if you have the option) and dunk them in hummus. The nacho-flavored chips have two and a half times the fat, so it's really no contest.

DINNER

SAD		Spark Swaps		Calories Saved
6 fish sticks with frozen Tater Tots and 2 tablespoons tartar sauce	674 calories	Panko-Breaded Fish with Tomato Salad (page 205) ½ cup sautéed zucchini ½ cup cooked whole-wheat couscous 1 tablespoon tartar sauce (optional) 1 kiwi	412 calories	262

Fish Stick Rehab. If the only fish you're eating comes in stick form dunked in tartar sauce, you're missing out on an ocean's worth of lean protein. This dish keeps the crunch but uses Japanese breadcrumbs and very little added fat. Salty capers, fresh parsley, and lemon juice create a tangy sauce that captures all you love about tartar sauce, but without the mayonnaise. Cast your line, hook this keeper of a dish, and sink almost 1,600 milligrams of sodium and 27 grams of fat.

Couscous? Yes, yes! Whole-wheat couscous should be a regular fixture at dinnertime. It's ready in less than 15 minutes and requires approximately 30 seconds of hands-on work: just add 1 cup to a bowl of 1¼ cups boiling water, let sit 5 minutes covered, then fluff with a fork after the water is absorbed. Then add broth, citrus, herbs, or dried fruit to perk it up. Serve a scoop with your salads or serve it hot alongside any grilled meat. You can even turn leftovers into breakfast by reheating it and adding fruit, milk, and a drizzle of honey.

Spark Swap Panko. Panko are Japanese-style breadcrumbs. They're larger and lighter than traditional ones, and the key to light yet crunchy crusts, like the one on this fish. We also use them to coat Meg's Pan-Fried Chicken (page 200). Choose whole-wheat panko if you can find them, and scatter a handful atop casseroles to add crunch for only a few extra calories.

Turn low-fat cheese sticks into a fun appetizer by cutting them in two, dipping them in a mixture of flour, egg whites, and panko seasoned with Italian herbs, then baking them at 375°F for 10 minutes, or until the cheese is melted. Use the same technique to make your own chicken tenders or nuggets.

SNACK

SAD		Spark Swaps		Calories Saved
1 cup chocolate ice cream	285 calories	½ cup slow-churned ice cream	110 calories	175

Slow Food. When slow-churned ice cream hit the market a few years ago, it was a healthy eater's dream come true. Ice cream with the texture and flavor of old-fashioned ice cream, but with half the fat. It's true. Manufacturers devised a way to reduce the size of the fat particles and ice crystals in ice cream, which gives a creamy texture to lower-fat ice creams. We think it's a smart swap.

Portion Distortion. We know the comparisons above aren't equal. We're pitting a cup of full-fat ice cream against half as much of its slow-churned brethren. Ice cream is a food that is easy to dish up too much of. Reach for the smallest bowl in your cabinet—even a ramekin or a teacup. Ditch the soup spoon and use a regular spoon or even a dainty iced-tea spoon if you have one. That ½-cup portion will seem reasonable if it's not served in a giant bowl.

SAD Total	Spark Swaps Total	Deficit
3,275 calories	1,518 calories	1,757 calories

DAILY TOTALS

Calories: 1,518	**Sodium: 1,433 mg**	**Fiber: 25 g**
Fat: 32 g	**Carbs: 220 g**	**Protein: 90 g**

Fitness That Fits

STRENGTH TRAINING: AMRAP
Perform the exercises in the Spark Swaps Strength Workout (page 247) in the order listed, this time doing as many reps as possible (AMRAP) and every exercise for 1 full minute, fitting in as many controlled, good reps as you can. Move quickly to the next exercise (with little or no rest) until you've done them all. For exercises performed on one side at a time, perform 1 full minute on each side before switching. Then move on to the next exercise. Record your score (reps) for each move for later reference.

Calories Burned: about 100

FLEXIBILITY
Spend 5 to 10 minutes stretching all major muscle groups after your workout.

NEAT: 45 MINUTES
Daily Deficit: 1,857 calories
Week-to-Date Deficit: 5,895 calories

SPARK IT UP: CHALLENGE YOURSELF
Try 90 seconds or 2 minutes of each exercise.

MAKE IT WORK: SOME IS BETTER THAN NONE
Cut your workout down to 30 seconds per move.

Daily Reflection

HOW DID YOU FEEL TODAY?	Poor		OK		Excellent
	1	2	3	4	5
I made healthy food choices based on the Spark Swaps meal plan.					
I was physically active, following the Fitness That Fits workouts.					
I felt motivated to stick with the Spark Solution program.					
I am ready to take on tomorrow and all that it has in store for me.					

What were the highlights of your day? What were the challenges? How can you use today's highs and lows to make tomorrow better and easier?

Habits of Healthy Eaters

Cook at Home

As obesity rates have risen, we have become kitchen illiterate at alarming rates. Reacquainting ourselves with the kitchen—meaning the stove and oven, not just the microwave and refrigerator—is an important part of a healthy lifestyle, especially if you're trying to lose weight.

Now, you might say, "Who has the time to cook dinner, let alone plan meals?" In our overscheduled, always-on-the-go society, mealtimes blur together and the kitchen goes largely unused. According to government data, in 1965 we spent two hours a day preparing meals; today we spend less than half that amount. The advent of timesaving appliances is partially responsible, but our reliance on restaurants and heat-and-eat frozen and packaged foods is indisputably to blame.

Meals prepared at home are more nutritious, put you in control of your eating habits, and are much more budget friendly than even the cheapest of fast-food meals. Dinner doesn't have to be fancy. It doesn't have to take hours. Even Chef Meg spends less than an hour making dinner for her family most nights, yet they regularly have a home-cooked meal.

With a little organization and a simple meal plan, you can reclaim the kitchen as the most important room in the house, like Ella did. Now 112 pounds lighter, Ella went from eating out every other day, and ordering twice as much food as her friends, to cooking every day. "Like, really cooking," she says. "I have learned to love spending time in the kitchen, trying to use veggies and fruits in new and exciting ways."

DAY 5

INSIDER TIP

Keep Your Eye on the Prize

"Being a good example for my kids matters to me. My daughter tells me she wants to run with me when she gets older (she is just under four) and that makes me feel like a million bucks."

—Marissa, 90 pounds lost

MIND-SET MAKEOVER

Stress can lead to overeating for many of us. If life gets hard today, pause and breathe. Close your eyes, if you can, and count to five as you inhale, hold for one count, then exhale for a count of five. Increase the count by one with each breath, until you've reached a count of ten. Whatever was bothering you likely will have passed, and you've averted a potential binge.

METABOLIC MAKEOVER

Chew carefully. We forget sometimes that digestion begins in the mouth, not the stomach. Thoroughly chewing your food and pausing between bites means that you will not only taste your meals more, but also give yourself more time to realize when you're full and help your digestive system get the most nutrients out of your food.

BREAKFAST

SAD		Spark Swaps		Calories Saved
Breakfast burrito: 1 13-inch flour tortilla 2 large eggs ¼ cup shredded cheddar cheese 2 sausage patties Coffee with 2 tablespoons half-and-half	635 calories	Mexican Breakfast Burrito (page 161) ½ cup cantaloupe cubes	309 calories	326

Burrito Overload. Flour tortillas have devolved into the carb equivalent of Mary Poppins's bag. Ever seen what you can fit inside those dinner-plate-size wraps? We recently saw an Italian burrito filled with pasta, meat, sauce, and spinach-artichoke dip. The finished product was so large you needed both hands.

The standard breakfast burrito isn't quite as heavy, but you'll still be loosening your belt after downing this breakfast. Even with a side of melon, our version is less than half the calories of the other.

Perfectly Wrapped. Unless you plan to use them to wrap a double portion, skip the 13-inch tortillas. Choose 7-inch whole-grain or whole-wheat wraps instead. You can even find a low-carb version, if you prefer those.

On the Go. Burritos freeze well, and they're perfect for busy mornings. Do yourself a favor and make a big batch, then stash them in the freezer.

LUNCH

SAD		Spark Swaps		Calories Saved
BLT sandwich	565 calories	Better BLT (page 172) 1 cup fresh strawberries 1 cup skim milk 2 dark chocolate kisses	490 calories	75

Bacon Intervention. We have no problem with bacon. What's troubling is the trend of piling it on anything imaginable (bacon sundaes? woven bacon cups?) and in large quantities. That was our starting point for the Better BLT. We wanted to keep the bacon, but in a more reasonable portion, to show that two slices of a low-sodium variety impart more than enough smoky taste for even the most fervent of bacon lovers.

Avocado Exchange. Mayonnaise adds much-needed moisture to the traditional BLT, but ours has a savory red pepper sauce with a Greek-yogurt base and avocado added for richness. Mayonnaise has only 3 more grams of fat, but avocado contains healthier fats.

SNACK

SAD		Spark Swaps		Calories Saved
16 ounces dark beer	196 calories	1 12-ounce can light beer	103 calories	93

Smart Sips. Alcohol calories are empty calories and add nothing to your diet nutritionally. So, when you're out for your weekly happy hour, consider your drink carefully. A can of beer is 12 ounces, rather than the 16 ounces often served at bars, and dark beers pack more of a punch calorie-wise than their light (in calories, but also to a lesser extent in color) counterparts.

DINNER

SAD		Spark Swaps		Calories Saved
Homemade macaroni and cheese	446 calories	Baked Macaroni and Cheese (page 195) 1 thick slice tomato 1 cup steamed green beans	384 calories	62

Macaroni Makeover. Whether it comes from Grandma's kitchen or a box, macaroni and cheese is a dish that's hard to resist. Most varieties are based on a classic cream sauce with loads of cheese enveloping white-flour pasta. We swapped for a whole-wheat pasta with more fiber and used puréed white beans to maintain a creamy, buttery texture with less fat.

Less Cheese, More Flavor. We wanted a really strong flavor in this dish, so we chose extra-sharp cheddar rather than a mild variety. Choose more pungent, stronger cheeses (feta, sharp cheddar, blue) to use less but still get the flavor you crave in every bite.

Cut the Richness. A good rule of thumb is to pair a rich main dish with a simple side, or vice versa. We served this macaroni and cheese with a slice of tomato, the acidity of which cuts the richness of the cheese, and simple

steamed green beans, which also help reset the palate between all those creamy bites.

SNACK

SAD		Spark Swaps		Calories Saved
1 slice apple pie (⅛ pie)	296 calories	Hot Apple Tart (page 237) 1 cup skim milk	210 calories	86

New Math. By adulthood, most of us have mastered fractions. We can look at a circle and mentally calculate ¼, ⅛, etc. But when it comes to pie, doesn't it seem difficult to remember that lesson? That ⅛-pie slice gets a little wider and longer as we cut into the pie. And how easy is it to pass by a pie and cut "just a sliver" to even it out? That was the inspiration for this recipe and the Berry Cobbler Cup (page 230) on Day 3. Not only do you save time and calories by swapping pie crust for graham crackers, but you get a portion-controlled serving of the best part: the juicy, sweet filling, which we packed with apples and cinnamon.

Pick a Pie. This basic recipe works well for all your favorite fruit pies. Try peaches, cherries, or blueberries. Swap out the graham crackers for a vanilla wafer or a gingersnap.

SAD Total	Spark Swaps Total	Deficit
2,138 calories	1,496 calories	642 calories

DAILY TOTALS

Calories: 1,496	Sodium: 1,868 mg	Fiber: 33 g
Fat: 38 g	Carbs: 210 g	Protein: 80 g

Fitness That Fits

CARDIO: 20 MINUTES

Choose a different activity than Day 1 and accumulate minutes in two 10-minute chunks or all at once. Work "somewhat hard" (8 out of 10) so you are slightly breathless the entire time.

Our Pick: Zumba or another cardio dance class or DVD (150 calories burned)

FLEXIBILITY

Spend 5 to 10 minutes stretching all major muscle groups after your workout.

NEAT: 30 MINUTES

Daily Deficit: 792 calories
Week-to-Date Deficit: 6,687 calories

SPARK IT UP: THE POWER OF TEN

Add another 10 minutes to your workout. You're already sweaty and dressed for it, so why not? (Another 75 calories burned!)

MAKE IT WORK: MUSIC MOTIVATES

Turn on the radio or play music on your phone. Crank up something upbeat and dance for at least 10 minutes.

Make Tomorrow Easier

While the mac and cheese is baking, mix up the Better "Buttermilk" Biscuits dough (page 218) and roll them out. Bake them while you're eating dinner. The oven will still be hot, so it won't take long to preheat.

Daily Reflection

HOW DID YOU FEEL TODAY?	Poor		OK		Excellent
	1	2	3	4	5
I made healthy food choices based on the Spark Swaps meal plan.					
I was physically active, following the Fitness That Fits workouts.					
I felt motivated to stick with the Spark Solution program.					
I am ready to take on tomorrow and all that it has in store for me.					

What were the highlights of your day? What were the challenges? How can you use today's highs and lows to make tomorrow better and easier?

DAY 6

INSIDER TIP

Be Patient

"The first two weeks of my new lifestyle were all about proving to myself that I could do it—that I could change and break old habits. I didn't care about the results, at that point. I just wanted to be able to say that I was doing everything I could to be healthier. Once I took the pressure off of myself to see results, the results happened because of the healthier lifestyle."

—Lisa, 83 pounds lost

MIND-SET MAKEOVER

Think of yourself in twenty-five years, reflecting on what you've done with your life. Think of the path you're on now. Are you making your

future self proud? What can you do today to help live a life you can be proud of?

METABOLIC MAKEOVER

Breakfast is the most important meal of the day, yet we rarely take the time to enjoy it. Carve out fifteen minutes—if not today then tomorrow—to sit down and have your morning meal. Notice whether this has any effect on your hunger levels.

Habits of Fit People

Listen to Your Body

It may seem counterintuitive to the no-pain-no-gain philosophy so many subscribe to, but listening to how you feel really makes a difference in your workouts. Your body is more intelligent than you realize. If you're really listening, it will tell you when you're tired, hungry, stressed, or sick. It also gives you signs when you're sore, injured, or exhausted—all of which could be clues that you need to cut back on your current workout routine. The opposite is also true; I find that I can tell when I have energy to burn, which often happens if I'm slacking in the gym or having a really stressful workday. On those days, I want and need a good, tough workout to combat stress and use up my pent-up energy.

Here are some of the ways I listen to my body when it comes to fitness. Most of these are a combination of listening and knowing how to remedy a situation as it arises.

- *If it hurts, stop.*
- *If you're injured, take time for recovery.*
- *If you feel tired, do less.*
- *Make time for sleep.*

You might say, "My body never wants to exercise. I'm tired. Sore. Old. If I listen to my body, I'll never work out." You may feel that way now, especially if you're new to exercise or just getting back into the habit of working out.

BREAKFAST

SAD		Spark Swaps		Calories Saved
Diner disaster: sausage gravy and biscuits	483 calories	Slim Sausage Gravy (page 166) and Better "Buttermilk" Biscuits (page 218)	374 calories	109
		¾ cup fresh peach slices		
		1 cup skim milk		

Most likely, we feel this way because we've ignored our bodies for so long that we've lost the desire to exercise. As kids, we called it playing and it was fun. But as adults, it's called working out.

If you truly listen to your body, it wants to move and be strong and fit. Once you get in the habit, it will tell you that more often. It also gives you cues when it needs a little downtime from the gym. Put simply, listening to your body will help you stick with a workout routine, prevent injury, and make exercise more enjoyable, all of which will help you make exercise a lifelong habit.

"I'm learning to tell the difference between injury pain and just the fact that I'm using a part of my body differently. I will listen and act accordingly to be safe and be strong." —Elizabeth, 32 pounds lost

"Today is supposed to be a running day, but I just can't face it. I considered challenging myself to my fastest walking pace instead. I felt so much more motivated. I can run tomorrow, if I listen to my body today." —Lisa, who's maintaining her weight

"I've found that listening to my body also motivates me to get moving. There are days I've designated as rest days, where my body is just humming with energy and the idea of just sitting around bums me out. So even on those rest days, I listen to my body and go for a nice long walk, do a quick SparkPeople video, or something. Nothing too intense, but something to make my body—and its newfound energy source—happy." —Colleen, 21 pounds lost

—Nicole Nichols

A Taste of the South. A Southern favorite, biscuits and gravy offer almost no nutrition: refined carbs covered with a saturated-fat-laden sauce. We cut back on the sausage and added fiber to the biscuits, then gave the meal staying power with milk. Peaches on the side cut the richness.

LUNCH

SAD		Spark Swaps		Calories Saved
12-inch meatball marinara sub	1,120 calories	Greek Meatball Pita (Keftedes) (page 178) 1 cup Greek salad (any combo of onions, peppers, cucumbers, and tomatoes) with 2 tablespoons light balsamic vinaigrette and 1 tablespoon crumbled low-fat feta cheese	393 calories	727

Foot in Mouth. With rare exceptions, food should not be measured in feet. Any food that touts its length in feet (even one foot) is probably best avoided. That goes for subs, hot dogs, and licorice too. If you do find yourself at a sub shop faced with a bargain foot-long sandwich, split it with someone or save half for later.

Sink That Sub. Sandwiches are perfect lunch food. They're portable, handheld, and often a well-balanced meal. Not the meatball marinara sub. Loaded with enough meat for three meals and gobs of cheese, with nary a veggie in sight, this monstrosity will sink your lunch plans. We swapped it for meatballs from the other side of the Mediterranean and mixed in plenty of vegetables.

Meatball Makeover. When you're ready to start cooking your own recipes, pair your favorite meatballs (made with extra-lean beef or turkey) with a low-fat marinara and a hefty serving of grilled vegetables. Top with low-fat mozzarella cheese and stuff into half a whole-wheat pita for a fraction of the calories in the sub shop's version.

SNACK

SAD		Spark Swaps		Calories Saved
1 ¾-ounce bag cheddar popcorn	180 calories	1 1-ounce bag low-fat microwave popcorn (yields 3½ cups popped) with your choice of herbs and spices	130 calories	50

Pop Secret. Did you know that popcorn is a whole grain? It is, and when popped with little or no added fat, it's a great snack choice. Plain popcorn can be pretty plain, so spritz it with cooking spray, then sprinkle on your favorite herbs and spices. (Be sure to choose salt-free seasonings.)

Try one of these combos:
- cinnamon, ginger, and cardamom
- cumin and curry powder
- smoked paprika
- garlic powder
- Italian seasoning and 1 tablespoon finely grated Parmesan cheese
- black pepper and lime zest
- steak seasoning or other all-purpose seasoning blends

DINNER

SAD		Spark Swaps		Calories Saved
Beef roast with mashed potatoes and gravy	529 calories	Dijon-Herb Pork Tenderloin (page 198) Perfect Mashed Potatoes (page 225) 1 cup steamed green beans ½ cup unsweetened applesauce 1 cup skim milk	494 calories	35

Chef's Tip. Pork tenderloin is a busy cook's best friend. It cooks quickly and pairs well with most seasonings you'll probably have on hand, yet it seems fancier than, say, chicken breast.

Double Up. Chef Meg loves to cook two tenderloins at a time, then portion the second into single servings. She pairs the leftovers with a simple salad and a slice of crusty whole-wheat bread for quick suppers, shreds the meat for tasty burrito filling, or turns it into barbecue sandwiches (along with her Hot-and-Sweet Rainbow Slaw, page 221).

Better Beef Roasts. The classic beef roast can remain a part of your healthy recipes repertoire. Choose lean cuts of beef (such as eye or top round roasts), trim any visible fat, and stick to 3-ounce portions.

Perfect Potatoes. What better way to soak up all the tasty juices from the roast than with a side of creamy mashed potatoes? Ours, you won't be surprised by now to learn, contain no butter and no cream. We wanted the potato flavor to stand out, so we used slightly acidic sour cream along with a few other ingredients. We like to place the roast directly atop the ½-cup serving of potatoes.

SNACK

SAD		Spark Swaps		Calories Saved
Sundae cone	320 calories	Fruit-Stuffed Ice Cream Cone (page 235)	87 calories	233

Sundae Any Day. The appeal of the sundae cone is the contrast of flavors and textures. We kept that in mind as we created one you can eat regularly. We filled the cone with fruit instead of chocolate, scooped up low-fat vanilla frozen yogurt, and opted for a crunchy sugar cone. You can mix the fruit with the frozen yogurt, swap it for a different flavor, or even use slow-churned ice cream. For added crunch, top with a few chopped nuts or sprinkles, which make anything feel festive. The fresh fruit cuts the sweetness of the frozen yogurt, which in turn makes the fruit seem like a treat. Drizzle on a balsamic reduction (see next page) to fancy it up.

We can't wait to try raspberries with chocolate frozen yogurt and chopped mint.

Spark Swap Balsamic Reduction. Balsamic glazes, reductions, and sauces are popping up all over menus these days, and we're thrilled. Swap this simple sauce for greasy gravy, and you'll cut half the calories and all the fat. Simply pour ½ cup balsamic vinegar into a small saucepan and bring to a simmer, cooking until the mixture has reduced by half and has a syrupy texture. (Stand back! You don't want to inhale the strong vinegar fumes.) Spoon 1 tablespoon over meats, grilled vegetables, or even your favorite low-fat vanilla ice cream—trust us.

SAD Total	Spark Swaps Total	Deficit
2,632 calories	1,478 calories	1,154 calories

DAILY TOTALS

Calories: 1,478	Sodium: 1,519 mg	Fiber: 27 g
Fat: 40 g	Carbs: 180 g	Protein: 105 g

Fitness That Fits

STRENGTH TRAINING: TWO SETS OF TWELVE REPS
Perform the exercises in the Spark Swaps Strength Workout (page 247) in reverse order, moving quickly from one exercise to the next for one set, then repeat for a second set. For exercises performed on one side at a time, perform all reps on each side before switching. Then move on to the next exercise.

Calories Burned: about 108

FLEXIBILITY
Spend 5 to 10 minutes stretching all major muscle groups after your workout.

NEAT: 45 MINUTES
Daily Deficit: 1,262 calories
Week-to-Date Deficit: 7,949 calories

SPARK IT UP: SQUEEZE IN CARDIO
Add cardio intervals between your strength moves. Keep it simple: high knees, hopping in place, and jumping jacks will all get your heart rate up.

MAKE IT WORK: THERE'S ALWAYS TIME
If you're short on time, drop down to one set. When you feel your workout motivation waning, put on your workout clothes as soon as you get home. Getting dressed is half the battle when it comes to motivating yourself to work out.

Daily Reflection

HOW DID YOU FEEL TODAY?	Poor		OK		Excellent
	1	2	3	4	5
I made healthy food choices based on the Spark Swaps meal plan.					
I was physically active, following the Fitness That Fits workouts.					
I felt motivated to stick with the Spark Solution program.					
I am ready to take on tomorrow and all that it has in store for me.					

What were the highlights of your day? What were the challenges? How can you use today's highs and lows to make tomorrow better and easier?

DAY 7

INSIDER TIP

Out of Sight, Out of Mouth

"By filling my plate in the kitchen, the food was less accessible to get seconds. In fact, I would even put the leftovers in containers for lunches the next day before I sat down to eat. This worked like a charm."

—Yvonne, 209 pounds lost

MIND-SET MAKEOVER

Since you have the day off from official exercise and you're marking the halfway point in this two-week program, take some time to think about your goals. On SparkPeople.com, we encourage members to create a goal collage or online pinboard, with images to remind you of your goals. Today's a great time to make your goal collage. Include images of clothes you want to wear, things you want to do, and people who inspire you to stick with your goals. Add inspirational quotes, your personal mantras, and a date you'd like to reach your ultimate goal, if you have one. Be sure to hang it someplace where you'll see it at least daily.

METABOLIC MAKEOVER

Keep track of condiments. While they're a small part of most meals, condiments can make or break your calorie goals for the day. It's all too easy to add a dollop of butter or accidentally pour on too much syrup. Pull out your measuring spoons for these calorie-dense foods, and start to recognize what the serving sizes look like on your plate.

BREAKFAST

SAD		Spark Swaps		Calories Saved
3 6-inch pancakes, 3 pats butter, and ¼ cup syrup	792 calories	Protein Pancakes (page 162) with 1 teaspoon unsalted butter and 1 tablespoon real maple syrup 1 cup fresh blueberries 1 cup skim milk	398 calories	394

The Real Deal. Read the ingredients list on your pancake syrup, and you may or may not find actual maple. Most are made with corn syrup, and with artificial and natural flavorings added. Real maple syrup is pricier but worth it. The flavor is stronger, so most people use less. One tablespoon is more than enough to impart maple taste into every bite.

No After-Breakfast Naps. Ever feel like face-planting on your plate after a pancake breakfast? With all those refined carbs in the pancakes themselves, plus the sugary syrup on top, it's no wonder. Ours are made with whole-wheat flour (yeah, fiber!) and Greek yogurt to keep blood-sugar levels stable. Tart blueberries cut the sweetness, and a cup of milk washes it all down while also providing more protein and giving this meal real staying power.

Favorite Pancake Fillings. After the batter has been poured into the skillet, sprinkle on one of these fillings:

- 10 blueberries
- 10 raisins
- 10 chocolate chips
- 2 teaspoons chopped pecans or walnuts
- 2 tablespoons chopped fresh apple or peach
- 1 teaspoon brown sugar and a sprinkle of cinnamon (skip the syrup)

LUNCH

SAD		Spark Swaps		Calories Saved
Miso salad (made with 2 cups chopped iceberg lettuce)	75 calories	Shrimp Salad with Miso-Carrot Dressing (page 187) ½ cup cooked brown rice drizzled with ½ teaspoon each toasted sesame oil and low-sodium soy sauce ½ cup mandarin oranges packed in water or juice	423 calories	(348)

The Salad Diet. It's a tactic that most dieters have tried at one point in time. You eat salad two or three meals a day in an attempt to be a pious eater and cut calories. By Day 2, you're ready to bite someone's head off and eat everything in sight. What gives? Aren't salads the quintessential diet food? Yes, but . . .

Sides Versus Mains. For a salad to be a well-balanced meal, it should contain at least three food groups, including protein. A side salad will do little to ward off hunger.

Dining Out. When grabbing lunch on the go, sushi is a fine choice. Choose brown rice in your rolls, use low-sodium soy sauce sparingly, and opt for simple rolls with added vegetables. Inquire about anything that includes the word "spicy" (often loaded with mayonnaise) and avoid items marked "tempura" (deep-fried). Get the salad with seaweed or the steamed broccoli on the side for another serving of veggies.

Salad Becomes the Star. The ginger-miso dressing served at Japanese restaurants is just so good it's a shame it isn't served more readily. The basis for many recipes (including ours) is carrots. We kept the dressing, added shrimp for protein, and bulked up the salad with plenty of other veggies. Seasoned brown rice completes the meal.

SNACK

SAD		Spark Swaps		Calories Saved
½ cup fat-free cottage cheese	80 calories	½ cup 2 percent cottage cheese	102 calories	(22)

Trick Question. Why is the higher-calorie cottage cheese a better choice? Shouldn't we be focused on cutting calories? Repeat after me: don't fear fat.

Fat Equals Flavor. When it comes to cheese, we prefer low-fat to fat-free. Not only does the low-fat have better flavor and a more satisfying texture, it doesn't contain the fillers and additives the fat-free versions do. Cottage cheese made with 2 percent milk fat has so much more flavor than the fat-free variety, and for only 22 additional calories. Sprinkle with black pepper or paprika and savor every bite.

DINNER

SAD		Spark Swaps		Calories Saved
1 fried chicken breast with skin 1 biscuit 1 cup coleslaw	564 calories	Meg's Pan-Fried Chicken (page 200) Better "Buttermilk" Biscuits (left over from yesterday) with 1 tablespoon honey ½ cup Hot-and-Sweet Rainbow Slaw (page 221) ½ cup chopped, cooked carrots 1 cup skim milk	497 calories	67

Fake Frying. The appeal of fried foods is not the grease, it's the crunch. Did you know you can easily replicate that texture with your oven? That's what we did with Meg's Pan-Fried Chicken. We did the same thing with our Baked Garlic-Herb Fries (page 217) and the crispy tortillas on our Trim Taco Salad (page 192).

Southern Feast. We set out to prove that you can feast on a sampler of your favorite comfort foods and still stick to your calorie goals. We succeeded by keeping portions in check, cutting out excess fat, and bulking up the meal with a serving of veggies.

Go Skinless. Removing the skin from a piece of fried chicken saves 57 calories and 5 grams of fat. Skip the breading and save another 31 calories and 4 grams of fat. Do that at every Sunday supper and drop a pound while still eating family favorites.

SNACK

SAD		Spark Swaps		Calories Saved
2 chocolate-covered cherries	150 calories	Cherry-Pistachio Yogurt Sundae (page 232)	104 calories	46

Fast Bites. Treats like chocolate-covered cherries go down fast. Two bites and your dessert is gone. Since these caloric treats often come in large boxes, they're easy to overeat. If this is a treat you crave, slow down and savor every bite. Close your eyes, let the flavor develop in your mouth as you chew thoroughly, and pause between bites.

Snacks into Treats. Yogurt is not ice cream, but it can satisfy that same craving for something creamy. It feels more like a treat when you top it with sweet cherries and crunchy pistachios. Serve it in a pretty bowl with a dainty dessert spoon and it turns snack time into something special.

SAD Total	Spark Swaps Total	Deficit
1,661 calories	1,524 calories	137 calories

DAILY TOTALS

Calories: 1,524	Sodium: 1,824 mg	Fiber: 24 g
Fat: 33 g	Carbs: 202 g	Protein: 110 g

Fitness That Fits

REST DAY: NO CARDIO OR STRENGTH TODAY
Rest up, rebuild, and recover.

NEAT: 75 MINUTES
Daily Deficit: 137 calories
Week-to-Date Deficit: 8,086 calories, or 2.3 pounds!

SPARK IT UP: CHILL OUT
Fight the urge to work out today. Your body needs the rest. Focus on racking up those NEAT minutes and get yourself ready for Week 2.

MAKE IT WORK: PLAY CATCH-UP
If you had to miss a day of exercise this week, now's your chance to make it up. Do the workout you didn't have time for earlier.

Daily Reflection

HOW DID YOU FEEL TODAY?	Poor		OK		Excellent
	1	2	3	4	5
I made healthy food choices based on the Spark Swaps meal plan.					
I was physically active, following the Fitness That Fits workouts.					
I felt motivated to stick with the Spark Solution program.					
I am ready to take on tomorrow and all that it has in store for me.					

What were the highlights of your day? What were the challenges? How can you use today's highs and lows to make tomorrow better and easier?

Lucky Number Seven

Congratulations for completing Week 1! How do you feel? You've had twenty-one chances to prep healthy meals, fourteen opportunities to snack smarter, and seven times to decide to make today your healthiest day yet. Whether you're exceeding your own expectations or moving a little more slowly, you're still building healthy habits. If you have moments of doubt, remember that these small steps you're taking are creating a really strong foundation for big change. Our successful members were once in your shoes. Even they wondered at times, "Can I really do this?" Those moments of doubt were fleeting. Now they say, "If I can do this, anyone can."

So, how are you feeling?

Have you had any cravings?

How have you been sleeping?

Has your energy increased?

How does exercise feel?

Are you moving more?

What were your highlights this week?

What were your biggest challenges?

Weigh and measure yourself, using the instructions we shared on pages 54 to 55.

Now, let's prepare for Week 2. You'll need to shop for your meals, schedule your workouts, and set goals for the week.

Habits of Healthy Eaters

Prep Veggies Ahead of Time

Stepfanie loves to chop vegetables and finds the task to be among the most relaxing in the kitchen. However, it takes time, which she doesn't have most nights. The solution is to chop vegetables ahead of time, so dinner can be prepared more quickly. Most vegetables can be prepped a few days in advance without much loss of quality.

You've probably noticed that you're eating onions and peppers daily. They're low in calories but pack in tons of flavor. Chop some every few days, and you'll save time throughout the week.

Chop veggies based on how you'll use them. Onions are usually chopped or diced for recipes, while peppers should be chopped or left in strips for easy snacking. Cut carrots and celery into sticks, and break broccoli and cauliflower into florets.

This time-saving trick doesn't work for all veggies:

Bok choy: Do not prep ahead of time as it will "rust" as it starts to oxidize.

Lettuce, spinach, and other greens: Prep only what you'll use in a day or two.

Potatoes and sweet potatoes: Do not prep ahead of time. Potatoes will turn black, and sweet potatoes will leach starch.

Tomatoes: Cut only twenty-four hours ahead, and only if they'll be cooked.

Week 2

With one week of healthy living under your belt, you're probably starting to get the hang of this. We have full faith in you. You can do this! This week will build on the healthy habits you started last week.

Make sure you have a fully stocked fridge, your workout clothes are ready to go, and your water bottle is never far from your side. Thirst is often misinterpreted as hunger, so drinking plenty of water can help ward off phantom hunger.

DAY 8

INSIDER TIP

Choose Your Company

"I surround myself with like-minded people (healthy eaters and active friends) in order to sustain my lifestyle. If I stayed around people who thought getting drunk and watching TV for hours was recreation, I would have a hard time going out for a run. By developing my social circle with like-minded friends we can support each other in our endeavors to lead healthier lives."

—*Tammy, 70 pounds lost*

MIND-SET MAKEOVER

It's easy to get caught up in the aesthetic aspects of weight loss. Today, think about the reasons you're doing this that don't involve pounds, pants sizes, or bathing-suit season. Why are those reasons important to you?

METABOLIC MAKEOVER

Though it's not on the "menu," add a couple of intervals to your workout today. Change up your speed to keep your body guessing and burn more calories.

BREAKFAST

SAD		Spark Swaps		Calories Saved
1 large cheese and fruit Danish	527 calories	Sweet and Creamy English Muffin (page 169) ½ banana 1 cup skim milk	409 calories	118

Sweet Starts. If you prefer a sweet start to your day, this simple breakfast is perfect for you. A crunchy English muffin is topped with creamy ricotta cheese, sweet jam, and real fruit. This meal is ready in two minutes (less time than you'd probably spend waiting in line to buy a Danish) and can be eaten in the car or at the kitchen table. Grabbing a Danish twice a week would add 16 pounds a year.

Plan Ahead. Freeze the other half of the banana and use in smoothies.

Spark Swap Low-Fat Ricotta Cheese. Often labeled PART-SKIM, ¼ cup of low-fat ricotta cheese has just 85 calories, 5 grams of fat, and 7 grams of protein. It's great with both sweet and savory dishes. Mix it with pesto or roasted red peppers and toss with whole-wheat pasta; add a scoop of it to a bowl of berries with balsamic vinegar and basil; or spread it on a whole-wheat tortilla, spike with garlic, and top with grilled veggies and chicken for a single-serving white pizza. Use low-fat ricotta as a swap for cream cheese at breakfast, with fruit for a fun snack, or mixed with marinara for a quick, creamy sauce.

LUNCH

SAD		Spark Swaps		Calories Saved
Fast-food taco salad in a tortilla bowl	630 calories and 1,530 milligrams sodium!	Trim Taco Salad (page 192) 1 cup skim milk	456 calories	174

Beware of Edible Bowls. Aside from lettuce cups, we can't think of a single edible bowl that's reasonably sized and not loaded with calories. Bread bowls, tortilla bowls, and—the latest fad—bacon bowls are all oversize and quite dense. Serve your food in a regular bowl to get your meal off to a better start.

A Better Base. At most restaurants, taco salads start not with the lettuce but with the meat and cheese. The greens can seem like an afterthought. We turned our salad around by building a base of dark leafy greens before adding lean protein and plenty of veggies. Rather than top it with greasy chips, we baked a tortilla and cut it into strips for crunchy contrast and a serving of whole grains.

Whether you're eating Mexican food at home, a party, or a restaurant, turn to the taco salad as a way to try a little of everything without loading up on chips, greasy taco shells, or oversize tortillas.

SNACK

SAD		Spark Swaps		Calories Saved
1 package vending machine peanut butter crackers	200 calories	Peanut Butter Cracker Sandwiches: 4 low-fat whole-wheat crackers with 1 tablespoon natural unsalted peanut butter	155 calories	45

Spice It Up. A drizzle of honey, a few raisins or dried cranberries, or a sprinkle of cinnamon, pumpkin pie spice, or ginger can make over a boring snack.

Desktop Dining. Stash a box of whole-grain crackers and a jar of natural peanut butter in an out-of-the-way drawer or in the office kitchen, if that's an option. When hunger strikes, bypass the vending machine. Even the seemingly healthy options like peanut butter crackers are hiding ingredients you don't want: salt, sugar, and trans fats.

DINNER

SAD		Spark Swaps		Calories Saved
Fettuccine Alfredo from an Italian chain restaurant	1,220 calories	Alfredo Pasta with Broccoli (page 193) Tomato Salad: 1 medium tomato, sliced and drizzled with 1 teaspoon each olive oil and balsamic vinegar 1 cup fresh strawberries	406 calories	814

The Secret's in the Sauce. Choose sauces that sneak in some extra vegetables or protein, like this one does. Add some grated Parmesan cheese on top instead of stirring it into the sauce, so you can really taste it.

Take shortcuts in the kitchen, not on your walk. If you need to get dinner on the table fast, use jarred sauce (low in sugar and salt) and frozen veggies.

Eyeball It. How do you measure pasta? One cup of cooked pasta is about the size of a baseball.

Spark Swap Fat-Free Evaporated Milk. Chef Meg's favorite swap for heavy cream and whole milk is fat-free evaporated milk, which is richer than skim milk and has a velvety texture. As you know, removing fat from food takes away that satisfying texture, but evaporated milk has had some of the water removed, so its texture resembles that of 2 percent milk. While we wouldn't suggest drinking this as one of your two daily servings of dairy, this milk has a longer shelf life and makes a great base for cream sauces.

SNACK

SAD		Spark Swaps		Calories Saved
Ice cream sandwich	140 calories	Chocolate Fro-Yo Sandwich (page 234)	99 calories	41

Single-Serve Sweets. If you're prone to overeating, having an entire box of treats at your disposal can prove too tempting. That's why we love these quick DIY desserts. You can make one sandwich at a time, using your favorite flavor of slow-churned ice cream or frozen yogurt, plus whatever else you have on hand. Though they take less than two minutes to make, that's enough time to talk yourself out of a second serving, should the craving arise.

SAD Total	Spark Swaps Total	Deficit
2,717 calories	1,525 calories	1,192 calories

DAILY TOTALS

Calories: 1,525	**Sodium: 1,207 mg**	**Fiber: 32 g**
Fat: 45 g	**Carbs: 203 g**	**Protein: 94 g**

Fitness That Fits

CARDIO: 30 MINUTES
Choose any activity and accumulate minutes in three 10-minute chunks, two 15-minute chunks, or all at once. Work "somewhat hard" (8 out of 10) so you are slightly breathless the entire time.

Our Pick: elliptical machine (375 calories burned)

FLEXIBILITY
Spend 5 to 10 minutes stretching all major muscle groups after your workout.

NEAT: 45 MINUTES
Daily Deficit: 1,567 calories
Week-to-Date Deficit: 1,567 calories

SPARK IT UP: LET GO

Get a core workout while you do your cardio: don't hold on to the handles of the elliptical.

MAKE IT WORK: BE FLEXIBLE

Worried you won't have time for your workout? Swap the Alfredo sauce on tonight's pasta dish for one of the quick-fix sauces in the recipes section, such as the Ten-Minute Garden Harvest Pasta Sauce (page 227) or the Creamy Roasted Red Pepper Pasta Sauce (page 220). You'll save ten minutes on dinner prep time, which you can use for a quick cardio workout.

Daily Reflection

HOW DID YOU FEEL TODAY?	Poor		OK		Excellent
	1	2	3	4	5
I made healthy food choices based on the Spark Swaps meal plan.					
I was physically active, following the Fitness That Fits workouts.					
I felt motivated to stick with the Spark Solution program.					
I am ready to take on tomorrow and all that it has in store for me.					

What were the highlights of your day? What were the challenges? How can you use today's highs and lows to make tomorrow better and easier?

DAY 9

INSIDER TIP

You Have to Want to Succeed

"Find a solid support system and make sure you have the right mind-set going in. Don't do it for your husband or your boss. Do it for you and for the right reasons. Don't think of it as a short-term venture. Make it a lifelong process."

—Lisa, 64 pounds lost

MIND-SET MAKEOVER

Take a minute sometime today to collect all the negative thoughts or feelings you've been experiencing this week. In one deep exhale, let them all leave your body and mind for good. What could you accomplish without the negativity in your life? How does negativity affect your success in all areas of life, particularly your health?

METABOLIC MAKEOVER

Don't underestimate the importance of stretching, especially if you sit all day. Rather than reach for snacks or caffeine to get you through the afternoon, take a minute or two to stretch. Even stretching your arms overhead and doing a couple of neck rolls can make a tremendous difference.

BREAKFAST

SAD		Spark Swaps		Calories Saved
Sausage-egg muffin	450 calories	Spicy Tomato-Egg Muffin (page 167) 16 grapes 1 cup skim milk	361 calories	89

Muffin Makeover. One thing's for sure about the fast-food sausage-and-egg breakfast. It's not skimping on the protein, with 21 grams. However, it also has 27 grams of fat—about two meals' worth. Our version replaces greasy sausage with a spicy sauce, plenty of low-fat cheddar cheese, and tomato to contrast the richness.

Habits of Fit People

Find Something Fun

For those of you just starting, exercise can seem daunting, and for too many people it's a necessary evil. You know you should be doing it, and you know it has all sorts of benefits, from helping you lose weight to improving your sleep, but often just knowing that it's good for you isn't enough. A workout becomes work, and you'd rather be doing something else. You probably have a long list of specific exercises or workouts you hate (mine includes the treadmill, most gym machines, and exercising alone). Instead of forcing yourself to do these, why not take the time to explore what you like, then create a workout program based around that?

When you're having fun, banishing boredom, learning new skills, or simply enjoying yourself, exercise becomes something you want to do, not something you have to do. There are lots of nontraditional activities and hobbies that can be fun and fitness-oriented. You could try rock climbing, Nintendo Wii, ballroom dancing, martial arts, swimming lessons, joining an adult sports league, playing with your kids, dancing around the house to your favorite tunes—anything that gets your body moving. My own workout program involves very few activities that I don't enjoy. I've discovered that I like Spinning classes (the group environment and great music motivates me), Pilates (it takes major focus and concentration), hiking and walking outdoors (it doesn't feel like exercise), and strength training at the gym (because I like to push myself). I also enjoy a good workout DVD now and then. I know I'm more likely to work out and push myself if I take a class at the gym than if I do it on my own too. Because these activities are fun for me, I don't dread my workout time; I look forward to it.

Plan Ahead. Make the sauce the night before, along with a batch of hard-boiled eggs. By the time the muffin toasts, you can assemble the remaining ingredients.

If you want to exercise regularly, you should find something you enjoy (or can tolerate at the very least). When you look forward to your workout, there's nothing stopping you from doing it. Here's what works for other people:

"I discovered Zumba eleven months ago and love it. I have tried the gym and frankly got bored. But I love to dance. So today I am going to try salsa." —Frances, 66 pounds lost

"I got a puppy! He was so full of energy, I had to walk him a lot just to keep him happy. He needed about three miles a day no matter what the weather. It's so much fun, it doesn't feel like work at all." —PJ, blog reader

"I pushed my bike into the living room. Now I watch my favorite TV shows while riding my recumbent bike." —Jenny, blog reader

"Initially, I hated exercise. Now I absolutely can't see not doing something. I have found many activities I enjoy and like to challenge myself: water aerobics, dancing, Wii Fit, and walking. I am not very strong, so I stick to the basics." —Teresa, blog reader

"I started out with running, but I really had to push myself to go for a run. Then I discovered that I could walk briskly almost as fast as I could run and I enjoyed it a whole lot more." —Lisa, 30 pounds lost

"Exercise is my reward for the day. I usually schedule it to fall at the end of the day in the late afternoon. The early part of the day is usually for 'mind' work and mundane things that have to be accomplished. Exercise is the release for the day—where I don't have to think, just do." —Paula, 5 pounds lost and maintaining a healthy weight

"I found the recumbent (stationary) bicycle, and it is so worth the money. I went from couch potato to riding every day. As SparkGuy says, 'Do ten minutes.' So I did, and do, at least that much." —Shary, 76 pounds lost

—Nicole Nichols

LUNCH

SAD		Spark Swaps		Calories Saved
8-inch Philly cheesesteak with all the trimmings	609 calories	Lean Philly Cheesesteak (page 179) 1 carrot, cut into sticks 1 tablespoon light ranch dressing	426 calories	183

Lunch on the Go. Finding time to run out and grab lunch is a challenge, which makes food trucks so convenient. They're right there, with food that's ready quickly, and it's affordable. At 600 calories each, a typical Philly cheesesteak is going to fill you up and knock you out. If you do find yourself staring down a cheesesteak, ask for light or no cheese, load up on veggies, and only eat part of the bun (ask for a dry bun).

Choose Your Dressing. If full-fat dressings are your favorite, you can still have them; just be sure to measure your portions. Or consider half low-fat and half regular. Lighten up your ranch but keep the flavor by mixing a store-bought seasoning packet into plain Greek yogurt in place of mayonnaise.

SNACK

SAD		Spark Swaps		Calories Saved
One serving pizza rolls (6 rolls)	200 calories	Cheater's Caprese Salad: 1 low-fat string cheese, chopped ½ cup chopped tomatoes 3 torn basil leaves ½ teaspoon olive oil	86 calories	114

Consider Your Cravings. When you crave something, stop for a minute and consider it. Would a similar yet healthier food suffice? That was the inspiration for this snack, which has all that pizza flavor without the fat.

DINNER

SAD		Spark Swaps		Calories Saved
1 cup canned chili with ¼ cup grated cheddar cheese, 2 tablespoons sour cream, and 1 ounce tortilla chips	647 calories	Speedy Turkey Chili (page 210) 1 toasted corn tortilla ½ cup fresh mango slices 1 cup skim milk	474 calories	173

Call On Chili. Though you could let your chili simmer all day, there's no need. You can get a hearty dish on the table in less than thirty minutes with this recipe. Everything is in one pot, so there's little mess, and there will be plenty of leftovers. Plus, as with most soups and stews, this chili is even better the next day. Consider doubling the batch and freezing single servings for cold nights and quick lunches.

Toasted tortillas are a quick side dish, but take them up a notch by squeezing on a bit of lime juice and sprinkling with cumin, smoked paprika, or chili powder. Or cut into wedges and dunk in your chili.

Swap It Up. Instead of turkey, you could use extra-lean chicken breast chunks or ground beef, or even lean pork or turkey sausage. Crumbled firm tofu would work too. Use any variety of beans you have on hand, and play around with the spice combos. Just make sure you add all your dried herbs and spices before adding the liquid, to maximize their flavors.

SNACK

SAD		Spark Swaps		Calories Saved
1 slice lemon meringue pie (⅛ pie)	360 calories	½ cup lemon sorbet	110 calories	250

What Are You Craving? Snack number one for the day taught you to think about your cravings and identify healthier swaps. Here's another chance.

Instead of lemon meringue pie, would lemon sorbet do? Cool and tangy, with a hint of sweetness, it's perfect on its own or with a sprinkle of mint.

Sorbet Sundae. Crumble a vanilla wafer in the bottom of a small dish, top with the sorbet and a dollop of light whipped topping.

SAD Total	Spark Swaps Total	Deficit
2,266 calories	1,457 calories	809 calories

DAILY TOTALS

Calories: 1,457	Sodium: 1,820 mg	Fiber: 32 g
Fat: 40 g	Carbs: 172 g	Protein: 94 g

Fitness That Fits

STRENGTH TRAINING: TWO SETS OF FIFTEEN REPS
Perform the exercises in the Spark Swaps Strength Workout (page 247) in the order listed, moving quickly from one exercise to the next for one set, then repeat for a second set. For exercises performed on one side at a time, perform all reps on each side before switching. Then move on to the next exercise.

Calories Burned: about 108

FLEXIBILITY
Spend 5 to 10 minutes stretching all major muscle groups after your workout.

NEAT: 60 MINUTES
Daily Deficit: 917 calories
Week-to-Date Deficit: 2,484 calories

SPARK IT UP: YOU'LL NEVER REGRET A WORKOUT
Add an extra 10 minutes to your warm-up today for a bonus cardio workout. And remember: strength training doesn't burn as many calories as

cardio does, but it's just as important. It's easy to fall into the mind-set that more calories burned equals a better workout, but forget about that. Cardio and strength are apples and oranges; they're both beneficial, so make sure you include both in your workout plan.

MAKE IT WORK: GET THE KIDS INVOLVED
Tonight's dinner is ready, thanks to the slow cooker. Exercise doesn't have to be something you do away from your kids. Take everyone outside to play, if weather permits, and do these exercises in the backyard while the little ones play.

Make Tomorrow Easier

Make Quick and Easy Granola (page 165) tonight, so it's ready for tomorrow's breakfast. And prep the chicken for tomorrow's lunch, if you don't have some ready.

Daily Reflection

HOW DID YOU FEEL TODAY?	Poor		OK		Excellent
	1	2	3	4	5
I made healthy food choices based on the Spark Swaps meal plan.					
I was physically active, following the Fitness That Fits workouts.					
I felt motivated to stick with the Spark Solution program.					
I am ready to take on tomorrow and all that it has in store for me.					

What were the highlights of your day? What were the challenges? How can you use today's highs and lows to make tomorrow better and easier?

DAY 10

INSIDER TIP

Do It for Yourself

"You must be your own hero. No one will do it for you. But reach out for help when you need it. Learn how to efficiently track your food and make it a part of every day. Find the little, happy rewards in each day. Learn that saying no to yourself is actually how you say yes to a healthy lifestyle."

—*Tina, 90 pounds lost*

When Life Doesn't Go as Planned

In weight loss and in life, we're all unique. The Spark Solution understands that. Your starting weight, height, activity level, gender, and age can all have an effect on your weight loss. While our plan was carefully created to balance the needs of most people, some might need to make some tweaks.

Not to worry. We're one step ahead of you and have the solution to common weight-loss issues:

What if I'm not losing any weight? *If the scale hasn't budged, be patient. Sometimes we notice loose clothes, lost inches, and other indicators of weight loss before the scale starts to move. Stay positive and focus on the other positive changes you've implemented.*

Women are generally smaller than men and therefore burn fewer calories throughout the day. If you're not losing weight eating 1,500 calories daily, you'll need to drop to about 1,200 calories—but no lower. Stick to the lowest number of daily servings in each food group: three vegetables, two fruits, five grains or starchy vegetables, two proteins, two dairy, and one fat. If you continue to see no change in the scale or with body measurements, contact your doctor.

What if I'm only losing half a pound to a pound a week? *If you're a woman, shorter than five feet two, or over fifty, you might burn fewer calo-*

MIND-SET MAKEOVER

After today you'll be two-thirds of the way through the program and well on your way to reaching your goal. Today, spend thirty seconds thinking about one of your most important goals, in any area of life. See yourself reaching this goal. What will you feel like? How will this change your life?

METABOLIC MAKEOVER

Stick to one portion. If you're served more, you'll eat more, according to a 2004 study published in the journal *Obesity*. Sit down to a giant portion at home or when dining out, and you're likely to eat 43 percent more

ries throughout the day. There's nothing wrong with losing at this slower rate, so continue with the program as usual. Be patient and stick with it.

__What if I'm losing more than 2 pounds a week?__ People who have more weight to lose (100 pounds or more) will see greater results early on, so this rate of weight loss might soon taper off. If you feel good, stick with the program. But if you're losing more than 2 pounds (or 1 percent of your body weight if you're 100 pounds or more overweight) and not feeling so hot, you should add 200 to 300 additional calories to your day by adding extra servings of vegetables, fruits, grains or starchy vegetables, and fat.

Signs that you need additional calories include:

- *fatigue*
- *dizziness*
- *lightheadedness*
- *loss of energy*
- *difficulty focusing*

This is common in people with physically demanding lifestyles and in some men, who generally require more calories than women, especially if they are larger or quite tall. If you continue to experience these symptoms, contact your doctor.

calories. If you ate that much more at dinner tonight, you'd cut into your calorie deficit by 205 calories.

BREAKFAST

SAD		Spark Swaps		Calories Saved
1 cup puffed rice cereal 8 ounces skim milk	186 calories	Quick and Easy Granola (page 165) 1 medium banana 1 cup skim milk	408 calories	(222)

Diet Downfall. You try to save calories with a small breakfast of a healthy cereal. But you're starving by ten in the morning because you chose one with little protein and fiber (another Diet Downfall). How do you remedy this?

A Better Breakfast. Our breakfasts are smaller than the other meals of the day but not by much, in an attempt to keep your blood sugar stable and your hunger in check. This granola is more filling than puffed rice, and we bulk it up with fruit and milk.

LUNCH

SAD		Spark Swaps		Calories Saved
Crispy chicken sandwich with a small order of fries	730 calories	Tomato-Basil Chicken Sandwich (page 191) 1 cup green bell pepper strips 1 tablespoon salad dressing (your choice) ½ cup cantaloupe cubes	375 calories	355

Drive Past the Drive-Through. Remember that small breakfast we talked about? Restricting at breakfast often leads to overeating later in the day,

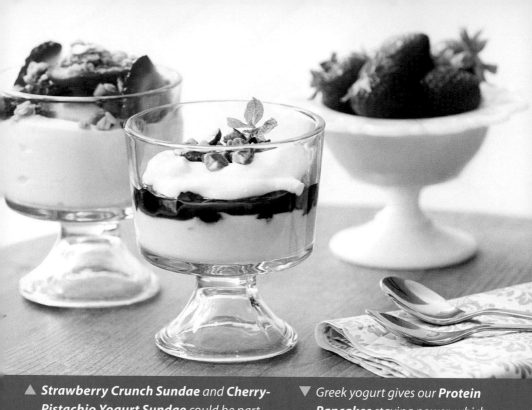

▲ **Strawberry Crunch Sundae** and **Cherry-Pistachio Yogurt Sundae** could be part of a healthy breakfast or an after-dinner treat (see pages 238 and 232).

▼ Greek yogurt gives our **Protein Pancakes** staying power, which means you'll be full until lunchtime (see page 162).

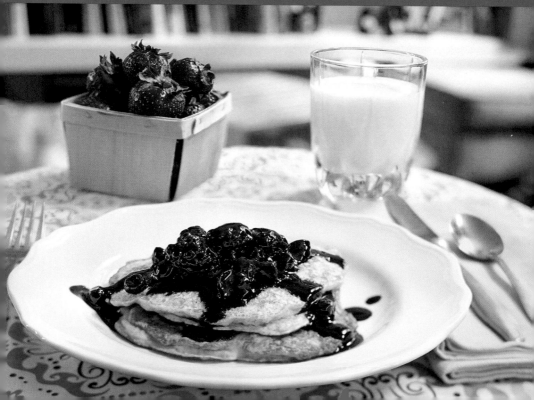

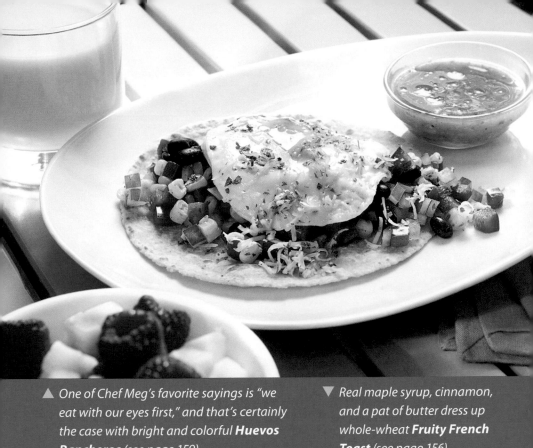

▲ One of Chef Meg's favorite sayings is "we eat with our eyes first," and that's certainly the case with bright and colorful **Huevos Rancheros** (see page 159).

▼ Real maple syrup, cinnamon, and a pat of butter dress up whole-wheat **Fruity French Toast** (see page 156).

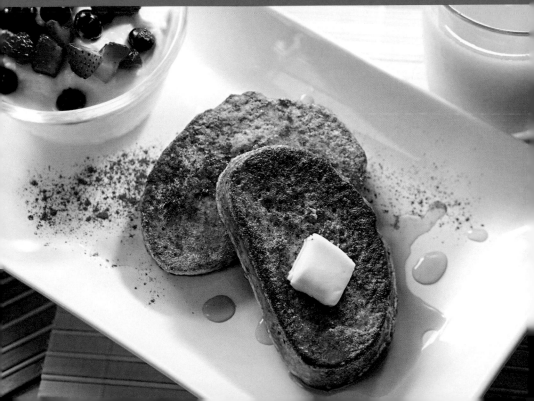

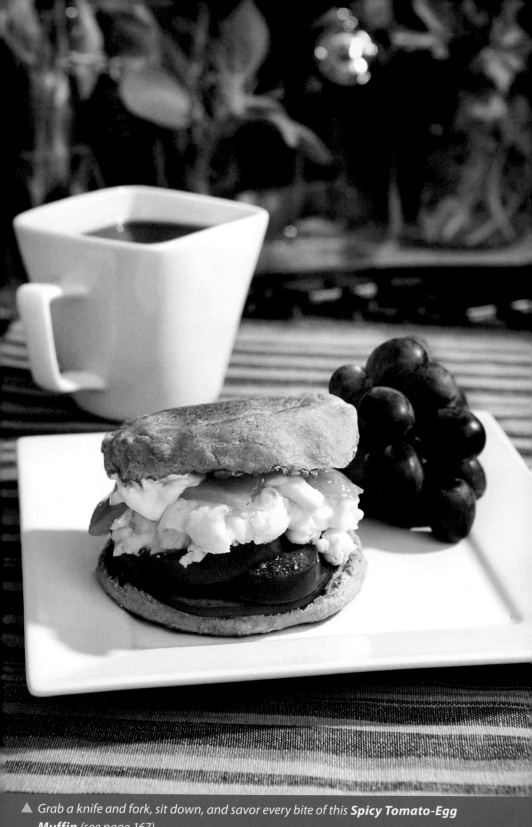

▲ *Grab a knife and fork, sit down, and savor every bite of this* **Spicy Tomato-Egg Muffin** *(see page 167).*

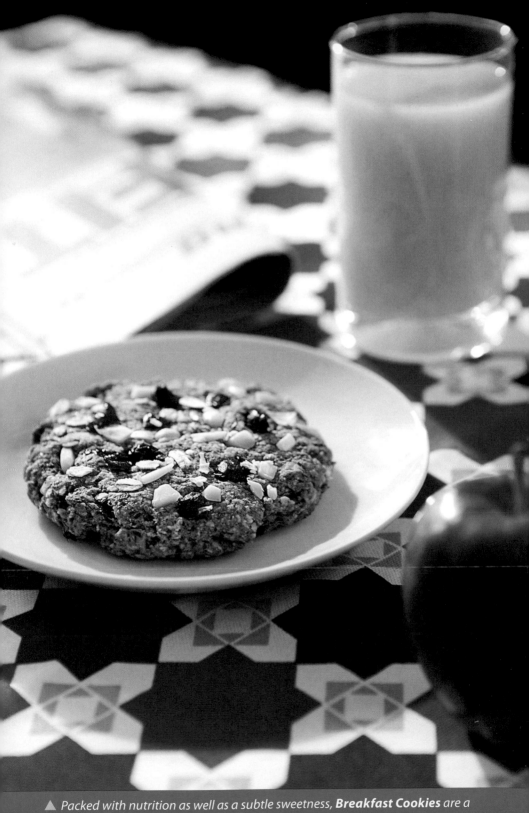

▲ *Packed with nutrition as well as a subtle sweetness, **Breakfast Cookies** are a necessity for busy mornings (see page 152).*

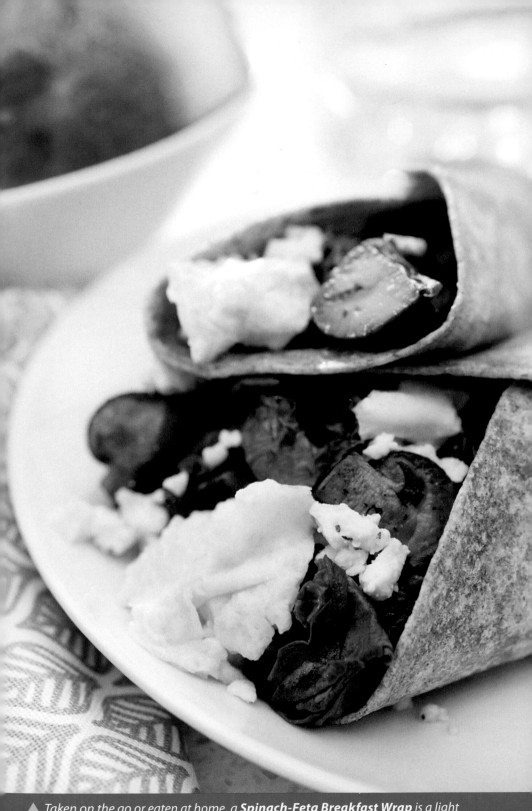

▲ Taken on the go or eaten at home, a **Spinach-Feta Breakfast Wrap** is a light yet filling breakfast (see page 168).

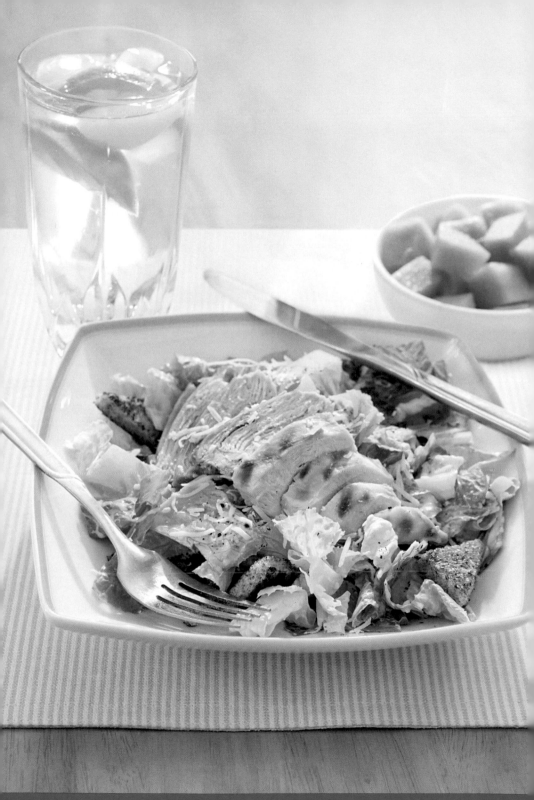

▲ The **Lighter Chicken Caesar Salad** is a study in contrasting flavors and textures (see page 182).

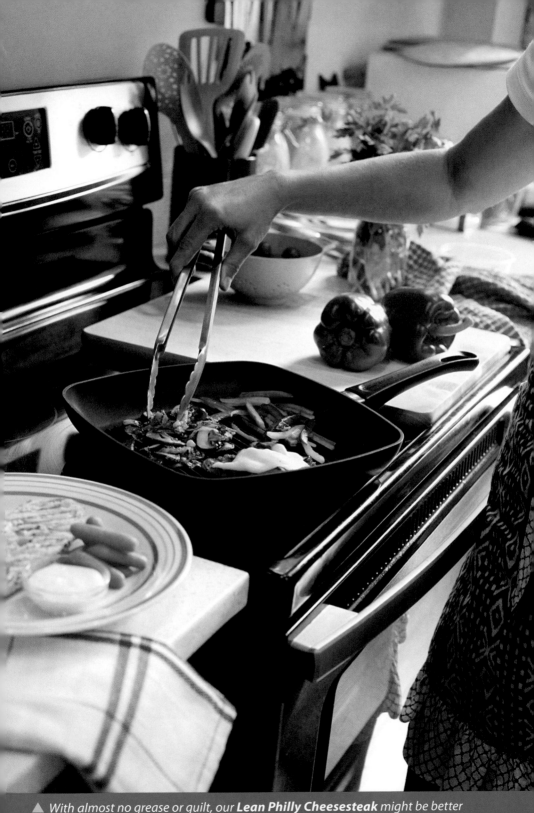

▲ With almost no grease or guilt, our **Lean Philly Cheesesteak** might be better than the original (see page 179).

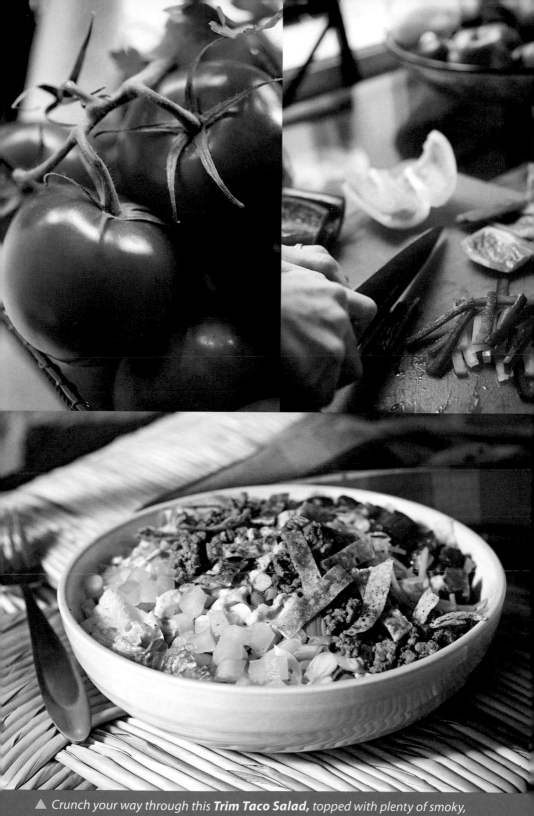

▲ Crunch your way through this **Trim Taco Salad,** *topped with plenty of smoky, creamy avocado dressing (see page 192).*

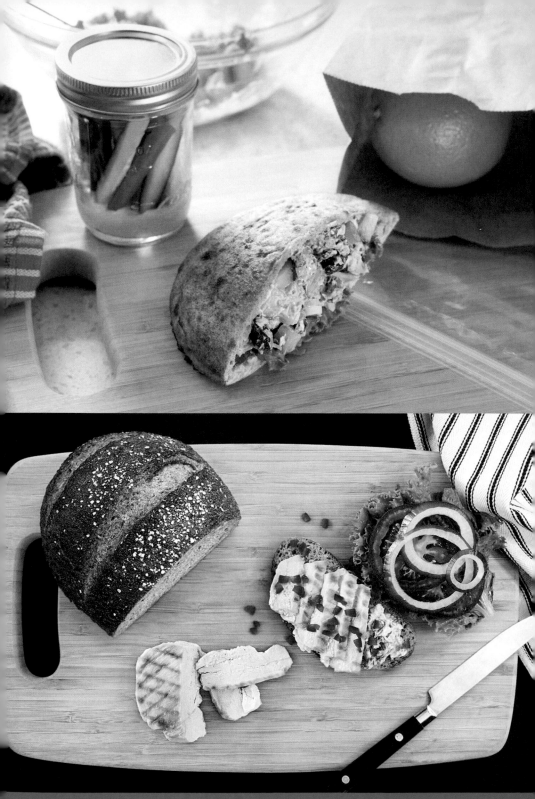

*Pack a **Curried Tuna Salad** (top) or **Tomato-Basil Chicken** (bottom) sandwich and look forward to lunchtime (see pages 176 and 191).*

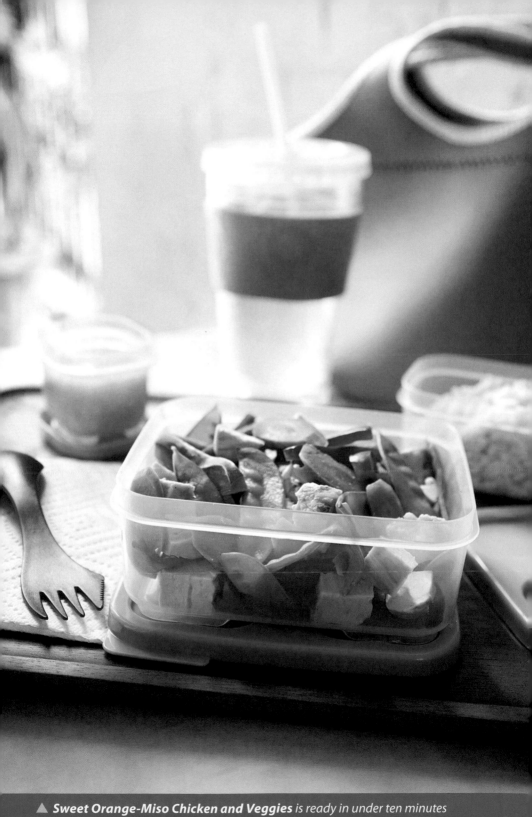

▲ *Sweet Orange-Miso Chicken and Veggies* is ready in under ten minutes
(see page 189).

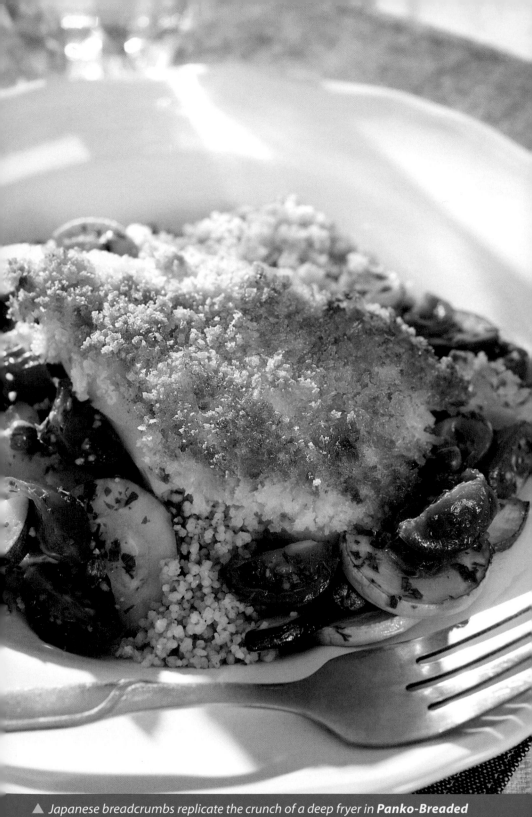

▲ Japanese breadcrumbs replicate the crunch of a deep fryer in **Panko-Breaded Fish with Tomato Salad** *(see page 205).*

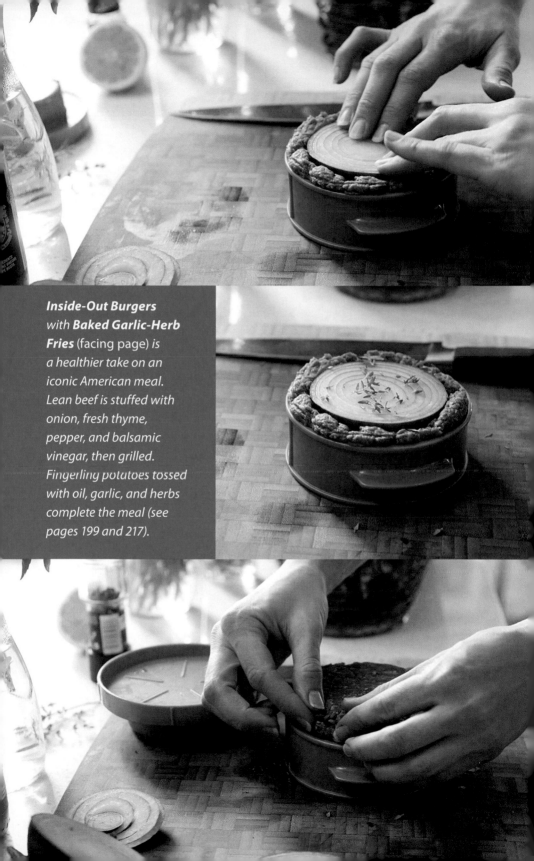

Inside-Out Burgers with **Baked Garlic-Herb Fries** (facing page) is a healthier take on an iconic American meal. Lean beef is stuffed with onion, fresh thyme, pepper, and balsamic vinegar, then grilled. Fingerling potatoes tossed with oil, garlic, and herbs complete the meal (see pages 199 and 217).

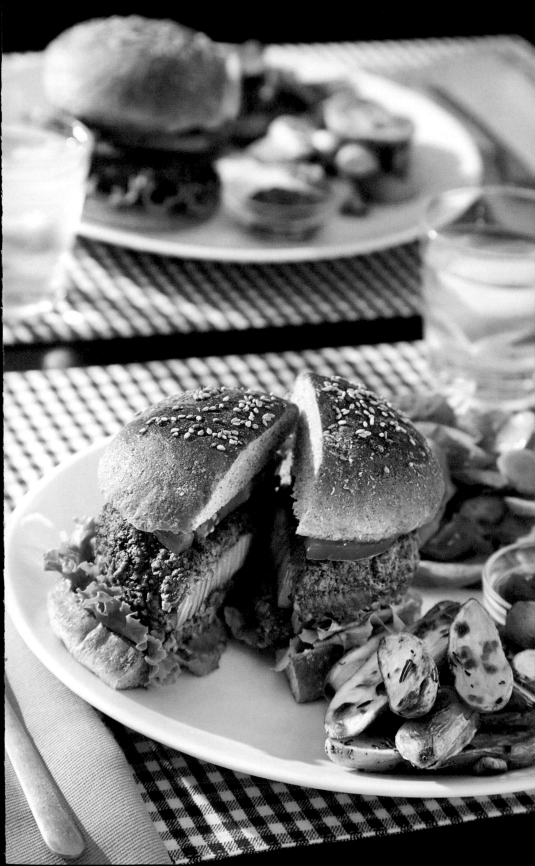

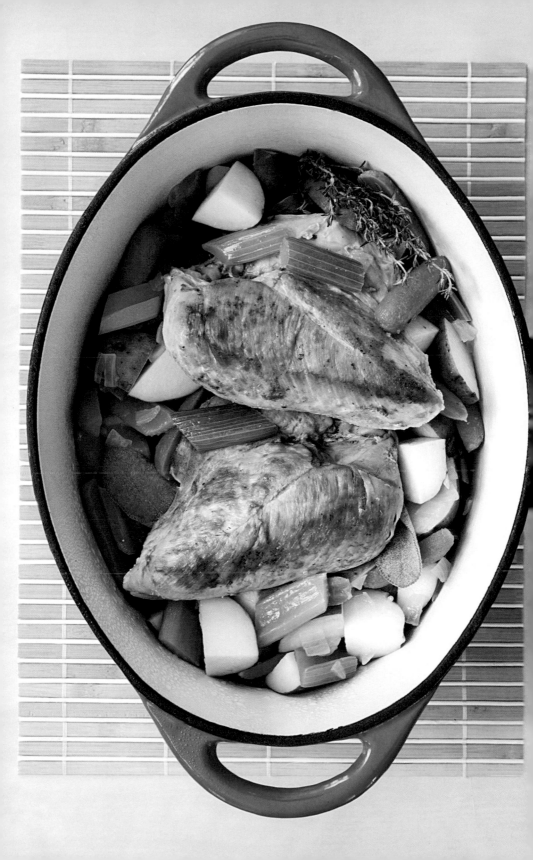

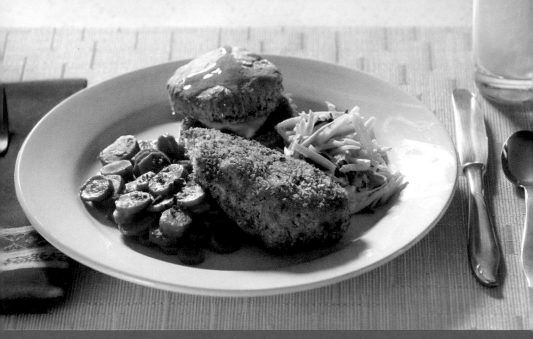

One-Dish Dinner: Roasted Chicken and Vegetables (facing page) *is a lighter version of a Sunday supper. It's ready in an hour, with only ten minutes of hands-on work (see page 203).* **Meg's Pan-Fried Chicken** *with* **Better "Buttermilk" Biscuits** *and* **Hot-and-Sweet Rainbow Slaw** *(above) is our spin on a Southern classic (see pages 200, 218, and 221).*

▼ **Alfredo Pasta with Broccoli** *has so much creamy sauce in every bite, yet not a drop of heavy cream was used in the recipe (see page 193).*

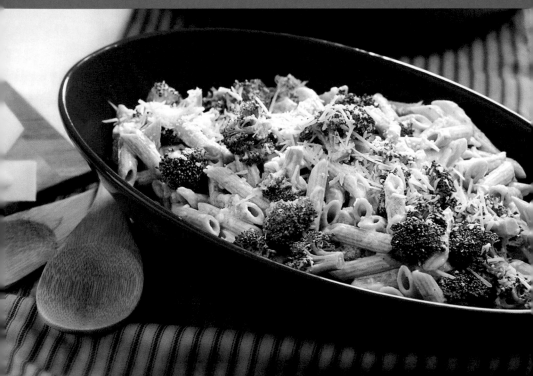

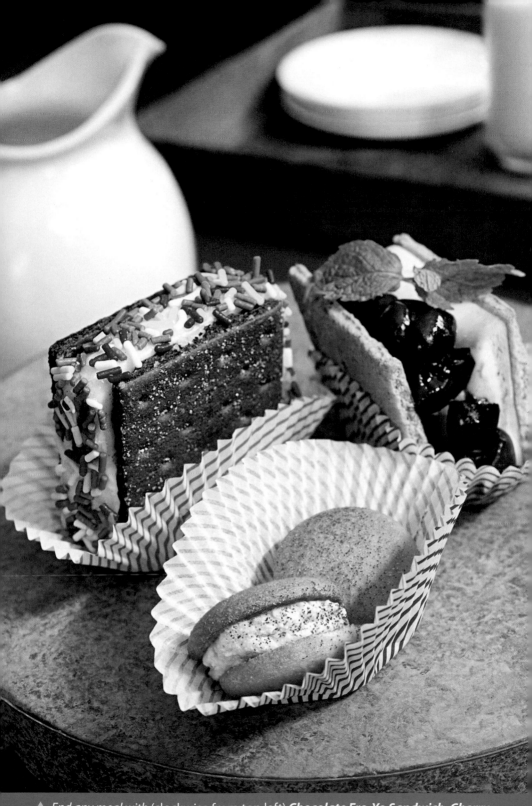

▲ *End any meal with* (clockwise from top left) **Chocolate Fro-Yo Sandwich, Cherry Fro-Yo Sandwich,** *and* **Tiramisu Sandwiches** *(see pages 234, 232, and 238).*

which is why the SAD option today is a fried chicken sandwich with fries. With the Spark Swaps breakfast you'll stay full until it's time to eat lunch, so you'll be able to resist the lure of the fast-food drive-through.

Lunchtime Classic. Chicken sandwiches are a staple on restaurant menus everywhere, so we thought we'd give this one a makeover. We started with grilled or roasted chicken on a whole-wheat bun or bread. Then we added lettuce, tomato, and creamy avocado, plus a tomato-basil sauce that's just as good as a sauce for pasta salad. On the side we pair green pepper strips with your choice of salad dressing.

SNACK

SAD		Spark Swaps		Calories Saved
1 ounce potato chips	152 calories	1 ounce baked potato chips	120 calories	32

Keep the Crunch. While we don't want to advocate spending too much time in the chips aisle, we would like to point out that there are some much healthier options these days. There are chips made with whole grains, legumes, or even vegetables, and plenty of baked options. What's great about the baked chips, in addition to the lower calorie count and less fat, is that you usually get more chips per serving.

Small Swaps Add Up. Say potato chips are your favorite snack, and that you like to eat them daily. Just by making the switch from fried to baked, you could save 3 pounds a year.

DINNER

SAD		Spark Swaps		Calories Saved
Beef lo mein (one serving, from a restaurant)	662 calories plus more than a day's worth of sodium: 2,417 milligrams!	Thai Peanut Noodles (page 213) 1 cup skim milk	476 calories	186

This dish is easier on the waistline and the wallet than a take-out version, and it's ready in twenty minutes. Swap in almond butter, change up the veggies, and ramp up the heat—do whatever you need to make this recipe your own.

Downsize It. Tonight, serve your dinner on a smaller plate. A 2006 study in the *American Journal of Preventive Medicine* found that you'll eat less when your plate or bowl fits your portion size, without a lot of empty space. This is a simple habit to stick with. When packing leftovers or lunches, choose containers that don't leave much extra room.

Dinner in a Hurry. Save more time by picking up pre-chopped vegetables from the grocery store salad bar or chopping them in the morning.

SNACK

SAD		Spark Swaps		Calories Saved
1 slice pineapple upside-down cake	366 calories	1 serving Grilled Pineapple with Toasted Coconut (page 236)	114 calories	252

Sweet Without Sugar. Grilling fruit intensifies its flavor, similar to the effect of caramelizing the pineapple in the upside-down cake. We use no added sugar, then top with coconut milk and unsweetened coconut flakes for a tropical treat that's quite light.

Once you've mastered grilled pineapple, try grilling peaches, plums, or pears.

SAD Total	Spark Swaps Total	Deficit
2,096 calories	1,493 calories	603 calories

DAILY TOTALS

Calories: 1,493	**Sodium: 1,041 mg**	**Fiber: 39 g**
Fat: 35 g	**Carbs: 232 g**	**Protein: 79 g**

Fitness That Fits

CARDIO INTERVALS: 45 MINUTES

Choose any form of cardio and alternate between high intensity and low intensity using this guide: 3 minutes of "moderate" intensity (6 out of 10), followed by 2 minutes of "somewhat hard" intensity (8 out of 10), then 1 minute of "all-out" intensity (9 out of 10). Repeat this sequence of intervals 7 times (42 total minutes). Warm up before and cool down after for 3 minutes each.

Our Pick: cycling at 13 miles per hour, with intervals at 15 miles per hour (486 calories burned)

FLEXIBILITY

Spend 5 to 10 minutes stretching all major muscle groups after your workout.

NEAT: 30 MINUTES

Daily Deficit: 1,089 calories
Week-to-Date Deficit: 3,573 calories

SPARK IT UP: CLIMBING HIGH

Find a hill in your neighborhood and ride up and down it on a bike a few times during your workout.

MAKE IT WORK: PLAN B

Weather not cooperating? Ride on a stationary bike or do a workout DVD instead.

Make Tomorrow Easier

Bake the Breakfast Casserole Cups (page 151) tonight and reheat in the morning.

Daily Reflection

HOW DID YOU FEEL TODAY?	Poor		OK		Excellent
	1	2	3	4	5
I made healthy food choices based on the Spark Swaps meal plan.					
I was physically active, following the Fitness That Fits workouts.					
I felt motivated to stick with the Spark Solution program.					
I am ready to take on tomorrow and all that it has in store for me.					

What were the highlights of your day? What were the challenges? How can you use today's highs and lows to make tomorrow better and easier?

DAY 11

INSIDER TIP

Always Be a Step Ahead

"Plan ahead. Grill a bunch of meat, chop veggies, portion it, and put it in ready-to-take containers. That way, when you leave the house you grab and go."

—Tia, dropped six dress sizes

MIND-SET MAKEOVER

Every time you start to say something negative about yourself today, pause and consider what you would say to a friend in that same situation. We spend a lot of time beating ourselves up, and it only makes your weight-loss journey that much more arduous. The only way to reach your goals is

to learn to treat yourself with love and respect. Though it won't happen overnight, you can start with these small steps.

METABOLIC MAKEOVER

Today your lunch and dinner includes foods that are high in water content and fiber, which can help with satiety. Starting your meal with a salad, broth-based soup, fruits, or vegetables can slow you down and help you assess your hunger, and studies have shown you'll eat less by including these foods.

BREAKFAST

SAD		Spark Swaps		Calories Saved
Breakfast bake with sausage, cheese, eggs, and hash browns	435 calories	Breakfast Casserole Cups (page 151) 1 slice whole-grain toast with 1 teaspoon unsalted butter and 2 teaspoons all-fruit jam 1 cup skim milk	407 calories	28

Family Recipe Redux. Breakfast casserole is one of those dishes you find on buffet tables at holiday brunches—delicious but packed with calories. We portioned ours into muffin tins, cut out a few ingredients, and added tomatoes. Make a double batch and freeze some to make mornings easier.

LUNCH

SAD		Spark Swaps		Calories Saved
Deluxe grilled cheese sandwich and tomato bisque from a neighborhood bistro	1,094 calories	Grilled cheese sandwich using whole-wheat bread and 1 ounce shredded low-fat cheddar 1 cup lentil-vegetable soup	372 calories	722

Super Soups. Today's lunch takes some help from the supermarket. Canned soups are a quick, healthy lunch, but they're not very filling. We recommend using them as the basis for a meal, not your entire meal. Feel free to choose another type of soup using the following recommendations:

- Choose broth-based soups, not creamy ones.

- Opt for low-sodium soups.

- Consider adding your own lean protein to veggie-based soups.

- Bulk up soups by adding a cup of frozen veggies or fresh spinach.

- Lentil and bean soups, like the one we chose today, are often low in calories and high in fiber.

- Read the label. A serving is typically one cup (eight ounces), but a can contains two or more servings.

- Keep a couple of cans of soup, along with a can opener, in your desk at the office for days you forget to pack a lunch.

Great Grilled Cheese. You can reinvent grilled cheese at home with whole-wheat bread, cheese of your choosing, and plenty of add-ons that add flavor with few calories.

- Use good bread. Choose bakery bread that's firm not spongy. This isn't a time for pitas, Sandwich Thin varieties, or flatbread, none of which will grill as easily. Whole-wheat is best, but avoid seeded whole-grain breads; the nuts and seeds can sometimes burn.

- Use shredded cheese, which melts more evenly. A little bit goes a long way; use about an ounce. Grate it yourself for better results.

- Coat the bread evenly with cooking spray or unsalted butter. Just a little won't add many calories, but it will taste amazing. One teaspoon of room-temperature butter should be enough to coat both sides of bread, for 34 calories. (Don't use margarine; it's more likely to burn.)

- Keep the heat set to medium-low. Start out on high and you'll end up with burned bread and cold cheese.

- Use a nonstick skillet so the cheese doesn't stick to the pan. You also won't have to use as much cooking spray or butter in the pan, which is not only healthier but also may prevent a soggy sandwich.

- Choose gooey cheese—mozzarella, jack, provolone, cheddar, and fontina are all great grilling cheeses. Hard cheeses like Parmesan and Asiago and creamy cheeses like goat and feta don't melt as well.
- Cook two minutes per side, then cover the skillet until the bread is toasted and the cheese melts. Covering helps the cheese melt before the bread burns.

Desktop Dining. Tuck 1 ounce of cheese into half a pita and microwave for about 30 seconds. It's not a grilled cheese sandwich, but it will do in a pinch.

SNACK

SAD		Spark Swaps		Calories Saved
2 ounces mini chocolate chip cookies	280 calories	2 fig Newtons (1.1 ounces)	100 calories	180

Vending Machine Showdown. The time has come. You forgot a snack, you're hungry, and your only option is the vending machine. The cookies are calling out to your sweet tooth, but which ones should you choose? Fig bars are one of the better options you'll find in most vending machines. They pack fiber and very little fat into a sweet package. For only 100 calories, you'll keep your sweet tooth in check.

DINNER

SAD		Spark Swaps		Calories Saved
Beef tacos: 2 shells, ¼ cup grated cheddar cheese, 4 ounces 80 percent lean ground beef, and 2 tablespoons sour cream	655 calories	Twenty-Minute Fish Tacos with Homemade Pico de Gallo (page 215) 1 cup fresh spinach topped with half of the pico de gallo and ½ teaspoon olive oil	380 calories	275

Taco Night. Have you ever eaten tacos from an authentic Mexican restaurant or taco truck? The first thing you might notice is the size, and the lack of toppings. While Americanized versions of tacos load up a plate-size tortilla with every topping imaginable, most authentic tacos are quite simple: meat, perhaps some pickled veggies or cabbage, and a slice of avocado or a sprinkle of mild white cheese. We took the middle ground with these fish tacos. Fish lightens up an old favorite, and fresh pico de gallo gives salsa a starring role. We turned half of the pico into a salad by adding spinach and some olive oil.

Not a fish fan? Check out the recipe's variations for making either chicken or bean tacos.

SNACK

SAD		Spark Swaps		Calories Saved
1 large cinnamon roll with icing (made from a refrigerated dough)	310 calories	1 slice toasted cinnamon-raisin bread with 1 tablespoon low-fat cream cheese 1 cup skim milk	200 calories	110

Outsmart Your Sweet Tooth. Rather than diving into a cinnamon roll, choose something that's similar yet healthier. The cream cheese offers the creaminess you crave, but it allows the sweetness of the bread and raisins to shine through.

SAD Total	Spark Swaps Total	Deficit
2,774 calories	1,459 calories	1,315 calories

DAILY TOTALS

Calories: 1,459	Sodium: 1,806 mg	Fiber: 27 g
Fat: 40 g	Carbs: 197 g	Protein: 84 g

Fitness That Fits

STRENGTH TRAINING: AMRAP

Perform the exercises in the Spark Swaps Strength Workout (page 247) in the order listed, doing as many reps as possible (AMRAP) and every exercise for 1 full minute, fitting in as many controlled, good reps as you can. Move quickly to the next exercise (with little or no rest) until you've done them all. For exercises performed on one side at a time, perform 1 full minute on each side before switching. Then move on to the next exercise. Your goal today is to beat last week's score for each exercise.

Calories Burned: about 200

FLEXIBILITY

Spend 5 to 10 minutes stretching all major muscle groups after your workout.

NEAT: 60 MINUTES

Daily Deficit: 1,515 calories
Week-to-Date Deficit: 5,088 calories

SPARK IT UP: WORK AND PLAY

Take your NEAT up a notch by dancing as you do your chores. Dancing burns 100 calories in 15 minutes (though we can't say for sure how many calories singing while you do it burns!).

MAKE IT WORK: TACOS IN LESS TIME

Skip the tortillas to save some calories, and use canned beans instead of fish if you're short on time. You can also grab your favorite jarred salsa, but be sure to bulk it up with extra chopped peppers and onions—which you chopped earlier this week, right?

Make Tomorrow Easier

Bake Better Banana Bread (page 230) after dinner tonight, but avoid the temptation of slicing into it.

Daily Reflection

HOW DID YOU FEEL TODAY?	Poor		OK		Excellent
	1	2	3	4	5
I made healthy food choices based on the Spark Swaps meal plan.					
I was physically active, following the Fitness That Fits workouts.					
I felt motivated to stick with the Spark Solution program.					
I am ready to take on tomorrow and all that it has in store for me.					

What were the highlights of your day? What were the challenges? How can you use today's highs and lows to make tomorrow better and easier?

DAY 12

INSIDER TIP

Living Comes First

"I just remember that I have to live my life. I can't set expectations that I will never eat chocolate cake again, because I can't meet those expectations. I set reasonable goals that are achievable and expectations for myself to where I don't feel like a failure all the time. I have definitely missed goals for myself and it has taken me almost two years to lose the weight I have, but I have seen a consistent loss, which I attribute to reasonable goal setting and rewards for myself."

—*Christy, 101 pounds lost*

MIND-SET MAKEOVER

Think back to the last time you got off track with your diet. What caused you to get derailed from your good intentions? Imagine rewinding the memory, but taking a different path where you make better choices. Think of this exercise the next time you're in danger of falling off the wagon.

METABOLIC MAKEOVER

Breaking the soda habit is tough, but the payoffs are immediate. Swapping a daily 20-ounce regular soda for a diet one cuts enough calories to amount to a 31-pound weight loss in a year. When the craving strikes, think *31 pounds a year* and reach for a calorie-free beverage instead.

BREAKFAST

SAD		Spark Swaps		Calories Saved
Banana nut muffin	540 calories	1 slice Better Banana Bread (page 230) served with 1 tablespoon low-fat cream cheese 2 tablespoons raisins 1 cup skim milk mixed with 2 tablespoons light chocolate syrup	421 calories	119

Mega Muffin. Picture the muffin tin you likely have in your kitchen. Now picture the muffin that's staring at you from the counter at the coffee shop. How many of your homemade muffins would it take to equal that monster-size treat? Three? Four? Better bypass it and make homemade banana bread, which even when paired with tasty toppings and a glass of chocolate milk still has fewer calories than that muffin.

LUNCH

SAD		Spark Swaps		Calories Saved
Fast-food Cobb salad	660 calories	Cobb Salad (page 175) 4 low-fat whole-wheat crackers	398 calories	262

Either/Or. The classic Cobb salad perfectly illustrates our either/or, not all-or-nothing, philosophy. Check out the recipe for all the delicious details. We focused on keeping flavor while cutting fat, ditching some traditional ingredients while adding some new ones.

Spark Swap Smoked Paprika. Bacon is tasty. No doubt about it. But its smokiness comes in a very dense package calorically. In many recipes, we skip the bacon and reach for smoked paprika, which adds the smoky flavor we crave but with almost no calories. We wouldn't ever ditch the bacon in our BLT, but we did use smoked paprika in its place in our Cobb salad, for example. Sprinkle paprika on popcorn or in cheese omelets. Stir it into sauces or add it in place of Canadian bacon in the Baked Macaroni and Cheese (page 195).

SNACK

SAD		Spark Swaps		Calories Saved
1 large apple	125 calories	1 small apple with 2 teaspoons natural unsalted peanut butter	125 calories	0

Stick-to-Your-Ribs Snacks. Give your snack a fighting chance to fight hunger. Give it some protein. We opted for a smaller apple and some natural peanut butter to boost this snack.

DINNER

SAD		Spark Swaps		Calories Saved
1 dozen buffalo wings	600 calories	Slow-Cooker Buffalo Chicken Casserole (page 208) 16 grapes 1 cup skim milk	470 calories	130

Keep What Works. Did you know that just three buffalo wings have 10 grams of fat? (Who eats just three?) This casserole has all the spice, creaminess, and tang of wings, but with a fraction of the fat. We kept all the components of hot wings—chicken, spiciness, celery, and blue cheese—but ditched the buttery, salty sauce.

SNACK

SAD		Spark Swaps		Calories Saved
1 14-ounce root beer float	300 calories	Root beer float alternative: 1 12-ounce can diet root beer soda with ½ cup slow-churned ice cream	100 calories	200

Soda Sometimes. Drinking soda regularly is a habit that's easy to break, and it can make an immediate impact on your weight. Every once in a while it's fine to enjoy one—diet, preferably—and why not turn it into an old-fashioned treat? If you don't care for the taste of artificial sweeteners, look for the zero-calorie sodas sweetened with stevia, which is a naturally sweet plant.

Start to think of soda differently. Soda is a treat, like ice cream, cake, or popcorn at the movies. Its purpose is to satiate a craving for something sweet, not hydrate you or quench your thirst on a regular basis.

SAD Total	Spark Swaps Total	Deficit
2,225 calories	1,514 calories	711 calories

DAILY TOTALS

Calories: 1,514	Sodium: 1,212 mg	Fiber: 24 g
Fat: 36 g	Carbs: 204 g	Protein: 107 g

Fitness That Fits

CARDIO: 30 MINUTES

Choose a different activity than Day 8 and accumulate minutes in three 10-minute chunks, two 15-minute chunks, or all at once. Work "somewhat hard" (8 out of 10) so you are slightly breathless the entire time.

Our Pick: Spinning or indoor cycling (262 calories)

NEAT: 45 MINUTES
Daily Deficit: 973 calories
Week-to-Date Deficit: 6,061 calories

SPARK IT UP: DINNER'S MAKING ITSELF
Tonight's dinner is ready, thanks to the slow cooker. Take advantage of that extra time by squeezing in another 10 or 20 minutes of exercise. Our pick: intervals of walking and running, or just increase your pace as you walk.

MAKE IT WORK: TAKE THE FIRST STEP
If you couldn't find time to work out earlier in the day, go for at least a 10-minute walk while dinner waits on you. Chances are, once you've started walking you won't want to stop.

Daily Reflection

HOW DID YOU FEEL TODAY?	Poor		OK		Excellent
	1	2	3	4	5
I made healthy food choices based on the Spark Swaps meal plan.					
I was physically active, following the Fitness That Fits workouts.					
I felt motivated to stick with the Spark Solution program.					
I am ready to take on tomorrow and all that it has in store for me.					

What were the highlights of your day? What were the challenges? How can you use today's highs and lows to make tomorrow better and easier?

DAY 13

INSIDER TIP

You Can Overcome Pessimism

"I'm not always positive. In fact, I can be quite the negative person. I tend to always look at the negatives first, so I found a way to turn that into my fuel to fight for me. The more I fought for myself and saw my winning results, the more I saw my true beauty shine through (and started seeing the positives). For someone who never truly liked myself, being able to name numerous things that I now love about me, that's huge."

—Emily, 77 pounds lost

MIND-SET MAKEOVER

Imagine that you've reached your goal weight and a friend asks you for advice on how to live a healthier lifestyle. How does it feel to have others look up to you? How would you help others make positive changes in their own lives based on your experience?

METABOLIC MAKEOVER

Slow down and savor your food. Aim to spend thirty minutes or more eating dinner, which can help you save 70 calories at each meal (because you'll have time to notice when you've had enough), or 7.3 pounds a year, according to a 2008 study in the *Journal of the American Dietetic Association*.

BREAKFAST

SAD		Spark Swaps		Calories Saved
Huevos rancheros from a Mexican chain restaurant	970 calories	Huevos Rancheros (page 159) 1 cup fresh mango slices	326 calories	644

Mexican Makeover. As with tacos, authentic huevos rancheros are much simpler than the versions we see on most restaurant menus: corn tortillas topped with eggs and spicy tomato sauce, sometimes with beans or avocado on the side. We kept the tortilla, added beans for extra protein along with a mango salsa for a sweet and savory start to the day. This meal is filling and fun, but it's quick enough for a weekday morning.

"Free" Food. The restaurant version of this dish is not only covered with cheese and served on fried tortillas, but it also comes with beans and rice on the side. Remember that just because something appears on your plate doesn't mean you have to eat it. Ask for a box and take the beans and rice to go if you prefer, or better yet, ask the server to replace it with veggies like lettuce and tomato.

LUNCH

SAD		Spark Swaps		Calories Saved
2 frozen meat-and-cheese croissants	601 calories	Cheesy Chicken Pouch (page 174) 1 cup skim milk ½ cup fresh pear slices	460 calories	141

Slimmer Sandwiches. Bursting with cheese and meat wrapped in a buttery crust, those pocket croissant sandwiches sure are tasty. But they're small and come two to a box, making it tempting to eat the whole package. We kept the idea but swapped out that crust and used leaner protein and less cheese. And, of course, we added vegetables. The result is a hot, cheesy sandwich that even kids will like.

Out of sight, out of mind works with food. If you have certain trigger foods—such as the "pocket" sandwiches or the candy on your desk—keep them away from you. Find a healthy swap for your trigger food or only buy controlled portions of that item. A 2006 study in the *International Journal of Obesity* found that removing high-calorie foods reduced unnecessary snacking throughout the day.

SNACK

SAD		Spark Swaps		Calories Saved
3 mini quiches	350 calories	2 slices lean deli ham 1 hard-boiled egg	105 calories	245

Party Planning. You have a great dinner planned, but first you have a birthday party to attend. You know there will be plenty of finger food—mostly pub grub. You have a plan in place: a protein-packed snack to ward off a growling belly until your late dinner, plus a club soda with lime.

DINNER

SAD		Spark Swaps		Calories Saved
Grilled salmon with pineapple glaze from a fast-casual take-out restaurant	450 calories	Sweet-and-Spicy Glazed Salmon (page 212) 1 cup steamed asparagus spears (about 8) 1 medium sweet potato, baked and topped with 1 teaspoon unsalted butter 2 packed teaspoons brown sugar	466 calories	(16)

Special Sauce. Salmon is packed with heart-healthy fats like omega-3s, and it's delicious to boot. It pairs well with sweet sauces, but ours keeps the sweetness in check and balances it with a bit of heat. Paired with a sweet potato and asparagus, this is a meal that won't send your blood sugar soaring.

Swifter Sweet Potatoes. While you shouldn't chop sweet potatoes ahead of time, you can prep a large batch a couple of times a week. Roasted sweet potatoes (whole, wedges, or cubes) are delightful reheated or cold, and they are a quick, healthy addition to any meal or snack. To prepare: pierce with a fork several times, then microwave on the "potato" setting or bake at 400°F for 45 minutes, until tender.

SNACK

SAD		Spark Swaps		Calories Saved
16 ounces frozen margarita	340 calories	5 ounces red wine	106 calories	234

Party Planning. Say you're at that party and your belly is content, thanks to the protein-rich snack earlier. You decide you want to stay a while and have a drink. By choosing the wine over the sugary margarita once a week, you'll cut 3 pounds a year while still enjoying happy hours and birthday parties. (Stick with club soda over the margarita to save 5 pounds.)

SAD Total	Spark Swaps Total	Deficit
2,711 calories	1,463 calories	1,248 calories

DAILY TOTALS

Calories: 1,463	Sodium: 1,278 mg	Fiber: 28 g
Fat: 35 g	Carbs: 174 g	Protein: 106 g

Fitness That Fits

STRENGTH TRAINING: THREE SETS OF TEN REPS
Perform the exercises in the Spark Swaps Strength Workout (page 247) in reverse order, moving quickly from one exercise to the next for one set, then repeat for a second set. For exercises performed on one side at a time, perform all reps on each side before switching. Then move on to the next exercise.

Calories Burned: about 120

NEAT: 60 MINUTES
Daily Deficit: 1,369 calories
Week-to-Date Deficit: 7,430 calories

SPARK IT UP: YOUR HEALTH COMES FIRST
Break the habit of putting your social life first. Consider skipping the party
if you haven't yet worked out for the day. That goes for tonight and any
night. Working out is a valid excuse to miss a party, albeit not a fun one.

MAKE IT WORK: COMMIT TO BE FIT
If it comes down to a choice of a post-party dinner or a workout, choose
the workout. Pick up cooked grilled salmon fillets at the supermarket on
the way home, and keep it simple with a squeeze of lemon and a sprinkle
of fresh herbs.

Daily Reflection

HOW DID YOU FEEL TODAY?	Poor		OK		Excellent
	1	2	3	4	5
I made healthy food choices based on the Spark Swaps meal plan.					
I was physically active, following the Fitness That Fits workouts.					
I felt motivated to stick with the Spark Solution program.					
I am ready to take on tomorrow and all that it has in store for me.					

What were the highlights of your day? What were the challenges? How
can you use today's highs and lows to make tomorrow better and easier?

DAY 14

INSIDER TIP

Never Give Up

"Don't give up on yourself. None of us is perfect, and every day we must challenge ourselves. This doesn't mean we don't have failures; it just means we pick ourselves up and keep going without regrets."

—*Teri, 30 pounds lost*

MIND-SET MAKEOVER

Stress can have profound effects on the waistline. A 2006 study in the journal *Physiology and Behavior* found that when stressed we're more likely to reach for high-fat foods. The study found that 71 percent of those who eat more under stress categorized themselves as dieters.

Today, since you have a "rest day," use the time you would spend exercising to instead de-stress. Read a book, take a bubble bath, call a friend—anything that helps you deal with stress. (Though you're probably already noticing that exercise is a great stress reliever, don't skimp on your rest.)

METABOLIC MAKEOVER

Choose your eating environment carefully. A quiet atmosphere can assist in weight loss. A 2004 study in the journal *Nutrition* found that eating in a noisy restaurant, with large groups of people around (such as in the office cafeteria) or with music or the television blaring in the background, can lead to overeating. Tonight at dinner, see what happens when it's just you, your fellow dining partners, and the food.

BREAKFAST

SAD		Spark Swaps		Calories Saved
Stuffed french toast with berries and whipped cream	808 calories	Fruity French Toast with Greek Yogurt (page 156) 1 cup skim milk	427 calories	381

Overstuffed. "Stuffed" is a word to be avoided on restaurant menus. In this case, the stuffed french toast is thick-cut white bread with creamy filling and sweetened berries. More like dessert than breakfast, this dish is more than half your day's calories. In France, this classic breakfast dish is called *pain perdu,* or "lost bread"; we'd like to lose it too!

Better Berries. Greek yogurt stands in for the cream filling, berries are sweet enough on their own, and our french toast is made with fiber-rich whole-wheat bread.

LUNCH

SAD		Spark Swaps		Calories Saved
1 slice New York–style pizza	730 calories	Mexican Pizza (page 184) ⅓ avocado	388 calories	342

A Slimmer Slice. A good rule of thumb is to not eat anything larger than your plate, or your head, and a slice of New York–style pizza is larger than both. If you do dig in, cut a piece that's more reasonable and share the rest with a friend.

Pizza Diversity. Though we headed south of the border for this pizza swap, you can top a whole-wheat tortilla with traditional pizza toppings too. This Mexican Pizza recipe is a fun diversion from both pizza and tacos and is loaded with veggies and lean protein.

SNACK

SAD		Spark Swaps		Calories Saved
1 cup peaches canned in syrup	103 calories	½ cup 2 percent cottage cheese ¼ cup fresh peach slices	120 calories	(17)

Skip the Syrup. For this snack, you can choose canned, fresh, or thawed frozen peaches, but don't reach for fruit packed in syrup, which is loaded with added sugars. If that's the only fruit available, drain and rinse it; otherwise, avoid it.

Friendly Fat. Your body needs fat, remember? We like to pair a bit of it with veggies and fruit to help your body fully metabolize vitamins and minerals. Plus, the pairing of creamy cottage cheese with sweet peaches is a contrast you'll love.

DINNER

SAD		Spark Swaps		Calories Saved
1 chicken drumstick with barbecue sauce and a loaded baked potato	503 calories	Carolina-Style Barbecue Chicken (page 197) ¾ cup Lemon Roasted Cauliflower (page 223) 1 small baked russet potato 1 tablespoon low-fat sour cream	436 calories	67

The Dark Side. Dark meat is no longer off-limits. It contains 1 gram of fat per ounce, just 3 more calories per ounce than white meat, and provides a greater amount of certain minerals. Choose white meat more often than dark, and always remove the skin and trim the visible fat.

The Skinny on Sauces. Most bottled barbecue sauces are packed with sugars. Chef Meg opted for a vinegar-and-mustard-based sauce that's balanced with some sweetness. We paired it with Lemon Roasted Cauliflower and a baked potato for a healthier twist on a barbecue feast.

SNACK

SAD		Spark Swaps		Calories Saved
Chocolate lava cake	475 calories	Chocolate Fondue (page 233) with ½ cup fresh strawberries (about 3 large)	80 calories	395

Choose Chocolate. You'll never hear us saying to avoid chocolate, but we look for ways to add other nutritious foods alongside it. We swapped one melty chocolate dessert for another. Fondue, especially paired with fruit, is easily portion controlled to keep chocolate servings in check.

SAD Total	Spark Swaps Total	Deficit
2,619 calories	1,451 calories	1,168 calories

DAILY TOTALS

Calories: 1,451	Sodium: 1,763 mg	Fiber: 27 g
Fat: 36 g	Carbs: 184 g	Protein: 105 g

Fitness That Fits

REST DAY: NO CARDIO OR STRENGTH TODAY
Rest up, rebuild, and recover.

NEAT: 90 MINUTES
Daily Deficit: 1,168 calories
Week-to-Date Deficit: 8,598 calories, or 2.5 pounds
Fourteen-Day Deficit: 16,684 calories, or 4.8 pounds

SPARK IT UP: LOOSEN UP

While you shouldn't skip your rest day entirely, if you'd like to move your body a bit, head out for a 30-minute walk or do some gentle yoga, to get the blood flowing and loosen your muscles. After yesterday's strength session, your body will appreciate it.

MAKE IT WORK: GET A HEAD START ON NEXT WEEK

Use your rest days to your advantage. Get caught up on anything in your personal or professional life that might interfere with your workouts or your time to prepare healthy meals and snacks. And schedule next week's workouts in your planner so you'll continue to make them a priority.

Daily Reflection

HOW DID YOU FEEL TODAY?	Poor		OK		Excellent
	1	2	3	4	5
I made healthy food choices based on the Spark Swaps meal plan.					
I was physically active, following the Fitness That Fits workouts.					
I felt motivated to stick with the Spark Solution program.					
I am ready to take on tomorrow and all that it has in store for me.					

What were the highlights of your day? What were the challenges? How can you use today's highs and lows to make tomorrow better and easier?

Congratulations! You've completed the first two weeks of the Spark Solution. Can you believe that you started this journey just fourteen days ago? Let's look back on all you've accomplished before we talk about what comes next. Check off each goal you reached and add any others we left off the list.

In two weeks, did you ...

lose at least 4 to 6 pounds of body fat, not water weight?

create a deficit of more than 16,000 calories?

develop the skills and kitchen confidence to prepare healthy, delicious meals with ease?

increase your cardio activity?

start to build fat-burning muscle through our simple strength routines?

After two weeks of eating this way, do you notice that ...

your sugar cravings are less frequent or intense?

you're consuming less caffeine?

you're eating—and enjoying—your vegetables?

you're satisfied between meals and snacks?

After two weeks of exercise, are you ...

huffing and puffing less?

adding more minutes or miles to your workouts?

feeling better during your strength workouts?

Have you ...

noticed clearer skin and healthier nails?

felt like you have more energy?

found your desire to binge or overeat diminishing?

slept better—and longer—than before?

started to feel satisfied rather than stuffed after meals?

felt better about yourself in ways you never thought possible?

realized that healthy living makes you feel great?

Can you believe that you . . .

worked out twelve of the last fourteen days (for almost five hours total)?

moved your body an additional nine hours?

made forty-two healthy, delicious meals?

What else have you noticed?

_____

_____

_____

_____

_____

_____

Maybe you've reached all those goals, or maybe you're not quite there yet. No worries. Celebrate today (but not with food!), and stick to the Spark Solution plan whether you've seen moderate or dramatic results. You're not done yet. Skip ahead to Part 4 to learn what's coming in Week 3, Week 4, and the rest of your life. (And remember, you'll find the recipes and your workout plans in Part 3.)

Tools for
Success

Spark Swaps Recipes

When we set out to create a meal plan for the Spark Solution, we turned to our resident healthy cooking expert, Chef Meg Galvin. A runner, full-time culinary instructor, and mom to three active teenage boys, she is passionate about food that's healthy and delicious. Though she trained in haute cuisine, she cooks much more simply at home—she makes many of these same meals for her own family. Chef Meg eats like it's her job (because it is her job), but she certainly doesn't look like it. She credits the principles of the Spark Solution for helping her stay on track and still have energy to get up before dawn to run most mornings.

We know you're busy, but you've chosen to make your health a priority. That means finding the time to assemble a meal. You don't need to be a chef, and you don't need to know the difference between sauté and sear. These recipes are quick, easy, and made with familiar ingredients that can fit into any budget.

About the Recipes

Most of the breakfast and lunch recipes are single servings, unless noted. In some cases the breakfast recipes serve more, because it was difficult to make a smaller batch, but we offer tips for freezing or repurposing the leftovers. Snacks are also perfectly portioned just for you. The dinners serve four.

When we surveyed our members about their eating habits, we found that they spend five to fifteen minutes making breakfast, lunch, or snacks, and thirty to forty-five minutes cooking and prepping dinner. We designed

our recipes to reflect those habits. Plus, we share tips on finding shortcuts and saving time in the kItchen.

As you prepare these recipes, tailor them to suit your needs, as long as you're not adding calorie-dense ingredients or salt. Cut back on the pepper, double up on the veggies, or swap the herbs. When it comes to fruits and veggies, use what's in season and what's on sale. For bread products, you can swap out our suggestions for what you have on hand, as long as the calories are similar. If we suggest a pita but you like Sandwich Thins, eat those instead. If you have bread on hand for breakfast but no English muffins, use it. With these meals, the bread serving should be about 120 calories or less, so read labels.

We use fresh herbs unless noted. To substitute dried, use half as much as the recipe calls for. We frequently use fresh citrus as a way to replace salt, but you can swap in bottled citrus to save time. Jarred ginger and garlic are also big time savers, especially if you don't use those ingredients very often. To ease your meal planning, we've included comprehensive shopping lists in the appendixes (see page 355).

Start the Day Off Right: Breakfasts

Bacon-Swiss Scramble

We chose this dish for Day 1 for its simplicity and its tastiness. It's ready in only five minutes, and you'd never guess this is a better-for-you breakfast.

> **Prep Time:** *1 minute*
> **Cooking Time:** *5 minutes*
> **Yield:** *serves 1*

> SPARK SWAPS TIPS

Swap mushrooms, onions, or tomatoes for the spinach, if desired.

Cook up a batch of bacon on the weekend and portion it out for use throughout the week.

1 large egg plus 1 egg white
1 slice reduced-sodium bacon, cooked and crumbled

**½ ounce low-fat Swiss cheese (2 tablespoons shredded or
   ½ deli slice)
1 cup (about 3 ounces) fresh spinach**

*Coat a small nonstick skillet with cooking spray, place it over medium heat,
then add the spinach along with a tablespoon of water. Cook for 1 minute,
stirring often, until the spinach is bright in color and slightly wilted. Add the
crumbled bacon and the eggs and continue cooking until the eggs are set,
stirring often. Then stir in the cheese and remove from heat. The residual heat
from the eggs will melt the cheese.*

Nutrition Information per Serving

Calories: 138.9	*Sodium: 206.2 mg*	*Fiber: 0.7 g*
Fat: 8.1 g	*Carbs: 1.6 g*	*Protein: 15.1 g*
Cholesterol: 195.0 mg		

Breakfast Casserole Cups

*Though the ingredients might vary slightly, every family has a recipe like this,
which combines all your favorite breakfast foods. We kept this version in a
single-serving size, but you could easily modify this to feed a crowd. If your
own recipe has different ingredients (bread instead of potatoes, sausage or
ham in place of bacon, Swiss cheese swapped for cheddar), go ahead and
adjust this recipe accordingly. You can also ditch the meat and add chopped,
cooked broccoli.*

> **Prep Time:** *5 minutes*
> **Cooking Time:** *20 minutes*
> **Yield:** *serves 1 (2 casserole cups)*

> SPARK SWAPS TIPS

You don't need to peel the potato, but since grated potatoes will turn brown quickly, wait
until you have all the other ingredients in the bowl before preparing the potato.

**1 egg white, lightly beaten
1 slice reduced-sodium bacon, cooked and crumbled**

4 grape or cherry tomatoes, quartered
2 tablespoons shredded low-fat sharp cheddar cheese
Pinch of black pepper
Pinch of cayenne pepper
½ medium russet potato, grated (about ½ cup)

Preheat the oven to 400°F. Coat two wells of a muffin tin with cooking spray.

In a small bowl, combine all the ingredients, then pour the mixture into the prepared wells of the muffin tin. Bake for 20 minutes.

Remove from the oven and let the cups rest for a minute. Use a knife to loosen the edges of each cup. Serve immediately.

Nutrition Information per Serving

Calories: 174.2	*Sodium: 266.5 mg*	*Fiber: 2.5 g*
Fat: 4.7 g	*Carbs: 21.2 g*	*Protein: 12.3 g*
Cholesterol: 10.6 mg		

Breakfast Cookies

Cookies for breakfast? Yep. Especially when they're packed with heart-healthy fats and plenty of fiber and protein, with no added sugar. Not only are they a great on-the-go breakfast, but they're also a mighty fine snack.

Prep Time: *5 minutes*
Cooking Time: *13–15 minutes*
Yield: *serves 2*
Serving Size: *1 cookie*

> SPARK SWAPS TIPS

Instead of reaching for the sugar bowl, we use reduced-sugar raspberry jam for sweetness. Use strawberry, grape, or any kind of reduced-sugar jam you like.

1 tablespoon ground flaxseeds
¼ cup water
¼ cup whole-wheat flour
¼ teaspoon baking soda

1 tablespoon natural unsalted peanut butter
½ cup old-fashioned oats
1 tablespoon chopped almonds
1 tablespoon dried cranberries
½ teaspoon vanilla extract
2 teaspoons reduced-sugar raspberry jam

Preheat the oven to 375°F. Line a small baking sheet with parchment paper or a silicone pan liner, or grease with cooking spray.

In a small bowl, whisk the ground flax with the water, then let sit for 3 minutes, until gelatinous in texture. In a medium mixing bowl, combine the flour and baking soda. Stir in the flax mixture, peanut butter, oats, almonds, cranberries, vanilla, and jam until just combined. The mixture will be thick.

Divide the dough in half and roll into balls. Place the balls on the prepared baking sheet and flatten so that each is about four inches in diameter. Bake 13 to 15 minutes, or until the cookies are slightly firm. Cool for a few minutes before eating.

Nutrition Information per Serving

Calories: 227.7	*Sodium: 242.9 mg*	*Fiber: 6.2 g*
Fat: 8.1 g	*Carbs: 32.9 g*	*Protein: 8.7 g*
Cholesterol: 0.0 mg		

Creamy Cinnamon Cups

These were a kitchen experiment that serendipitously yielded a tasty, slimmed-down cinnamon roll. Creamy ricotta cheese stands in for all that icing, while flax and pecans add crunch. Cinnamon sweetens without any added sugar.

Prep Time: *5 minutes*
Cooking Time: *10–12 minutes*
Yield: *serves 1 (2 cups)*

1 serving whole-wheat pancake batter, prepared according to package directions (about ¼ cup)

2 tablespoons part-skim ricotta cheese
1 tablespoon ground flaxseeds
1 teaspoon cinnamon
1 tablespoon chopped pecans
1 packed teaspoon brown sugar

Preheat the oven to 350°F. Coat two wells of a muffin tin with cooking spray.

In a small bowl, combine the ricotta, flaxseeds, and cinnamon. Pour 2 table-spoons of the prepared batter into each cup, then fill with half of the ricotta mixture. Top with the chopped nuts and brown sugar.

Bake 10 to 12 minutes, or until the sides start to brown. Allow to cool for a couple of minutes before removing from the muffin tin. Serve immediately.

Nutrition Information per Serving

Calories: 198.5	*Sodium: 89.9 mg*	*Fiber: 4.2 g*
Fat: 5.1 g	*Carbs: 23.1 g*	*Protein: 6.7 g*
Cholesterol: 14.9 mg		

Egg Cups (Mini "Quiches") with Brown Rice Crust

Turn leftovers into breakfast with these perfectly portioned egg cups. This is a great use for the small bits of vegetables that weren't eaten at dinner last night. Brown rice stands in for a high-fat pie crust, which has little nutritional value.

Prep Time: *8 minutes*
Cooking Time: *15 minutes*
Yield: *serves 2*
Serving Size: *2 quiches*

> SPARK SWAPS TIPS

To freeze, allow the cups to cool completely, then place them in a ziplock bag. To reheat, microwave on high for 2 to 3 minutes.

2 large eggs
1 cup cooked brown rice
3 green onions, green and white parts chopped separately

1 bell pepper, chopped
¼ teaspoon black pepper
¼ teaspoon nutmeg
1 tablespoon plus 1 teaspoon shredded Parmesan cheese

Preheat the oven to 400°F. Coat four wells of a muffin tin with cooking spray.

In a small mixing bowl, combine one egg white with the rice and the green tops of the onions. Divide the mixture among the four wells and use the bottom of a small measuring cup to pack down the rice.

In the same mixing bowl, whisk the remaining egg and yolk and combine with the white parts of the onions, bell pepper, black pepper, and nutmeg. Divide the egg mixture among the four rice crusts, then sprinkle each with 1 teaspoon cheese.

Bake 13 to 15 minutes, or until the eggs are set and no longer jiggly. Allow to cool for 3 minutes before removing from the muffin tin, then serve.

Nutrition Information per Serving

Calories: 169.4	*Sodium: 134.2 mg*	*Fiber: 3.1 g*
Fat: 6.7 g	*Carbs: 18.5 g*	*Protein: 9.9 g*
Cholesterol: 187.4 mg		

Eggs Florentine Muffin

Simple enough for a workday breakfast yet decadent enough for a weekend brunch. Monterey jack cheese is mild and creamy enough that, when melted, it becomes a stand-in for the cream sauce in the original.

Prep Time: *3 minutes*
Cooking Time: *10 minutes*
Yield: *serves 1*

> SPARK SWAPS TIPS

Not a fan of poached eggs? Fry (using cooking spray) or scramble them instead. Add zing to the dish with a smear of Dijon mustard on one side of the toasted muffin.

1 large egg
1 tablespoon white vinegar
2 cups (about 6 ounces) fresh baby spinach
2 tablespoons shredded Monterey jack cheese
Pinch of nutmeg (optional)
1 whole-wheat English muffin, split and toasted

Crack the egg into a small bowl. Set aside.

Fill a small saucepan halfway with water. Add the vinegar and place the saucepan over medium heat. Bring it to a simmer. When small bubbles start to form around the edge, use the end of a wooden spoon to stir the water in a circular motion, then reduce the heat slightly.

Holding the edge of the bowl at the level of the water, slide the egg into the center of the simmering water. The water around it should be swirling slightly. Cook for 3 minutes, then use a slotted spoon to remove the egg. Set it aside on a plate.

While the egg is cooking, microwave the spinach on high for 1 minute, then wring out the spinach in a paper towel to remove excess moisture. Place atop half of the muffin. Top with the cheese and nutmeg, then add the egg and the other muffin half.

Nutrition Information per Serving

Calories: 259.4 *Sodium: 413.2 mg* *Fiber: 4.4 g*
Fat: 10.7 g *Carbs: 25.5 g* *Protein: 17.4 g*
Cholesterol: 197.6 mg

Fruity French Toast with Greek Yogurt

French toast is not inherently unhealthy; it's the butter and maple-flavored syrup we drown it in that's not so great. This version is simple: frothy egg whites and cinnamon, then a sprinkle of powdered sugar. Served with fresh berries and vanilla Greek yogurt, this version is light yet filling.

Prep Time: *5 minutes*
Cooking Time: *4 minutes*

Yield: *serves 1 (includes 1 slice french toast, 1 cup yogurt, and ½ cup fruit)*

> SPARK SWAPS TIPS

For french toast, choose the stalest bread you have in the house. Soft bread will soak up too much egg and get soggy.

1 egg white
¼ teaspoon cinnamon
1 slice whole-wheat bread
¼ teaspoon powdered sugar
½ cup mixed berries
1 cup fat-free vanilla Greek yogurt

In a flat dish, whip the egg white and cinnamon with a whisk or a fork until foamy.

Coat a nonstick skillet with cooking spray and place over medium-high heat. Dip both sides of the bread in the egg mixture, then place it in the heated pan. Cook for 2 minutes on each side.

Serve on a plate, sprinkled with powdered sugar, along with the berries and yogurt.

Nutrition Information per Serving

Calories: 340.7	*Sodium: 291.8 mg*	*Fiber: 5.1 g*
Fat: 2.5 g	*Carbs: 52.3 g*	*Protein: 27.7 g*
Cholesterol: 0.0 mg		

Ham and Cheese Stuffed Pancakes

Though we think of pancakes as a sweet breakfast, in their most basic form they're almost savory. Here we turned ordinary whole-wheat pancake batter into a stuffed sandwich that my three teenage boys (and their friends) love. What they don't know is how much better for you this version is than the fast-food version.

Prep Time: *5 minutes*
Cooking Time: *5 minutes*
Yield: *serves 4*
Serving Size: *1 stuffed pancake*

> SPARK SWAPS TIPS

Choose a skillet that's large enough to accommodate two pancakes at a time.

What's the secret to perfectly round pancakes? Use a ring mold or metal cookie cutter. Coat the inside with cooking spray, place it in the pan, and pour in your batter. Make your own ring mold: remove the top and bottom of a clean tuna can.

1 cup whole-wheat pancake mix
1 large egg
⅔ cup skim milk
1 tablespoon canola oil
4 slices (about 2 ounces) low-sodium deli-sliced ham
4 tablespoons shredded low-fat cheddar cheese

Combine the pancake mix, egg, milk, and oil in a medium bowl.

Coat a griddle or large skillet with cooking spray and place it over medium-high heat. When hot, pour about 2 tablespoons of the batter on the griddle (or into the skillet) and allow it to spread. Top with a slice of ham and 1 tablespoon of the cheese. Top with another 2 tablespoons of the batter. Cook 2 to 3 minutes, then flip and cook another 2 minutes. Repeat with the remaining ingredients.

To keep the pancakes warm, spread them in a single layer on a baking sheet and place in the oven on low heat.

To freeze, allow the pancakes to cool completely before placing them in a freezer bag. Reheat the still-frozen pancakes in a toaster oven on medium for 4 to 6 minutes or a microwave on high for 2 minutes, flipping halfway through.

Caution: The cheese will be quite hot, so allow it to cool a bit before eating.

Nutrition Information per Serving

Calories: 222.3	*Sodium: 531.0 mg*	*Fiber: 2.3 g*
Fat: 6.3 g	*Carbs: 29.4 g*	*Protein: 11.8 g*
Cholesterol: 59.8 mg		

Huevos Rancheros

This meal is fast and fun, and a great way to spice up a dull morning or bring a brunch favorite to the work week.

Huevos rancheros is a pretty simple meal: corn tortillas, eggs, and spicy tomato sauce. Many versions, however, don't stop there; they also include chili (with meat), refried beans, loads of cheese, and other high-calorie toppings. We loaded ours up too, but with fresh mango salsa, creamy black beans, and plenty of vegetables.

> **Prep Time:** *5 minutes*
> **Cooking Time:** *10 minutes*
> **Yield:** *serves 1*

> SPARK SWAPS TIPS

We used chipotle chili powder for added smokiness, but you can use any chili powder plus a pinch of smoked paprika.

No fresh mango? Use frozen or swap in corn kernels.

Salsa verde is made not from green tomatoes but from tomatillos, a tart relative of the tomato that's common in Mexican cuisine, plus cilantro, onions, and various hot peppers. Can't find it? Swap in your favorite salsa.

Craving cheese? Top the tortilla with 2 tablespoons grated low-fat cheddar or pepper jack.

1 6-inch corn tortilla
¼ teaspoon chili powder, divided
¼ cup chopped red onion
½ bell pepper, chopped
2 tablespoons canned low-sodium black beans, drained and rinsed
2 tablespoons chopped fresh mango
Zest and juice of ½ lime
¼ teaspoon ground cumin
1 large egg
2 teaspoons low-sodium salsa verde
1 tablespoon chopped fresh cilantro

Place a medium skillet over medium heat.

Coat both sides of the tortilla with cooking spray, then sprinkle it with a pinch (⅛ teaspoon) of the chili powder. Heat the tortilla for 30 seconds on each side, then place it on a plate.

Away from the heat, coat the skillet again with cooking spray, then return it to the burner. Sauté the onion, pepper, and beans for 3 to 4 minutes, until the veggies start to soften. Add the mango, lime zest and juice, cumin, and remaining ⅛ teaspoon of chili powder. Cook for 2 minutes. Pour the mixture over the tortilla.

Coat the skillet with cooking spray again and return to the heat. Fry the egg until the yolk is set, then slide it on top of the veggie-and-bean mixture, and garnish with the salsa verde and cilantro. Serve immediately.

Nutrition Information per Serving

Calories: 218.3	*Sodium: 185.9 mg*	*Fiber: 5.5 g*
Fat: 6.1 g	*Carbs: 31.0 g*	*Protein: 10.9 g*
Cholesterol: 185.0 mg		

Lemon-Ricotta Pancakes with Warm Summer Berries

The secret ingredient that gives the ricotta cheese a lift in flavor is fresh thyme. It will remind you that although this dish looks like dessert, it tastes like breakfast.

We first made these pancakes when strawberries were in season, but use any berry you like.

Prep Time: *8 minutes*
Cooking Time: *5 minutes*
Yield: *serves 2*
Serving Size: *2 pancakes with ½ cup strawberries*

> SPARK SWAPS TIPS

When swapping dried herbs for fresh, cut the amount in half, as drying the herbs intensifies their flavors.

Ricotta cheese is good for more than just lasagna. The soft cheese is rich in protein (7 grams in ¼ cup) and adds richness to these pancakes.

½ cup whole-wheat pancake mix
¼ cup part-skim ricotta cheese
Zest and juice of 1 lemon, kept separate
¼ teaspoon vanilla extract
1 teaspoon chopped fresh thyme
1 cup fresh strawberries, hulled and sliced

In a small bowl, stir together the pancake mix, ricotta, lemon zest, all but 1 teaspoon of the lemon juice, vanilla, and thyme until just combined. Add water 2 tablespoons at a time until the batter is thin enough to pour.

Coat a large skillet (or griddle) with cooking spray and place over medium-high heat. Pour the batter ¼ cup at a time into the hot skillet. Cook for 1 to 2 minutes, or until bubbles form and pop, then flip the pancake and cook another 1 to 2 minutes. Divide the cooked pancakes between two serving plates.

To the still-warm pan, add the chopped strawberries and the reserved teaspoon of lemon juice. Heat the strawberries, then top each plate of pancakes with half of the strawberries.

Note: These pancakes can be frozen or refrigerated for up to four days.

Nutrition Information per Serving

Calories: 194.9	*Sodium: 342.7 mg*	*Fiber: 4.5 g*
Fat: 3.1 g	*Carbs: 35.3 g*	*Protein: 7.9 g*
Cholesterol: 9.5 mg		

Mexican Breakfast Burrito

A hot breakfast need not be reserved for weekend mornings. Even on hectic workdays, you can make time for these quick, portable breakfast burritos.

Prep Time: *5 minutes*
Cooking Time: *5 minutes*
Yield: *serves 1*

> SPARK SWAPS TIPS

To freeze, allow the burrito to cool, then wrap it in plastic wrap or place it in a small ziplock bag. To reheat, microwave it on high for 4 minutes.

1 large egg plus 1 egg white
1 7-inch whole-wheat tortilla
¼ cup canned low-sodium black beans, drained and rinsed
¼ teaspoon chili powder
¼ teaspoon ground cumin
1 tablespoon low-fat shredded cheddar cheese
1 tablespoon low-sodium salsa

In a small bowl, whisk the eggs. Set aside.

Place the tortilla on a plate, cover it with a damp towel, and microwave it on high for 30 seconds.

Coat a small skillet with cooking spray and place it over medium heat. Sauté the beans with the chili powder and cumin for 2 minutes. Stir in the eggs and cook until the eggs are set, about 2 minutes.

Fill the center of the tortilla with the beans and eggs, then top with the cheese and salsa. To wrap the burrito, fold up one end, then both sides. Serve immediately, or wrap it in foil to take on the go.

Nutrition Information per Serving

Calories: 281.2	*Sodium: 493.4 mg*	*Fiber: 4.8 g*
Fat: 7.1 g	*Carbs: 36.9 g*	*Protein: 21.0 g*
Cholesterol: 186.4 mg		

Protein Pancakes

Boxed pancake mixes are great for quick breakfasts, but you can also whip up pancakes in a jiffy without one. As a bonus, these pancakes have a serving of protein, thanks to the Greek yogurt and egg. They are heartier than traditional varieties but just as delicious.

Prep Time: *5 minutes*
Cooking Time: *10 minutes*
Yield: *serves 2*
Serving Size: *2 pancakes*

1 large egg
⅔ cup fat-free plain Greek yogurt
1 teaspoon lemon juice
½ teaspoon vanilla extract
⅓ cup whole-wheat flour
¼ teaspoon baking soda
Pinch of salt

In a medium mixing bowl, whisk together the egg, yogurt, lemon juice, and vanilla with 1 tablespoon of water. In a small mixing bowl, combine the flour, baking soda, and salt. Gently fold the dry ingredients into the wet until just combined.

Heat a large skillet (or griddle) over medium heat, then coat it with cooking spray. Pour ¼ cup batter into the skillet, using the back of a spoon to spread it out. Cook for 2 to 3 minutes, or until bubbles form around the edge and pop. Flip and press the cooked side to push out the batter on the bottom. Cook another 2 minutes. Repeat with the remaining batter. Serve hot with fresh fruit or a tablespoon of maple syrup.

Nutrition Information per Serving

Calories: 145.0	*Sodium: 284.2 mg*	*Fiber: 2.4 g*
Fat: 2.9 g	*Carbs: 17.8 g*	*Protein: 13.2 g*
Cholesterol: 92.5 mg		

Quick Berry Muffins

These muffins are fast—mix all the ingredients in one bowl, and then they go straight into the oven. The secret ingredient is pancake mix. No need for eggs

or oil; Greek yogurt will replace them both. I tested this recipe with peaches and blueberries, but use your favorite fruit.

Prep Time: 5 minutes
Cooking Time: 15–17 minutes
Yield: serves 2
Serving Size: 2 muffins

> SPARK SWAPS TIPS

If using frozen fruit, thaw and drain it before adding it to the muffin mix.

½ cup whole-wheat pancake mix
2 tablespoons old-fashioned oats
2 packed teaspoons brown sugar
½ teaspoon cinnamon
2 tablespoons fat-free plain Greek yogurt
2 tablespoons skim milk
½ cup blueberries or 1 peach, chopped

Preheat the oven to 400°F. Line four wells of a muffin tin with paper baking cups and coat the cups with cooking spray.

In a small bowl, combine the pancake mix, oats, brown sugar, cinnamon, yogurt, and skim milk, then gently fold in the fruit. The batter will be thick. Divide it among the four prepared baking cups and bake 15 to 17 minutes, or until a toothpick inserted in the center comes out clean. Cool slightly before eating.

Save the other two for snacks. Let them cool completely, then store them in a ziplock bag or airtight container.

Nutrition Information per Serving

Calories: 198.5	Sodium: 377.9 mg	Fiber: 4.1 g
Fat: 0.7 g	Carbs: 42.6 g	Protein: 7.9 g
Cholesterol: 0.3 mg		

Quick and Easy Granola

This granola is ready in a snap with no need to preheat the oven. It's quite versatile. Use it as a cereal in ½-cup portions. Eat as a snack (¼-cup portions) or as a topping for yogurt or fruit (2-tablespoon servings).

Prep Time: *5 minutes*
Cooking Time: *5 minutes*
Yield: *serves 4*
Serving Size: *heaping ½ cup*

> **SPARK SWAPS TIPS**

Cut the cranberries in half or quarters with scissors so you get a bite of fruit in every spoonful.

Avoid rush-hour hunger-induced madness. Store ¼-cup snack-size servings of this granola in small airtight containers. Keep one in your bag or your car but the rest out of reach (in the trunk, if you're a car commuter) to avoid temptation. It's that good.

1 tablespoon natural unsalted peanut butter
1 packed tablespoon brown sugar
1 teaspoon cinnamon
2 cups old-fashioned oats
2 tablespoons sliced or chopped raw almonds
2 tablespoons dried cranberries
2 tablespoons unsweetened coconut flakes (optional)

In a large mixing bowl, combine the peanut butter, brown sugar, cinnamon, oats, and almonds. Using a wooden spoon, mash the peanut butter into the dry ingredients until it's completely incorporated.

Place the mixture in a microwave-safe 9-inch glass dish and cook on high for 5 minutes, stirring halfway through. Remove the dish from the microwave and stir in the cranberries and coconut (optional). Allow to cool completely before storing. The granola will keep for up to one month in an airtight container.

Nutrition Information per Serving

Calories: 214.1	*Sodium: 1.1 mg*	*Fiber: 5.1 g*
Fat: 6.6 g	*Carbs: 31.9 g*	*Protein: 6.8 g*
Cholesterol: 0.0 mg		

Slim Sausage Gravy

Who said you can't have biscuits and gravy on a diet meal plan? You can with this slimmed-down version. A little sausage goes a long way, and we used a special ingredient (mushrooms!) to stretch the flavor of the meat without much fat.

Prep Time: *10 minutes*
Cooking Time: *15 minutes*
Yield: *serves 1*

> SPARK SWAPS TIPS

Choose baby bella mushrooms for the best "meaty" flavor. And boost the nutrition by stirring in chopped greens (try kale) along with the other veggies.

We serve this with Better "Buttermilk" Biscuits (page 218). The biscuit recipe yields six servings: one for breakfast, one for a snack, and the rest for dinner. They freeze well if you have leftovers.

1 ounce reduced-fat breakfast sausage*
2 tablespoons chopped white or yellow onion
½ cup chopped mushrooms (about 2 ounces)
1½ teaspoons whole-wheat flour
Pinch of red pepper flakes
⅓ cup skim milk

* We used reduced-fat pork sausage. You might prefer chicken or turkey sausage—we also tested the recipe with chicken sausage—but be sure to choose a variety with reduced fat and/or low sodium.

Coat a small skillet with cooking spray and place it over medium heat. Add the sausage, breaking it up in the pan with the back of a wooden spoon. Brown lightly, then stir in the onions and mushrooms and sauté for 3 to 4 minutes, or until the mushrooms are dark brown. Add the flour and pepper flakes, and stir constantly for 1 minute. Pour in the milk, and stir until the gravy is thick and smooth. Serve immediately over a Better "Buttermilk" Biscuit (page 218) or toast.

Nutrition Information per Serving

Calories: 125.4	*Sodium: 218.3 mg*	*Fiber: 1.4 g*
Fat: 5.8 g	*Carbs: 10.6 g*	*Protein: 9.0 g*
Cholesterol: 19.2 mg		

Spicy Tomato-Egg Muffin

Taking this sandwich to go? Cook your egg until the yolk is hard (or scramble it) to avoid making a mess. If you don't like spice, swap the hot sauce for a pinch of smoked paprika, which will add depth without the heat.

Prep Time: *5 minutes*
Cooking Time: *5 minutes*
Yield: *serves 1*

> SPARK SWAPS TIPS

Watching your sodium? Skip the Canadian bacon.

Sauce
1 tablespoon fat-free plain Greek yogurt
2 drops hot sauce
Sandwich
1 slice (½ ounce) Canadian bacon
2 tablespoons shredded low-fat cheddar cheese
Pinch of black pepper
2 ¼-inch-thick slices tomato
1 whole-wheat English muffin, split and toasted
1 large egg

For the sauce, in a small dish combine the yogurt and hot sauce, then set aside.

Place a small nonstick skillet over medium heat. Cook the Canadian bacon for 1 minute on each side. Sprinkle the cheese and pepper on the bacon, and cook until the cheese melts, about 2 minutes, then remove and place it atop one half of the English muffin. Place the tomato slices atop the bacon.

Coat the skillet with cooking spray again, then cook the egg for 2 to 3 minutes, or until it cooks to a desired hardness. Place it atop the tomatoes. Spoon the sauce over the egg, then top with the second half of the muffin. Serve immediately.

Nutrition Information per Serving

Calories: 242.1	*Sodium: 559.2 mg*	*Fiber: 3.3 g*
Fat: 7.5 g	*Carbs: 25.5 g*	*Protein: 17.5 g*
Cholesterol: 193.0 mg		

Spinach-Feta Breakfast Wrap

Try adding chopped tomatoes or peppers, or goat cheese in place of feta. If you want to cut more calories or prefer toast on the side, cook the eggs omelet-style, then add the filling and roll it up like a burrito.

Prep Time: *3 minutes*
Cooking Time: *5 minutes*
Yield: *serves 1*

> SPARK SWAPS TIPS

To freeze, allow the wrap to cool, then store in a ziplock bag or plastic wrap. To reheat, microwave on high for 4 minutes.

1 7-inch whole-wheat tortilla
¼ cup sliced mushrooms
¼ teaspoon black pepper
2 cups (about 6 ounces) fresh spinach
1 large egg plus 1 egg white, lightly whisked
2 tablespoons crumbled low-fat feta cheese

Place the tortilla on a microwave-safe plate and heat on high for 1 minute.

Coat a small skillet with cooking spray, then place it over medium heat. Sauté the mushrooms and pepper for 2 minutes. Stir in the spinach and sauté for another 1 to 2 minutes, or until wilted. Add the eggs and cook, stirring often, until they are set, about 2 minutes.

Place the egg scramble in the center of the tortilla, then top it with the crumbled feta. To wrap, fold up one end, then both sides. Serve immediately, or wrap in foil to take it on the go.

Nutrition Information per Serving

Calories: 264.4	*Sodium: 531.5 mg*	*Fiber: 2.7 g*
Fat: 9.3 g	*Carbs: 26.7 g*	*Protein: 18.5 g*
Cholesterol: 197.6 mg		

Sweet and Creamy English Muffin

Skip the buttery Danish but keep the creamy, sweet taste you crave. This simple breakfast is a keeper. Try it with fresh or dried figs, orange marmalade, and fresh thyme for something unexpected.

Prep Time: *2 minutes*
Cooking Time: *1 minute*
Yield: *serves 1*

> SPARK SWAPS TIPS

If berries aren't in season, thaw frozen berries in the microwave. The added sauce will make this breakfast seem even more like a pastry.

If you're taking this on the go, use a whole-wheat pita to avoid leakage.

1 whole-wheat English muffin, toasted
¼ cup part-skim ricotta cheese
1 tablespoon all-fruit spread
½ cup fresh berries

Spread the ricotta and the jam on the English muffin. Top with the berries, and serve immediately.

Nutrition Information per Serving

Calories: 269.3	*Sodium: 301.2 mg*	*Fiber: 4.7 g*
Fat: 6.2 g	*Carbs: 41.8 g*	*Protein: 13.6 g*
Cholesterol: 19.1 mg		

Sweet Potato Hash

Red flannel hash is a staple at greasy-spoon diners, with its combo of salty corned beef, fried potatoes, and beets to give it that signature color. We slashed the fat in half and bulked ours up with veggies that aren't fried.

Prep Time: *15 minutes*
Cooking Time: *20 minutes*
Yield: *serves 1*

> SPARK SWAPS TIPS

We swapped out the beets because we know not everyone likes those ruby red veggies. If you're a fan, use half a small sweet potato and one small beet, diced, for a bright pink breakfast.

1 small sweet potato (about 4 ounces)
1 ounce reduced-fat breakfast sausage*
½ cup red onion, sliced
½ bell pepper, sliced (about ½ cup)
1 clove garlic, minced
Pinch of red pepper flakes
Pinch of black pepper
1 tablespoon red wine vinegar
1 cup packed (about 3 ounces) fresh baby spinach
1 large egg, cooked to your preference**

* This 1 ounce equals about 1½ links of sausage. We used reduced-fat pork sausage. You might prefer chicken or turkey sausage—we also tested the recipe with chicken sausage—but be sure to choose a variety with reduced fat and/or low sodium.

** We recommend "frying" an egg in a small skillet coated with cooking spray over medium heat while the hash cooks. You could also poach it or add it to the pan just before wilting the spinach to create a scramble.

Pierce the unpeeled sweet potato with a fork several times, then place it on a microwave-safe dish, and cook it on high for 3 to 5 minutes, or until it's slightly tender in the center. Allow it to cool for 5 minutes, then chop it into ½-inch cubes, keeping the skin on.

While the sweet potato is in the microwave, coat a large skillet with cooking spray and place it over medium heat. Sauté the sausage and onion until the sausage is lightly browned, about 3 minutes. Add the bell pepper, garlic, red pepper flakes, and black pepper and sauté another 3 minutes, stirring occasionally. Add the vinegar, stirring to remove any browned bits from the pan. Add the chopped sweet potato to the pan and sauté another 4 minutes, to give the sweet potato some color. Add the spinach, cover, and let it cook until the spinach just wilts, about 1 minute.

Spoon the hash onto a plate and top with the cooked egg before serving.

Nutrition Information per Serving

Calories: 260.6	Sodium: 318.1 mg	Fiber: 5.4 g
Fat: 11.1 g	Carbs: 26.9 g	Protein: 15.4 g
Cholesterol: 202.5 mg		

Three-Minute Crustless Quiche

If my students knew I was microwaving eggs, they'd faint from shock. I confess this was a new technique for me, but it works. The trick is to get to know your microwave. Stay close by, and start with sixty seconds, then add ten-second increments until your eggs are almost cooked. Appliances vary, and the eggs will continue to cook after you remove them from the microwave.

Serve this dish at brunch and call it Quiche au Micro-Ondes (Microwave Quiche). Doesn't that name prove that food sounds fancier and more appetizing in French? The technique is simple, and you can start playing around with flavor combos: bell peppers and spicy pepper jack cheese with chicken sausage; broccoli and cheddar cheese with ham; tomatoes, basil, and Parmesan cheese . . . Turn leftovers into breakfast in under two minutes! It's a great recipe for hotels, dorms, offices, or anywhere you might not have access to a stove.

> **Prep Time:** *5 minutes*
> **Cooking Time:** *3 minutes*
> **Yield:** *serves 1*

> SPARK SWAPS TIPS

Shredded cheese can dry out quickly. Buy cheese in blocks and grate it yourself. Not only will you save money, but the cheese will also melt better and have a stronger flavor.

Olive oil takes the place of the heavy cream traditionally used in quiche and eliminates the spongy texture common in microwaved eggs.

> **2 cups (about 6 ounces) fresh spinach, roughly chopped**
> **1 slice Canadian bacon**
> **1 large egg plus 1 egg white**
> **1 teaspoon olive oil**
> **Pinch of black pepper**
> **Pinch of nutmeg**
> **2 tablespoons shredded low-fat cheddar cheese**

Place the spinach in a microwave-safe bowl. Cover the bowl with a paper towel, then put the bacon on top of the towel. Cover the bacon with another paper towel. Microwave on high for 60 seconds. Slice the bacon into strips. Wring out the spinach in the paper towel to remove excess moisture.

In a medium mixing bowl, whisk together the cooked spinach, eggs, oil, pepper, nutmeg, and cheese, then add the bacon.

Coat the same microwave-safe bowl with more cooking spray, then add the egg mixture. Microwave on high for 90 seconds, or until the eggs are approximately 75 percent set. Allow the quiche to cool for a minute before serving.

Nutrition Information per Serving

Calories: 183.2 *Sodium: 437.5 mg* *Fiber: 1.5 g*
Fat: 11.3 g *Carbs: 3.3 g* *Protein: 15.9 g*
Cholesterol: 193.1 mg

Look Forward to Lunch

Better BLT

Even low-sodium bacon is plenty salty for this sandwich, and by chopping it, you spread that smoky goodness into every bite. A tangy yogurt sauce hides additional vegetables, and avocado stands in for mayonnaise for a dose of heart-healthy fat. In summertime, when tomatoes are at their freshest, I can't get enough of this lunch.

Prep Time: *5 minutes*
Cooking Time: *2 minutes*
Yield: *serves 1*

> SPARK SWAPS TIPS

Don't want to dirty extra dishes? You can stir together the sauce rather than puréeing it and skip the step of tossing the lettuce in the dressing.

Dressing

**1 tablespoon low-fat sour cream or fat-free plain Greek
  yogurt**
½ red bell pepper, diced

½ teaspoon Dijon mustard
¼ teaspoon black pepper
½ teaspoon red wine vinegar
Sandwich
    2 slices reduced-sodium bacon
    ¼ avocado, mashed*
    1 cup chopped Romaine lettuce
    ½ small tomato, sliced
    1 whole-wheat Sandwich Thin, toasted

* Choose avocados that feel heavy for their size with skin that isn't dried out. We prefer Hass for flavor and texture. If you're purchasing avocados to eat immediately, the flesh should give slightly when you press your thumb into the skin. If you're buying them a few days ahead, choose fruit with firm flesh. Once ripe, avocados can be refrigerated for a couple of days.

To cut, place the avocado on a cutting board and insert a small knife into the middle of the fruit until you hit the pit. Follow that line around the entire avocado, then twist the two halves in opposite directions. Slice the avocado while it's still in the skin, then scoop the flesh out with a spoon. To store the remaining avocado, keep the pit in it, sprinkle the avocado with lime or lemon juice, and wrap it tightly in plastic. Use or freeze it within twenty-four hours.

To prepare the dressing, purée the yogurt, bell pepper, mustard, black pepper, and vinegar in a blender and set aside.

Place the bacon on a microwave-safe plate between two paper towels and microwave for 90 seconds, until the slices are crisp. Allow the bacon to cool, then chop it and mix it with the mashed avocado.

Toss the lettuce with half of the dressing, then pile it on the bottom half of the Sandwich Thin. Top with the tomato slices, the avocado-bacon mix, and the rest of the dressing. Alternately, you can serve the second half of the dressing as a dipping sauce on the side.

Nutrition Information per Serving

Calories: 308.6	*Sodium: 479.1 mg*	*Fiber: 10.7 g*
Fat: 16.8 g	*Carbs: 33.7 g*	*Protein: 13.1 g*
Cholesterol: 20.9 mg		

Cheesy Chicken Pouch

This recipe came at Becky's special request as a replacement for those boxed pastry sandwiches found in the freezer section. While those aren't too high in calories, they have loads of added salt and almost no veggies. These are simple to make, especially if you use leftover sautéed veggies. This is a great recipe for picky kids and teens.

> **Prep Time:** *5 minutes*
> **Cooking Time:** *15 minutes*
> **Yield:** *serves 1*

> SPARK SWAPS TIPS

Love cheese but have trouble controlling portions? Shredding it can help. A 1-ounce serving yields 1 standard deli slice or 2 cubes (about the size of a pair of dice) but ¼ cup shredded, which looks like more.

> **1 small zucchini, grated (about ½ cup)**
> **¼ cup chopped white or yellow onion**
> **½ cup sliced mushrooms**
> **¼ cup shredded Swiss cheese**
> **3 ounces cooked chicken breast, diced**
> **¼ teaspoon plus 1 pinch of smoked paprika**
> **¼ teaspoon black pepper**
> **1 whole-wheat flatbread or 7-inch tortilla**

Wrap the zucchini in two layers of paper towels or a lint-free tea towel and press down hard to remove any excess moisture. (Don't skip this step or your sandwich will be soggy.)

Coat a medium skillet with cooking spray and set it over medium heat. Sauté the onions and mushrooms for 3 minutes, then remove the skillet from heat.

In a small bowl, combine the onions and mushrooms with the zucchini, cheese, chicken, paprika, and pepper. Spoon the mixture into the middle of the flatbread or tortilla, fold up the ends and then the sides. Spray the wrapped pouch with cooking spray, then cook it in the same skillet on medium heat for 3 minutes on each side.

Serve immediately, or allow it to cool and then wrap it in aluminum foil before refrigerating. To reheat, microwave it unwrapped on high for 30 seconds to 1 minute.

Nutrition Information per Serving

Calories: 325.2	*Sodium: 456.1 mg*	*Fiber: 10.9 g*
Fat: 9.9 g	*Carbs: 27.0 g*	*Protein: 39.0 g*
Cholesterol: 69.3 mg		

Cobb Salad

A typical Cobb salad is a meal in a bowl, and its appeal is both its abundance and its simplicity. We wanted to keep some things the same: a large bowl of greens with vibrant ingredients contrasting flavors and textures. We made a few key changes, which help illustrate our either-or, not all-or-nothing, philosophy. We ditched one egg yolk to cut cholesterol. The original recipe had several high-fat foods: bacon, blue cheese, and avocado. We skipped the bacon in favor of a leaner protein but kept some smokiness by adding smoked paprika to the dressing. We left off the blue cheese and focused on the avocado, which adds fiber and serves as a source of healthy fat. We kept one yolk in our hard-cooked eggs to add some richness to the salad. Carrots add sweetness and crunch.

For a vegetarian option, swap the chicken for chickpeas.

Prep Time: *10 minutes*
Yield: *serves 1*

> SPARK SWAPS TIPS

If you're eating this away from home, store the dressing separately and dress the greens just before serving.

Crave a smokier flavor? Sprinkle a pinch of smoked paprika over the salad.

Dressing
2 tablespoons fat-free plain Greek yogurt
½ teaspoon Dijon mustard

¼ teaspoon black pepper
¼ teaspoon smoked paprika
1 teaspoon lemon juice
1 green onion, green and white parts chopped separately

Salad

2 cups Romaine lettuce, chopped or torn into bite-size pieces
1 large hard-boiled egg plus 1 hard-boiled egg white, chopped
3 ounces cooked chicken breast, diced
6 grape or cherry tomatoes, halved, or 1 Roma tomato, chopped
¼ cup sliced or diced red onion
1 medium carrot, grated or sliced (about ½ cup)
¼ avocado, cubed

To make the dressing, in a small bowl whisk together the yogurt, mustard, pepper, paprika, lemon juice, and white parts of the green onion.

In a medium bowl, toss the lettuce with half of the dressing. Top with the remaining ingredients—the chopped egg, chicken, tomatoes, onion, carrot, green onion tops, and avocado—and drizzle on the remaining dressing.

Nutrition Information per Serving

Calories: 337.5	Sodium: 305.0 mg	Fiber: 8.4 g
Fat: 13.7 g	Carbs: 20.4 g	Protein: 36.8 g
Cholesterol: 234.3 mg		

Curried Tuna Salad Sandwich

We gave this lean lunchtime staple an East Indian twist. A bit of curry powder spices it up, some dried cranberries add unexpected sweetness, and cucumber offers much-needed texture. A mix of olive-oil mayonnaise and fat-free plain Greek yogurt keeps the salad creamy yet low in fat.

Swap cooked chicken, diced firm tofu, canned salmon, canned shrimp, or hard-boiled eggs for the tuna.

Prep Time: *10 minutes*
Yield: *serves 1*

> SPARK SWAPS TIPS

English cucumbers, also called hothouse cucumbers, are long and slender with thin skins. They're often wrapped in plastic at the supermarket, which means they haven't been treated with waxes, so you can eat the skin. If you can't find an English cucumber, scrub the skin of another cucumber variety to remove the wax or peel it.

Desktop Dining. To avoid a soggy sandwich, keep the tuna salad and lettuce separate from the pita and assemble just before eating.

> 1 teaspoon olive-oil mayonnaise
> 1 tablespoon fat-free plain Greek yogurt
> ¼ teaspoon yellow curry powder
> 1 green onion, chopped
> ¼ English cucumber, diced (about ¼ cup)
> Pinch of black pepper
> 1 tablespoon dried cranberries
> 1 2.6-ounce pouch low-sodium chunk tuna, packed in water
>   and drained
> ½ whole-wheat pita
> ½ cup red leaf lettuce, chopped or torn

In a medium bowl, combine the mayonnaise, yogurt, and curry powder. Stir in the green onion, cucumber, pepper, and cranberries. Gently fold in the tuna, mixing until just combined.

Microwave the pita for about 20 seconds to soften it, then fill it with the lettuce and the tuna salad. Serve immediately.

Nutrition Information per Serving

Calories: 220.1	*Sodium: 348.8 mg*	*Fiber: 3.6 g*
Fat: 2.8 g	*Carbs: 25.2 g*	*Protein: 25.0 g*
Cholesterol: 31.6 mg		

Greek Meatball Pita (Keftedes)

We ventured across the Mediterranean for this meatball makeover. We swapped lamb (rich and delicious but quite pricey) for lean beef and added onion and herbs to impart flavor and moisture. The result is a sandwich just like Yaya used to make. Add red onion slices and chopped Roma tomatoes, if you prefer.

Prep Time: *5 minutes*
Cooking Time: *10 minutes*
Yield: *serves 1*

> SPARK SWAPS TIPS

When combining ground meat with other ingredients, handle the meat as little as possible. Overmixing can yield tough meat.

To speed cooking time, flatten the meatballs into patties. These patties fit perfectly into the pita.

To make the pita more pliable, microwave it for 20 seconds just before filling.

Desktop Dining. Keep the cooked meat, pita, and other ingredients separate, then reheat the meat and assemble just before eating.

Dressing
1 teaspoon finely chopped fresh parsley
1 teaspoon lemon zest
1 teaspoon lemon juice
1 tablespoon fat-free plain Greek yogurt
½ cup finely chopped cucumber

Meatballs
4 ounces 96 percent lean ground beef
2 tablespoons finely chopped white or yellow onion
1 teaspoon finely chopped fresh parsley
1 teaspoon finely chopped fresh mint or ½ teaspoon dried mint
Pinch of black pepper

Pita
½ whole-wheat pita
½ cup chopped Romaine lettuce

To prepare the dressing, in a small bowl combine the parsley, lemon zest, lemon juice, and yogurt. Set aside.

Place the cucumbers on a paper towel to allow any excess moisture to drain off.

In a separate small bowl, using a fork or your hands, mix the beef, onion, parsley, mint, and pepper until just combined. Form the mixture into two patties.

Coat a small skillet with cooking spray and set it over medium heat. Cook the patties for 5 minutes per side, until the beef reaches an internal temperature of 160°F using a quick-read thermometer. Remove the skillet from heat.

Mix the cucumber into the dressing, then spread it inside the pita. Add the lettuce and meat, and serve.

Nutrition Information per Serving

Calories: 255.1   *Sodium: 240.6 mg*   *Fiber: 5.4 g*

Fat: 4.7 g   *Carbs: 21.1 g*   *Protein: 30.6 g*

Cholesterol: 60.0 mg

Lean Philly Cheesesteak

Street trucks are such a temptation at lunchtime. The food just smells so good, but you know it's not good for you. We re-created one of our favorite lunch-truck specialties: the Philly cheesesteak. The trick to making the lean beef and veggies taste like the real deal is the fond, *the crust that develops on the bottom of the pan (from a French term meaning both "foundation" and "dregs"). Instead of leaving those tasty bits in the pan, we scrape them up to create a mouthwatering sauce. We used onions and mushrooms, but feel free to add bell peppers too. We chose a pita to hold all the tasty juices, but this is also delicious on a whole-wheat bun.*

Prep Time: *5 minutes*

Cooking Time: *7 minutes*

Yield: *serves 1*

> SPARK SWAPS TIPS

To make the pita more pliable, microwave it for 20 seconds.

For a fun twist on the original, serve the filling inside half a bell pepper that's been roasted or grilled until soft.

Desktop Dining. Skip the step of melting the cheese in the pan. Allow the meat and veggies to cool completely, then spoon the mixture into a resealable container and top with the cheese. Store the pita in a ziplock bag. Reheat the filling in the microwave and assemble the pita just before eating.

1 small white or yellow onion, sliced (about ½ cup)
½ cup sliced mushrooms
¼ teaspoon dried thyme
¼ teaspoon black pepper
2 ounces cooked extra-lean roast beef, thinly sliced*
1 slice provolone cheese (about 1 ounce)
½ whole-wheat pita

* We took some help from the prepared-food section of the supermarket and picked up some precooked roast beef. You can swap lean deli roast beef, but it will add more salt to the recipe.

Heat a small skillet over medium heat. Remove it from the heat to coat it with cooking spray. Then return it to the heat and add the onions, mushrooms, thyme, and pepper. Sauté for 5 minutes, until the onions turn golden brown.

Add a tablespoon of water to the skillet and stir well. Using a wooden spoon, scrape the browned bits off the bottom of the pan. Add the beef, and stir to combine. Top the mixture with the cheese. Cover and cook until the cheese melts.

Fill the pita with the mixture, and serve immediately.

Nutrition Information per Serving

Calories: 340.5	Sodium: 254.3 mg	Fiber: 3.6 g
Fat: 12.2 g	Carbs: 19.8 g	Protein: 38.8 g
Cholesterol: 75.0 mg		

Leftover-Lunchbox Burrito

Burritos are perfect for leftover lunches. After dinners when you don't have a full serving of anything left, combine the extras and turn them into a tasty burrito or wrap for tomorrow's lunch. Get creative. We love the combo of pork with salsa verde and white beans. Carrots and corn add crunch, while the spices and lime juice make this meal seem like much more than a sixty-second recipe.

Prep Time: *5 minutes*
Cooking Time: *1 minute*
Yield: *serves 1*

> SPARK SWAPS TIPS

Freeze the burrito filling in individual portions and reheat it in the microwave on high for 1 minute.

Have extra room in your calorie budget? Add ¼ mashed avocado or 2 tablespoons fat-free plain Greek yogurt or low-fat sour cream.

Desktop Dining. Store the tortilla separately from the filling, which takes only a minute to reheat in the microwave.

3 ounces roasted pork, diced*
2 tablespoons low-sodium salsa verde
¼ cup grated carrots
2 tablespoons corn kernels
¼ cup canned cannellini (white kidney) beans, drained and rinsed**
⅛ teaspoon ground cumin
⅛ teaspoon chili powder
Zest of 1 lime and 1 teaspoon lime juice (optional)
1 7-inch whole-wheat tortilla

* Pork tenderloin is a lean, versatile protein. Consider roasting one every few weeks, slicing the meat, and portioning it into individual servings for quick lunches and dinners. No time? Pick up a serving of roast pork from the prepared-foods section of the supermarket, or use any leftover lean protein you have on hand, such as chicken or turkey breast, roast beef, steak, or ground beef.

** If you can't find cannellini beans, use Great Northern or navy beans.

In a microwave-safe container, combine all the ingredients for the filling—the pork, salsa verde, carrots, corn, beans, cumin, chili powder, and the optional lime zest and lime juice. Microwave the mixture on high for 1 minute, then spoon it on the tortilla. Fold up one end, then both sides, and serve.

Nutrition Information per Serving

Calories: 435.8   *Sodium: 471.3 mg*   *Fiber: 8.2 g*

Fat: 10.8 g   *Carbs: 41.5 g*   *Protein: 41.9 g*

Cholesterol: 89.6 mg

Lighter Chicken Caesar Salad

Caesar dressing is packed full of flavorful ingredients: egg yolk, anchovies, and Parmesan cheese. However, it's also quite high in fat. With just a few simple swaps, this popular salad lost half the calories and 900 milligrams of sodium. At home, swap the croutons for a toasted whole-wheat tortilla rubbed with a garlic clove for a twist on pizza. You'll love the hot-and-cold combo. You can also swap the chicken for salmon, shrimp, or white beans.

Prep Time: *10 minutes*

Yield: *serves 1*

> SPARK SWAPS TIPS

Desktop Dining. Pack the croutons in a ziplock bag and the dressing and the salad in two separate resealable containers. Assemble just before eating.

Dressing

1 small clove garlic, minced

⅛ teaspoon Dijon mustard

½ teaspoon miso paste

2 teaspoons lemon juice

2 tablespoons fat-free plain Greek yogurt

Salad

2 cups Romaine lettuce, chopped or torn into bite-size pieces

3 ounces cooked chicken breast, diced

1 teaspoon shredded Parmesan cheese

Pinch of black pepper

1 whole-wheat Sandwich Thin or 1 slice whole-wheat bread, toasted and cubed

In a medium bowl, combine the garlic, mustard, and miso. Stir in the lemon juice and yogurt. Add the lettuce and chicken and toss to coat. Transfer the salad to a serving plate or resealable container. Top with the grated cheese and pepper. Add the toasted bread cubes just before serving.

Nutrition Information per Serving

Calories: 308.3

Fat: 5.5 g

Cholesterol: 72.9 mg

Sodium: 617.4 mg

Carbs: 28.5 g

Fiber: 7.3 g

Protein: 38.9 g

Loaded Sweet Potato

Baked potatoes—white or sweet—are a quick, easy side dish. The trouble is the toppings: sour cream, butter, cheese, bacon, and a few chives for good measure. We dumped those fatty toppings and stuffed a sweet potato with veggies, lean chicken breast, and a spicy-sweet chipotle orange sauce. Ready in ten minutes from mostly leftover ingredients, this meal is a welcome respite from lunchtime frozen meals.

Prep Time: *5 minutes*

Cooking Time: *10 minutes*

Yield: *serves 1*

> SPARK SWAPS TIPS

Don't forget to eat the skin of the potato! It's loaded with fiber.

Desktop Dining. Cook the sweet potato at home until it's almost tender, then finish cooking it in the microwave at the office. Reheat the veggies and chicken, and assemble your potato.

1 medium sweet potato (about 4 ounces)

2 tablespoons chopped white or yellow onion

¼ bell pepper, chopped (about ¼ cup)

2 tablespoons frozen corn
3 ounces cooked chicken breast, diced
¼ teaspoon black pepper
Sauce
1 tablespoon fat-free plain Greek yogurt
1 teaspoon orange zest
1 tablespoon orange juice
¼ chipotle pepper in adobo sauce, chopped

Pierce the sweet potato with a fork several times and place it in a microwave-safe dish. Microwave on high until tender, about 7 minutes.

Meanwhile, coat a skillet with cooking spray and place it over medium heat. Sauté the onion, bell pepper, corn, chicken, and black pepper for 3 minutes, or until the vegetables are tender.

To prepare the sauce, in a small bowl combine the yogurt, orange zest, orange juice, and chipotle pepper. Set aside.

Place the sweet potato on a serving plate. Slice it almost entirely in half and mash the flesh with a fork. Then fill the potato with the vegetables and chicken and top with the sauce.

Nutrition Information per Serving

Calories: 258.7	Sodium: 109.3 mg	Fiber: 5.3 g
Fat: 1.6 g	Carbs: 36.2 g	Protein: 26.0 g
Cholesterol: 49.3 mg		

Mexican Pizza

Whole-wheat tortillas are great stand-ins for portion-controlled pizza crusts. Though we took a south-of-the-border approach to this dish, you can top it with anything you want. Try chicken and barbecue sauce with sharp cheddar cheese, spinach, and onions; tomato sauce with basil and mozzarella cheese; or turkey pepperoni with roasted peppers and onions.

Prep Time: *5 minutes*
Cooking Time: *12 minutes*
Yield: *serves 1*

> SPARK SWAPS TIPS

Top with 1 cup chopped lettuce for added crunch and freshness.

Not a fan of wheat tortillas? Use 2 small corn tortillas instead.

Always wash citrus before zesting.

1 7-inch whole-wheat tortilla
½ cup canned low-sodium black beans, drained and rinsed
¼ teaspoon chili powder
¼ teaspoon ground cumin
2 tablespoons low-sodium salsa
½ bell pepper, chopped
3 tablespoons shredded low-fat cheese*
Zest of 1 lime (optional)
½ teaspoon lime juice
1 teaspoon fat-free plain Greek yogurt or low-fat sour cream

* We used Monterey jack and cheddar; you could use a Mexican blend or pepper jack too.

Preheat the oven to 400°F.

Coat both sides of the tortilla with cooking spray. Bake it on a small baking sheet for 6 minutes, flipping the tortilla halfway through.

In a small microwave-safe bowl, combine the beans with a teaspoon of water, the chili powder, and the cumin, and microwave for 90 seconds, then carefully mash the mixture with a fork. Spoon the beans on the tortilla, then top with the salsa and chopped pepper. Sprinkle on the cheese and the optional lime zest. Bake in the preheated oven for 5 to 6 minutes, or until the cheese bubbles.

While the tortilla is baking, mix the yogurt with ½ teaspoon lime juice. (Add an extra pinch of cumin, if you want.) When ready, cut the pizza into wedges, top with the lime "cream," and serve.

If you aren't going to serve this immediately, let the pizza cool, then store it in an airtight container. Top with the cream just before eating.

Nutrition Information per Serving

Calories: 293.1	Sodium: 572.3 mg	Fiber: 9.5 g
Fat: 3.3 g	Carbs: 53.8 g	Protein: 17.7 g
Cholesterol: 4.3 mg		

Sautéed Kale Salad

Let's be honest. Kale is not winning any veggie popularity contests. It's tough, the flavor can be strong, and it's so green and healthy. Don't discount this good-for-you green. Learn how to use its hardiness to your advantage. Where other greens would be slimy or mushy in this dish, kale keeps its bite yet becomes much more tender. The sweet, acidic balsamic vinegar mellows kale and the eggs add a creamy contrast.

Prep Time: *5 minutes*
Cooking Time: *5 minutes*
Yield: *serves 1*

> SPARK SWAPS TIPS

Desktop Dining. Prep the salad the night before, store it in an airtight container, and reheat it in the microwave for 30 seconds on high. Add the eggs just before eating.

1 teaspoon olive oil
¼ medium red onion, sliced (about ¼ cup)
½ teaspoon Dijon mustard
½ bunch kale, tough stems removed, leaves chopped into bite-size pieces (about 1½ cups)
2 teaspoons balsamic vinegar
½ teaspoon black pepper
1 Roma tomato, chopped
2 hard-boiled eggs, one yolk discarded, chopped

Heat the olive oil in a large skillet over medium heat. Sauté the onion for 3 minutes, until soft, then stir in the mustard, 2 tablespoons of water, and the kale. Sauté another 30 seconds, or until the kale is just wilted. Add the vinegar, pepper, and tomatoes, stir well, and remove from the heat. Transfer the salad to a serving dish, top with the eggs, and serve warm.

Nutrition Information per Serving

Calories: 204.9	*Sodium: 239.2 mg*	*Fiber: 4.8 g*
Fat: 10.5 g	*Carbs: 15.9 g*	*Protein: 14.5 g*
Cholesterol: 185.0 mg		

Shrimp Salad with Miso-Carrot Dressing

This salad was inspired by the complimentary salads often served at Japanese restaurants. The light starter usually contains little more than iceberg lettuce and a few shreds of carrot, but the dressing steals the show: the humble carrot is puréed with ginger and miso, plus a bit of sesame oil for an addictive yet light salad topper.

Here, we re-created that dressing but bulked it up. The iceberg is gone, and in its place are crunchy radishes, cucumbers, and more carrots. Who says a salad always needs lettuce? Topped with a serving of cooked shrimp—either left over from another meal or the ready-to-eat frozen variety—this salad becomes a light lunch.

> **Prep Time:** *10 minutes*
> **Yield:** *serves 1*

> SPARK SWAPS TIPS

Want greens? Add 1 cup packed (about 3 ounces) spinach or chopped Romaine lettuce.

Save time by using the slicing or shredding blades on a food processor to prep the veggies.

Scrape the skin off fresh ginger with the back of a spoon, then grate it using a microplane or the smallest side of a box grater. (You can also use jarred ginger.)

Desktop Dining. Store the dressing separate from the salad until just before eating.

Dressing

> **2 teaspoons white wine vinegar**
> **½ teaspoon miso paste**
> **¼ teaspoon toasted sesame oil**
> **1 teaspoon olive oil**
> **¼ teaspoon grated fresh gingerroot**
> **2 medium carrots, grated (about 1 cup)**
> **⅛ teaspoon black pepper**

½ cucumber, peeled (if not English variety) and diced or cut into strips (about 1 cup)
6 radishes, sliced (about ½ cup)
3 ounces cooked shrimp, peeled (about 4 medium shrimp)*

* If using frozen, ready-to-eat shrimp, first thaw it under cold running water.

To prepare the dressing, purée the vinegar, miso, sesame oil, olive oil, ginger, ¼ cup of the carrots, and pepper in a food processor or blender until smooth.

In a medium bowl, toss the remaining carrots with the cucumber and radishes in half of the dressing. Top with the shrimp, and drizzle with the rest of the dressing. Serve immediately.

Nutrition Information per Serving

Calories: 208.5	*Sodium: 381.3 mg*	*Fiber: 5.0 g*
Fat: 7.0 g	*Carbs: 16.8 g*	*Protein: 20.0 g*
Cholesterol: 165.8 mg		

Spinach Salad with Salmon and Creamy Dill Dressing

Spinach salads are a staple for dieters, but most versions are pretty bland. If you're relying on a salad but skipping the protein at lunchtime, you're bound to be starving by mid-afternoon. Here, we top a hearty portion of veggies with salmon for belly-filling protein and a dose of omega-3 fatty acids.

Prep Time: *5 minutes*
Yield: *serves 1*

> SPARK SWAPS TIPS

No leftover salmon? Use canned salmon instead. Be sure to check for bones, drain it well, and combine it with half of the dressing before adding it to the salad.

Desktop Dining. Prepare the dressing in a small resealable container. Store the spinach and vegetables separately from the salmon, and assemble everything just before eating.

2 tablespoons fat-free plain Greek yogurt
2 teaspoons lemon juice
½ teaspoon dried dill or 1 teaspoon fresh, chopped dill

2 cups packed (about 6 ounces) fresh baby spinach
½ cup sliced grape or cherry tomatoes (about 8)
½ cup sliced cucumber
½ cup grated or sliced carrots
Pinch of black pepper
3 ounces cooked salmon

To prepare the dressing, in a small bowl combine the yogurt, lemon juice, and dill.

In a medium bowl, toss the spinach, tomatoes, cucumbers, and carrots with half of the dressing. Top with the pepper, salmon, and the remaining dressing, then serve.

Nutrition Information per Serving

Calories: 294.8	*Sodium: 175.2 mg*	*Fiber: 3.6 g*
Fat: 9.7 g	*Carbs: 15.6 g*	*Protein: 36.6 g*
Cholesterol: 80.5 mg		

Sweet Orange-Miso Chicken and Veggies

While Asian cuisine is often a healthy choice, food-court Chinese is an exception to that rule. Deep-fried dark-meat chicken, sugary sauces, and white rice will land in your belly like a brick, ensuring an afternoon crash. Swap this better-than-takeout five-minute meal instead.

Prep Time: *2 minutes*
Cooking Time: *5 minutes*
Yield: *serves 1*

> SPARK SWAPS TIPS

The next time you steam brown rice or grill chicken, double the amount; both freeze well. Allow to cool completely and store single servings for easy lunches and quick dinners.

Save time with jarred minced garlic.

Desktop Dining. Make the sauce the night before, and store in a small resealable container. Store the rice, veggies, and chicken in a separate container. Pour on the sauce, reheat, and eat.

Miso

Miso is a tangy paste made from fermented rice, barley, soybeans, and my favorite, buckwheat. Though its primary flavor is salty, miso can be very subtle or complex with fruity, salty, and umami notes. The darker the miso, the more flavor and depth it will add to the dish.

Miso—like yogurt, kimchi, and sauerkraut—contains probiotics, which aid digestion by creating microbial balance in the GI tract. Those delicate probiotics lose their effectiveness if miso is boiled. I often use it in the raw state or in cooked dishes that require shorter cooking times.

I also prefer to use miso in place of salt in lots of my dishes, such as salmon, mushrooms, chicken, whole-wheat pasta, or even eggs. One tablespoon or so is all you need to impart a rich, salty flavor, and for just 30 calories and half a gram of fat. The sodium levels vary by brands, from 330 milligrams to 880 milligrams, so read labels and choose a brand that suits your dietary needs.

Miso is found in the refrigerated or health-food sections of your supermarket. It will keep in your refrigerator for up to one year.

At my house, we love it:

- *mixed with olive oil and spread on toasted bread, instead of butter*
- *swirled into soups*
- *tossed with steamed green beans for a creamy sauce consistency*
- *added to stews to boost flavor*

1 cup frozen stir-fry vegetables
3 ounces cooked chicken breast, diced
½ cup cooked brown rice
Zest and juice of 1 orange (about 2 tablespoons zest and
     ⅓ cup juice)
½ teaspoon miso paste
1 clove garlic, chopped
½ teaspoon cornstarch

In a medium bowl, microwave the vegetables on high until thawed and heated through, about 90 seconds. Stir in the chicken and rice and microwave for another minute. Assemble the mixture on a serving plate.

In a small saucepan set over medium-high heat, simmer the orange juice, miso, and garlic for 1 minute.

In a small dish, dilute the cornstarch with 1 tablespoon cold water. Add it to the saucepan along with the orange zest, and stir until the sauce thickens, about 1 minute. Pour the sauce over the chicken, rice, and veggies and serve.

Nutrition Information per Serving

Calories: 358.6   Sodium: 410.2 mg   Fiber: 4.0 g

Fat: 4.0 g   Carbs: 44.3 g   Protein: 31.5 g

Cholesterol: 65.7 mg

Tomato-Basil Chicken Sandwich

A lunchtime staple gets a sophisticated twist, but it's still ready in five minutes.

Prep Time: *5 minutes*

Yield: *serves 1*

> SPARK SWAPS TIPS

This sandwich is so simple, it almost doesn't need a recipe. We encourage you to start with a whole-wheat bun and chicken, and top it as desired. Get creative, but track those calories!

3 ounces cooked chicken breast

1 whole-wheat Sandwich Thin

Pinch of black pepper

1 thick slice tomato

1 large leaf lettuce

1 serving Tomato-Basil Aioli (page 228)

Place the chicken on the bottom half of the Sandwich Thin, sprinkle it with pepper, and layer it with the tomato, lettuce, and aioli sauce.

Nutrition Information per Serving

Calories: 250.4   Sodium: 358.4 mg   Fiber: 5.8 g

Fat: 2.6 g   Carbs: 24.6 g   Protein: 34.4 g

Cholesterol: 65.7 mg

Trim Taco Salad

Salads are inherently healthy, but any meal served in an edible carb-based receptacle is a bad idea, taco salads included. Fried tortilla shells add hundreds of unnecessary calories and little nutrition, and traditional taco seasoning is loaded with sodium. This version swaps in a crispy—not greasy—tortilla, extra-lean beef, and plenty of veggies.

> **Prep Time:** *5 minutes*
> **Cooking Time:** *6 minutes*
> **Yield:** *serves 1*

> SPARK SWAPS TIPS

Pressed for time? Swap the beef for ½ cup red beans. You can also skip the step of cooking the peppers, if you prefer them raw.

Have leftover ground beef, chicken, or steak? Use it instead.

Desktop Dining. Store the veggies and meat, dressing, lettuce, and tortilla strips all in separate containers and assemble just before eating. If you prefer to store everything in one container, pour in the dressing first, then the meat and veggies, and top with the lettuce. Keep the tortilla strips separate until you're ready to eat.

Dressing
   ¼ avocado
   ¼ teaspoon chili powder
   ¼ teaspoon ground cumin
   Zest and juice of 1 lime (about 1 teaspoon zest and
      2 tablespoons juice)
   1 tablespoon fat-free plain Greek yogurt

Topping
   1 6-inch corn tortilla
   4 ounces 96 percent lean ground beef
   ¼ teaspoon chili powder
   ¼ teaspoon ground cumin
   ½ bell pepper, chopped (about ½ cup)
   3 green onions, green and white parts chopped separately

Salad
   2 cups Romaine lettuce, chopped or torn into bite-size pieces
   2 tablespoons shredded low-fat cheddar cheese
   1 Roma tomato, chopped

To prepare the dressing, in a small bowl mash the avocado with a fork, then stir in the chili powder, cumin, lime zest, lime juice, and yogurt.

Place a small skillet over medium-high heat. Coat both sides of the tortilla with cooking spray and sprinkle with an additional pinch of chili powder and cumin, if desired. Cook for 30 seconds on each side, until toasted. Remove from the pan and set aside to cool.

Brown the ground beef in the same skillet over medium-high heat. Add the chili powder, cumin, bell pepper, and the whites of the green onion, and sauté for 3 minutes, or until the veggies are soft.

In a large serving bowl, toss the lettuce with half of the dressing. Top with the meat mixture. Drizzle on the remaining dressing, and top with the cheese, tomatoes, and greens of the onion. Slice the tortillas into strips and sprinkle on top of the salad just before serving.

Nutrition Information per Serving

Calories: 371.4	*Sodium: 233.1 mg*	*Fiber: 9.5 g*
Fat: 13.8 g	*Carbs: 28.6 g*	*Protein: 36.0 g*
Cholesterol: 63.1 mg		

Simple Suppers

Alfredo Pasta with Broccoli

There's more than one way to replicate the creamy, rich texture and taste of heavy cream. In fact, it's entirely possible to create an "Alfredo" sauce that contains not one drop of it. I swap in fat-free evaporated milk and puréed white beans, then use plenty of real Parmesan cheese.

Prep Time: *5 minutes*
Cooking Time: *15 minutes*
Yield: *serves 4*
Serving Size: *2 cups*

> SPARK SWAPS TIPS

In place of the broccoli, you could use sautéed red bell peppers, asparagus, cauliflower, or a mix of Italian-style frozen vegetables.

What's the secret to getting your sauce to stick to your pasta? Reserve ½ cup of the pasta cooking water. The starches that the pasta has deposited in the water will help thicken any sauce, binding it to the pasta. Add the water 1 tablespoon at a time until you reach the desired consistency.

You can prep the broccoli and sauce ahead of time but don't prep the pasta until you're ready to eat or it will absorb all the liquid and become mushy.

6 ounces whole-wheat spaghetti

10 ounces frozen broccoli florets or 1 pound fresh broccoli, stem peeled and chopped, crowns broken into florets

½ cup canned cannellini (white kidney) beans, drained and rinsed*

¾ cup fat-free evaporated milk

1 teaspoon olive oil

2 cloves garlic, chopped

¼ teaspoon black pepper

½ cup shredded Parmesan cheese, divided

* If you can't find cannellini beans, use Great Northern or navy beans.

Cook the pasta according to package directions. If using frozen broccoli, add it to the pasta about halfway through the cooking process. If using fresh broccoli, add it to the pasta 1 minute before removing the pasta from the heat. Drain when ready.

While the pasta is cooking, purée the beans and milk in a blender until smooth.

Heat the olive oil in a large skillet set over medium heat, then sauté the garlic for 2 minutes. Add the bean and milk mixture to the skillet with 1/3 cup of the pasta cooking water. Whisk the sauce until it starts to bubble, then reduce the heat and simmer for 2 minutes. Add the pepper and ¼ cup of the Parmesan, and continue to simmer for another 2 minutes.

Add the drained pasta and broccoli to the skillet, stirring to coat with the sauce. Portion 2 cups of the pasta and broccoli onto each serving plate, and sprinkle with the remaining ¼ cup of the cheese. Serve immediately.

Nutrition Information per Serving

Calories: 292.1   Sodium: 259.1 mg   Fiber: 8.2 g

Fat: 6.0 g   Carbs: 47.1 g   Protein: 17.9 g

Cholesterol: 10.1 mg

Baked Macaroni and Cheese

You'll forget all about boxed and frozen macaroni and cheese when you taste this one. Full of real ingredients, it's rich and creamy with less than 400 calories a serving plus a whopping 6 grams of fiber and 23 grams of protein. Just as with our Alfredo sauce (Alfredo Pasta with Broccoli, page 193), we added cannellini (white kidney) beans, which have a creamy texture and buttery flavor, to help thicken the sauce and add nutrition. Sharp cheddar cheese offers strong flavor, so we could use less of it. If you prefer your macaroni and cheese with extra sauce, skip the oven and serve it from the stovetop.

Prep Time: *5 minutes*

Cooking Time: *30 minutes*

Yield: *serves 4*

Serving Size: *1½ cups*

> **SPARK SWAPS TIPS**

We used cannellini (white kidney) beans, but you could use any white bean in this recipe.

For a smoother sauce, purée the beans in a blender with 1 cup of the milk.

In dishes where cheese is an integral ingredient rather than a topping, it is that much more important to choose the highest quality you can find. Buy a block and grate it yourself for best flavor and results.

Panko are Japanese-style breadcrumbs. Available in regular and whole-wheat, they're larger and lighter than traditional breadcrumbs and perfect for faux frying or a fat-free crunchy topping added to casseroles like this one. If you can't find them, substitute regular whole-wheat breadcrumbs.

6 ounces whole-wheat elbow macaroni (about 1½ cups dry)

1 tablespoon unsalted butter

2 tablespoons finely chopped white or yellow onion

1 clove garlic, minced

1 tablespoon whole-wheat flour

½ cup canned cannellini (white kidney) beans, drained, rinsed, and mashed or puréed

2 cups skim milk

1 cup shredded low-fat sharp cheddar cheese

½ teaspoon Dijon mustard

¼ teaspoon hot sauce

4 slices Canadian bacon (about 2 ounces), chopped

¼ cup panko (Japanese-style breadcrumbs)

Preheat the oven to 350°F. Grease an 8 × 10-inch baking dish with cooking spray.

Cook the macaroni according to package directions. Drain when ready.

Meanwhile, in a medium saucepan melt the butter over medium heat. Sauté the onion and garlic until the onion is tender, about 2 minutes. Add the flour and stir constantly for 1 minute, until the flour is slightly browned. Stir in the mashed beans, then slowly whisk in the milk, increasing the heat to medium-high to bring the sauce to a boil. Reduce the heat to medium again and simmer until the sauce has thickened, about 3 minutes. Stir in the cheese, mustard, and hot sauce, and remove from heat.

Add the pasta, coating it fully in the sauce, then pour the mixture into the prepared baking dish. Sprinkle with the Canadian bacon and panko, then spritz the top with cooking spray. Bake for 20 minutes, or until the cheese bubbles.

Nutrition Information per Serving

Calories: 343.8	*Sodium: 522.3 mg*	*Fiber: 5.8 g*
Fat: 7.1 g	*Carbs: 48.7 g*	*Protein: 22.5 g*
Cholesterol: 24.4 mg		

Carolina-Style Barbecue Chicken

Barbecue sauces are like snowflakes; no two are alike (though plenty of regions are known for their certain type of sauce). This version is less like the sweet, tomato-based variety that's become the most common. Rather, this sauce is based on recipes from North Carolina, with vinegar and mustard, which offer a tangy contrast to the rich meat. Brown sugar balances out the acid.

Dark meat, while higher in calories and fat than light meat, does have a place in a healthy diet. In fact, you get twice as much iron, zinc, and thiamine when choosing dark over white. Plus, the added fat keeps the meat extra juicy and tasty, so go ahead and choose chicken thighs from time to time, as long as you remove the skin and keep portions in check.

Prep Time: *5 minutes*
Cooking Time: *30 minutes*
Yield: *serves 4*
Serving Size: *2 thighs*

> SPARK SWAPS TIPS

This sauce gets quite sticky, so the foil saves you some cleanup time.

Sauce
3 tablespoons prepared yellow mustard
1 teaspoon Worcestershire sauce
2 packed teaspoons brown sugar
2 tablespoons red wine vinegar
2 cloves garlic, minced
Pinch of paprika

1½ pounds boneless, skinless chicken thighs (8 thighs)

Preheat the oven to 400°F. Line a baking sheet with aluminum foil, then coat it with cooking spray.

In a medium bowl, combine the sauce ingredients—the mustard, Worcestershire sauce, brown sugar, vinegar, garlic, and paprika—then add the chicken and stir until each thigh is thoroughly coated. Use tongs to transfer the chicken to the prepared baking sheet, leaving room between each piece. Bake for 30

minutes, or until the internal temperature reaches 180°F using a quick-read thermometer and the juices run clear.

Nutrition Information per Serving

Calories: 201.5   *Sodium: 256.7 mg*   *Fiber: 0.4 g*

Fat: 5.8 g   *Carbs: 3.7 g*   *Protein: 27.7 g*

Cholesterol: 114.5 mg

Dijon-Herb Pork Tenderloin

If you're intimidated by large cuts of meat, pork tenderloin is a good place to start. This lean protein cooks fast enough for a weeknight meal, and you can use the leftovers for lunches and quick dinners.

Prep Time: *5 minutes*
Cooking Time: *30 minutes*
Yield: *serves 4*
Serving Size: *3 ounces cooked pork*

> SPARK SWAPS TIPS

Searing the meat in a hot pan before finishing it in the oven will not only create a nicely browned exterior but also lock in moisture.

1 pound pork tenderloin, trimmed of any fat or silver skin*
2 teaspoons chopped fresh thyme
2 cloves garlic, chopped
½ teaspoon Dijon mustard
1 teaspoon olive oil
¼ teaspoon black pepper

* Silver skin is the shiny tendon that runs the length of the muscle in the pork tenderloin. It will not break down during cooking. To remove it, run the tip of a small knife along both sides of the tendon.

Preheat the oven to 375°F.

In a small bowl, combine the thyme, garlic, mustard, and olive oil.

Pat the meat dry with paper towels. Rub the meat with black pepper and coat it with cooking spray. Heat a large oven-safe skillet over medium-high heat, and sear the meat on the top and bottom, about 4 minutes per side. Spread the herb sauce over the pork and transfer the skillet to the oven. Roast for 20 minutes, or until the internal temperature reaches 145°F using a quick-read thermometer. Allow the meat to rest for 3 to 4 minutes before slicing it into thin strips and serving.

Nutrition Information per Serving

Calories: 199.4   *Sodium: 78.8 mg*   *Fiber: 0.1 g*

Fat: 6.6 g   *Carbs: 0.7 g*   *Protein: 32.0 g*

Cholesterol: 89.5 mg

Inside-Out Burgers

Lean beef can dry out easily, and it lacks the flavor of fatter cuts. So how do you create a burger you'll crave? You fill it with the good stuff. My son Ian specializes in "Juicy Lucys." He puts onions, mushrooms, peppers, and cheese inside a serving of extra-lean turkey or beef and grills it. The result? A burger that will satisfy even teenage boys. This version is slightly more sophisticated but just as simple. The balsamic vinegar and thyme add great flavor, and you'll find that you need little more than juicy tomatoes, crisp lettuce, and perhaps a smear of good quality mustard (or a squirt of ketchup).

Prep Time: *5 minutes*

Cooking Time: *10 minutes*

Yield: *serves 4*

Serving Size: *1 burger*

> SPARK SWAPS TIPS

To change up your burgers, use ¼ cup sautéed mushrooms with chopped fresh rosemary or fresh basil and chopped red bell pepper. You could also use 2 tablespoons shredded cheese.

1 pound 96 percent lean ground beef

1 teaspoon black pepper

1 small white or yellow onion, cut into four slices

1 teaspoon fresh thyme
2 teaspoons balsamic vinegar
4 whole-wheat Sandwich Thins, toasted
1 large tomato (3-inch diameter), cut into four slices
4 large lettuce leaves

Preheat an outdoor grill to 400°F or a skillet over medium heat.

Divide the beef into four equal portions, then flatten each into a 5-inch burger patty. Sprinkle the patties with black pepper, then top each with an onion slice, thyme, and vinegar. Fold up the sides of each patty, sealing the toppings inside.

Place the patties on the grill, or in the skillet, and cook 4 to 5 minutes per side, until the internal temperature reaches 160°F using a quick-read thermometer. Serve each burger on a Sandwich Thin with a slice of tomato and a leaf of lettuce.

Nutrition Information per Serving

Calories: 261.8	*Sodium: 324.9 mg*	*Fiber: 6.1 g*
Fat: 5.7 g	*Carbs: 25.7 g*	*Protein: 29.9 g*
Cholesterol: 60.0 mg		

Meg's Pan-Fried Chicken

The appeal of fried chicken is the crunch when you bite down on that crust into the moist meat inside. I ditched most of the fat and relied on herbs and spices for flavor. The Southern gal in me is proud of this recipe. You'll think you're on a screened-in porch with the colonel as your host when you bite into this pan-fried chicken. I'm from Kentucky, so I suppose we could call this dish Kentucky Pan-Fried Chicken.

Prep Time: *5 minutes*
Cooking Time: *15 minutes*
Yield: *serves 4*
Serving Size: *3 ounces cooked chicken*

> SPARK SWAPS TIPS

You'll want to prep the chicken in two batches to ensure a crunchy crust. Crowding all four pieces into the pan at once or breading them all and letting them sit will yield a soggy coating.

Why are we baking pan-fried chicken? We used a hot skillet to get a crispy coating on the meat, but if we kept the meat on the stovetop, the crust would burn before the inside reached a safe temperature. Finishing the dish in the oven yields perfect results every time.

We also love this meal as a biscuit sandwich. Split a biscuit, then top it with the chicken and slaw.

4 4-ounce chicken breasts, skin and fat removed
1 tablespoon whole-wheat flour
1 egg white, beaten until foamy
½ cup panko (Japanese-style breadcrumbs)*
1 teaspoon dried thyme
½ teaspoon sweet paprika
½ teaspoon onion powder
2 teaspoons olive oil

* Use whole-wheat breadcrumbs if you can't find panko.

Preheat the oven to 375°F. Coat a 9 × 13-inch baking dish with cooking spray.

Line up three flat dishes as a breading station. The first dish should hold the flour and the second the beaten egg white. In the third, combine the panko, thyme, paprika, and onion powder.

Coat a large skillet with cooking spray and place it over medium-high heat. Add 1 teaspoon of the olive oil.

Prep the chicken in two batches. Pat each piece of chicken dry with paper towels.

Dredge two pieces of chicken in the flour, then dip them in the egg white, and coat them with the breadcrumbs. Add them to the hot skillet and cook for 3 minutes per side, then transfer them to the baking dish.

Add the remaining teaspoon of oil to the skillet for the second batch. Repeat the breading and pan-frying process with the other two chicken breasts, then bake them in the preheated oven for 7 to 8 minutes, or until the meat is no

longer pink and reaches an internal temperature of 165°F using a quick-read thermometer.

Nutrition Information per Serving

Calories: 170.5	*Sodium: 87.8 mg*	*Fiber: 1.0 g*
Fat: 3.9 g	*Carbs: 4.6 g*	*Protein: 28.0 g*
Cholesterol: 65.7 mg		

One-Dish Dinner: Roasted Chicken and Vegetables

Roasted chicken and vegetables is so simple and comforting, but it's not exactly a quick-cooking meal. Rather than roast a whole chicken, we cooked a bone-in chicken breast, which we cooked in the same pot as the veggies. The chicken flavors the veggies, the veggies keep the chicken moist, and the whole meal is ready in under an hour.

Prep Time: *10 minutes*
Cooking Time: *45 minutes*
Yield: *serves 4*
Serving Size: *3 to 4 ounces cooked chicken, 2 cups vegetables, and 1 tablespoon sauce*

> SPARK SWAPS TIPS

This dish is supposed to have a rustic feel, so keep the veggies in large but similar-size pieces. You don't even need to cut the baby carrots.

4 split, bone-in, skinless chicken breasts (about 1½ pounds)
2 teaspoons canola oil
1 large white or yellow onion, roughly chopped (about 1 cup)
3 stalks celery, roughly chopped (about 1½ cups)
8 ounces baby carrots (about 1¾ cups)
1 pound waxy potatoes, such as Yukon Gold, quartered
    (about 4 medium)
4 sprigs fresh thyme
1 sprig fresh sage
1 bay leaf
¾ to 1 cup homemade or low-sodium chicken stock*

½ lemon, cut into wedges
2 teaspoons cornstarch

* The amount of stock you need will depend on the size of your chicken and your pot. You want enough stock to cover about half of the chicken.

Preheat the oven to 300°F.

Heat the oil in a Dutch oven set over medium heat. Add the chicken breasts, bone side up, and cook for 5 minutes to brown the flesh. Then move the chicken to one side of the pot, and add the onion, celery, and carrots to the other side. Cook for about 3 more minutes. Add the potatoes, thyme, sage, bay leaf, and stock. Keeping the bone side facing up, place the chicken on top of the vegetables. Turn the heat to medium-high, bring the mixture to a simmer, then remove the pot from heat. Add the lemon wedges, cover, and bake in the preheated oven for 30 minutes, or until the internal temperature reaches 165°F using a quick-read thermometer.

Transfer the chicken and veggies to another dish. Place the pot over high heat, and bring the leftover cooking juices to a simmer.

Meanwhile, in a small dish dilute the cornstarch with 2 teaspoons of cold water. Whisk the cornstarch mixture into the cooking liquid, and simmer for 2 minutes, until the sauce has thickened. Discard the herbs.

Carve the chicken into four equal portions and divide among four plates. Add 2 cups of vegetables to each plate. Serve immediately, with the extra sauce in a separate dish on the table.

Nutrition Information per Serving

Calories: 360.8	*Sodium: 151.1 mg*	*Fiber: 8.2 g*
Fat: 4.1 g	*Carbs: 49.7 g*	*Protein: 32.4 g*
Cholesterol: 65.7 mg		

One-Dish Dinner: Southwestern Chicken and Rice

This dish is a staple at Becky's house. In addition to being quite delicious, it's budget-friendly and easy to adapt. Simply swap in a different variety of salsa

and you have a whole new dish. Plus, it's easy enough for teens to make, and cleanup is a breeze since you've dirtied only one pan.

Prep Time: *5 minutes*
Cooking Time: *20 minutes*
Yield: *serves 6*
Serving Size: *1 cup*

> SPARK SWAPS TIPS

Add fresh or frozen spinach to the pan for an extra serving of veggies.

Turn leftovers into a second meal: add them to an omelet or use them as a burrito filling.

1 pound boneless, skinless chicken breasts, cut into bite-size pieces
1 teaspoon chili powder
1 teaspoon ground cumin
1½ cups low-sodium salsa
2 cups frozen corn kernels
1 15-ounce can low-sodium black beans, drained and rinsed
1½ cups uncooked instant brown rice
6 tablespoons shredded low-fat cheddar cheese
6 tablespoons low-fat sour cream or fat-free plain Greek yogurt

Coat a large skillet with cooking spray and place it over medium-high heat. Cook the chicken with the chili powder and cumin, stirring often, until it's lightly browned, about 3 to 5 minutes. Stir in the salsa, corn, beans, and rice. Add 2 cups of water, stir to combine, and bring the mixture to a boil. Then reduce the heat and simmer, covered, until the rice is tender, about 15 minutes.

Portion into serving bowls. Garnish each serving with 1 tablespoon of the cheese and 1 tablespoon of the sour cream or yogurt.

Nutrition Information per Serving

Calories: 301.2	*Sodium: 447.4 mg*	*Fiber: 7.4 g*
Fat: 4.4 g	*Carbs: 43.5 g*	*Protein: 28.4 g*
Cholesterol: 51.2 mg		

Panko-Breaded Fish with Tomato Salad

Believe it or not, fish sticks were the inspiration for this dish. We kept the crunchy crust, skipped the deep fryer, and instead of tartar sauce, we added capers, parsley, and lemon juice. Cherry tomatoes cooked in the same pan become a tangy, sweet side. Use any mild white-fleshed fish; we used perch, but sole or tilapia would also work well.

Prep Time: *10 minutes*
Cooking Time: *7 minutes*
Yield: *serves 4*
Serving Size: *3 ounces cooked fish with ½ cup tomato salad*

> SPARK SWAPS TIPS

Want an extra serving of vegetables? After cooking the tomatoes, sauté 4 cups fresh spinach in the same pan until just wilted. Serve the fish on top of the cooked greens.

**1 pound white-fleshed fish fillets, skin removed, cut into four
    equal portions**
1 tablespoon whole-wheat flour
¼ teaspoon black pepper
1 egg white, beaten until foamy
½ cup panko (Japanese-style breadcrumbs)*
2 teaspoons olive oil
**1 pint (about 2 cups) grape or cherry tomatoes, halved or
    quartered**
1 tablespoon capers, drained and rinsed
1 tablespoon lemon juice
½ bunch parsley, leaves only, chopped (about ¾ cup)

* Use whole-wheat breadcrumbs if you can't find panko.

Set up a breading station. Line up three flat-bottomed dishes or pie plates. Combine the flour and pepper in the first, place the egg white in the second, and the panko in the third.

While you heat the oil in a large skillet over high heat, pat the fish dry with a paper towel. Dip each piece of fish into the flour, then into the egg white, and

finally into the panko. Cook the fish in the skillet 2 minutes per side, then trans-
fer to a serving platter.

Add the tomatoes and capers to the still-hot pan and toss for 30 seconds, then
drizzle the lemon juice over the tomatoes, add the parsley, and stir to com-
bine. Pour the tomato mixture over the fish and serve immediately.

Nutrition Information per Serving

Calories: 153.6　　　*Sodium: 170.3 mg*　　　*Fiber: 0.9 g*
Fat: 4.9 g　　　*Carbs: 9.3 g*　　　*Protein: 18.5 g*
Cholesterol: 51.0 mg

Quick Chicken Enchiladas

My traditional enchilada recipe takes over an hour to prepare. This version
gets some help from the supermarket and uses leftovers to cut the cooking
time by two-thirds, with only ten minutes of hands-on work.

Prep Time: *10 minutes*
Cooking Time: *15 minutes*
Yield: *serves 4*
Serving Size: *2 enchiladas*

> SPARK SWAPS TIPS

When you start to control portions, how and where you use high-calorie ingredients becomes
that much more important. Rather than bury the cheese in the enchiladas, where its texture
and flavor will compete with the veggies and chicken, we put it on top so you can taste every
gooey bite.

Want more spice? Use pepper jack cheese.

2 cups (about 6 ounces) chopped fresh spinach
12 ounces cooked chicken breast, shredded or diced
½ cup canned cannellini (white kidney) beans, drained and
　　rinsed*
½ teaspoon ground cumin
¼ teaspoon chili powder

1½ cups low-sodium salsa
4 tablespoons chopped fresh cilantro
3 cloves garlic, smashed and chopped
1 large red onion, chopped (about 1 cup)
1 bell pepper, chopped (about 1 cup)
8 6-inch corn tortillas
½ cup shredded low-fat Monterey jack cheese
Zest and juice of 1 lime

* If you can't find cannellini beans, use Great Northern or navy beans.

Preheat the oven to 350°F. Coat a 9 × 12-inch baking dish with cooking spray.

In a medium microwave-safe bowl, microwave the spinach on high for 2 minutes, until wilted. Remove and wring out the spinach in a double layer of paper towels to remove excess moisture. Return the spinach to the bowl, and combine it with the chicken, beans, cumin, chili powder, ¼ cup of the salsa, and 3 tablespoons of the cilantro.

In a blender or small food processor, purée the garlic, onion, bell pepper, and remaining 1¼ cup of salsa.

Soften the tortillas by microwaving them on high for 30 seconds, then place them on a cutting board. Fill each with ½ cup of the chicken mixture. Roll up and place each in the baking dish, seam side down, repeating with all the tortillas. Spoon the puréed salsa over the enchiladas and cover with foil. Bake in the preheated oven for 10 minutes. Remove the foil, and sprinkle on the cheese. Bake another 5 to 10 minutes, uncovered, or until the cheese melts.

Sprinkle over the top the remaining cilantro, lime zest, and lime juice. Eat immediately or allow to cool completely and store in airtight containers.

Nutrition Information per Serving

Calories: 349.7	Sodium: 663.7 mg	Fiber: 7.9 g
Fat: 4.4 g	Carbs: 42.2 g	Protein: 37.1 g
Cholesterol: 68.7 mg		

Slow-Cooker Buffalo Chicken Casserole

Even buffalo wings have a place in our plan, with a few tweaks. We ditched the actual wings in lieu of lean chicken breast. We kept the heat, cut sodium by adding spices as well as hot sauce, and topped it with tangy blue cheese. We even kept the carrots and celery you might have with wings, but we added them to the main dish. To save time, we turned to the slow cooker. This meal is perfect for tailgating, potlucks, and busy weeknights.

> **Prep Time:** *10 minutes*
> **Cooking Time:** *6 hours*
> **Yield:** *serves 4*
> **Serving Size:** *2 cups*

> SPARK SWAPS TIPS

Hot sauce is packed full of salt. We chose to use spices to add flavor, then added a bit of hot sauce for tang.

1 pound boneless, skinless chicken breast, diced
1 white or yellow onion, diced (about 1 cup)
2 stalks celery, diced (about ½ cup)
1 medium carrot, diced (about ½ cup)
1 hot pepper, deseeded and mInced*
1 15-ounce can unsalted diced tomatoes (about 1½ cups)
2 cloves garlic, sliced
½ teaspoon hot or smoked paprika
¼ teaspoon cayenne pepper
2½ cups homemade or low-sodium chicken stock
2 cups instant brown rice
1 tablespoon hot sauce
¼ cup fat-free plain Greek yogurt
¼ cup crumbled blue cheese, for garnish

* Choose a pepper that's right for your heat preference. An Anaheim pepper is mild and that's what I used in this recipe.

In a slow cooker, stir together the chicken, onion, celery, carrot, hot pepper, tomatoes, garlic, paprika, cayenne, and chicken stock. Cover and cook on high for 3 hours or on low for 6 hours.

About 30 minutes before serving, remove the slow-cooker lid, stir in the rice, and cover.

Just before serving, in a small bowl stir the hot sauce and Greek yogurt into ½ cup of the hot casserole, then incorporate the casserole-yogurt mixture into the rest of the slow-cooker mixture. (This step prevents the yogurt from curdling.)

Top each portion with 1 tablespoon blue cheese before serving.

Nutrition Information per Serving

Calories: 351.2	*Sodium: 243.4 mg*	*Fiber: 4.4 g*
Fat: 5.2 g	*Carbs: 38.3 g*	*Protein: 35.9 g*
Cholesterol: 72.1 mg		

Slow-Cooker Veggie Lasagna

This dish is perfect for busy families. Make the dish the night before and store in the fridge. Have the kids put it in the slow cooker when they get home from school. On nights when you have a late game, a session with your trainer, or parent–teacher conferences, this veggie-filled dish is a lifesaver.

Prep Time: *10 minutes*
Cooking Time: *4½ hours*
Yield: *serves 4*
Serving Size: *about ½ cup*

> SPARK SWAPS TIPS

For more flavor, choose baby bella mushrooms.

Pressing the tofu will prevent your lasagna from getting too soggy. Place the tofu in a lint-free kitchen towel and squeeze out any excess water. The tofu will be mashed in the lasagna, so you don't need to worry if you smash it slightly beforehand.

1 large white or yellow onion, chopped (about 1 cup)
4 ounces mushrooms, quartered (1½ cups)
1 small eggplant, unpeeled and diced (about 8 ounces)
1 teaspoon salt-free Italian seasoning
**5 ounces (⅓ block) extra-firm tofu, drained, pressed, and
    mashed**

¼ cup shredded Parmesan cheese
⅓ bunch parsley, leaves only, chopped (about ½ cup)
2 cups no-salt-added pasta sauce
4 no-boil lasagna noodles, 2 broken in half
¼ cup shredded low-fat mozzarella cheese

Coat the insert of a slow cooker with cooking spray.

Heat a large skillet over high heat. Then remove it from heat and also coat it with cooking spray, before returning it to the heat. Sauté the onion, mushrooms, and eggplant until soft, about 4 or 5 minutes. Stir in the Italian seasoning, and remove the skillet from heat. Set aside.

In a small bowl, combine the tofu, Parmesan, and parsley. Set aside.

To assemble the lasagna, layer as follows: Pour ⅔ cup pasta sauce in the bottom of the slow cooker insert. Top with a third of the cooked vegetables and half of the tofu mixture. Place one whole uncooked noodle along the center, then place the two broken halves along either side of that. Ladle on another ⅔ cup pasta sauce, a third of the cooked vegetables, and the remaining tofu mixture and noodles. Add the remaining cooked vegetables and sauce, then top with the mozzarella. Cover with the lid, and slow cook on high for 3 hours.

Nutrition Information per Serving

Calories: 298.9	*Sodium: 307.4 mg*	*Fiber: 5.9 g*
Fat: 8.9 g	*Carbs: 41.9 g*	*Protein: 18.0 g*
Cholesterol: 7.7 mg		

Speedy Turkey Chili

Most quick chili recipes involve dumping cans and vegetables into a pot, simmering, and serving. The result can be a bit flat. With a few small tweaks, we created a twenty-minute chili that tastes like it simmered for hours. We sautéed the veggies, used red onion and a chili pepper for extra punch, and cooked the spices to maximize their impact. By puréeing half of the beans and tomatoes, we were able to thicken the chili without making you wait for dinner.

The problem with most quick chili recipes is that you lose the depth of flavor with the reduced cooking time. I swapped out traditional white onion for red to bring a sharp note, used a red chili pepper instead of a red bell pepper to give a "bite" to the dish, and threw in the technique of cooking the spices before adding the liquid. Chili in a flash.

Prep Time: *5 minutes*
Cooking Time: *20 minutes*
Yield: *serves 4*
Serving Size: *1½ cups*

> SPARK SWAPS TIPS

When foods are piping hot, the flavors dull slightly. Let the chili cool for a few minutes to allow the flavors to really shine. This soup freezes well, and it also gets better if you eat it the next day.

If you don't like the texture of beans, purée them all.

    1 15-ounce can low-sodium red or black beans, drained and rinsed
    1 15-ounce can no-salt-added diced tomatoes
    1 teaspoon vegetable oil
    8 ounces extra-lean ground turkey breast
    1 large red onion, chopped (about 1 cup)
    1 red Anaheim pepper*
    2 cloves garlic, sliced
    2 medium carrots, grated (about 1 cup)
    1 tablespoon dark chili powder
    1 teaspoon cumin seed

Toppings
    ½ avocado, diced
    ¼ cup fat-free plain Greek yogurt
    ¼ cup shredded low-fat cheddar cheese
    Hot sauce (optional)

* Also called California red chili peppers, Anaheim peppers are commonly used in New Mexican cooking. Though spicier than a bell pepper, these peppers are milder than a jalapeño. If you can't find them, swap in a poblano pepper.

If you prefer spicier chili, leave the seeds in the pepper. Otherwise, remove them using the back of a teaspoon.

In a blender or food processor, purée half of the beans and all of the tomatoes.

Heat the oil in a Dutch oven or large saucepan set over medium heat. Sauté the turkey, onion, pepper, and garlic for about 3 minutes, stirring often to break up the turkey meat. When the turkey is no longer pink, add the carrots, chili powder, and cumin seed, and cook another 3 minutes, or until the spices are fragrant and the carrots are soft. Add the puréed beans and tomatoes and remaining whole beans, along with 2 cups of water. Increase the heat to high, bring the pot to a boil, then lower to medium and simmer for 15 minutes.

Ladle 1½ cups into each serving bowl and allow to cool for a few minutes. Top with the avocado and 1 tablespoon each of the yogurt and the cheese. Sprinkle with hot sauce, if desired.

Nutrition Information per Serving

Calories: 334.9	*Sodium: 371.1 mg*	*Fiber: 10.2 g*
Fat: 8.1 g	*Carbs: 41.5 g*	*Protein: 26.4 g*
Cholesterol: 36.5 mg		

Sweet-and-Spicy Glazed Salmon

Barbecue sauce is one of the easiest ways to add flavor to any protein, but most bottled varieties are loaded with sugar. This sauce melds Asian flavors with those of the American South for a sauce that's well balanced between sweet and spicy. We used it on salmon, but you could also use it on chicken or firm tofu.

Prep Time: *5 minutes*
Cooking Time: *7 minutes*
Yield: *serves 4*
Serving Size: *3 ounces cooked salmon*

> SPARK SWAPS TIPS

Salmon often has pin bones that run down the center of the fish. To remove them, place the fish skin side down and use a pair of clean tweezers or needle-nose pliers to remove them. You can also ask to have them removed before you buy your fish.

You can use either fresh or frozen (thawed) salmon in this recipe.

Sauce

1 packed tablespoon brown sugar

1 teaspoon chili powder

Pinch of black pepper

½ teaspoon Sriracha (Thai chili sauce)

½ teaspoon grated fresh gingerroot

1 tablespoon all-fruit orange marmalade

1 pound salmon fillet, skin removed, cut into 4 equal pieces

In a small bowl, combine all the sauce ingredients—the brown sugar, chili powder, black pepper, Sriracha, ginger, and marmalade—and set aside.

Place a nonstick or cast-iron skillet over medium-high heat. Coat both sides of the fish with cooking spray and spread half of the sauce on the top side of the fillets. Place the fillets, sauced side up, in the skillet. Cook about 2 minutes. Flip and spread the rest of the sauce on the other side. Cook another 2 to 3 minutes, until the flesh feels firm.

Nutrition Information per Serving

Calories: 178.4	*Sodium: 65.4 mg*	*Fiber: 0.3 g*
Fat: 7.0 g	*Carbs: 6.9 g*	*Protein: 21.7 g*
Cholesterol: 60.4 mg		

Thai Peanut Noodles

Who needs takeout when you can make a huge noodle bowl loaded with veggies and tangy peanut sauce in only twenty minutes? If you're short on time, swap in a bag of frozen stir-fry veggies.

Prep Time: *10 minutes*

Cooking Time: *20 minutes*

Yield: *serves 4*

Serving Size: *2 heaping cups*

> SPARK SWAPS TIPS

Serrano chilies are hotter than jalapeños but nowhere near as hot as a habanero. If you like heat, keep the innards in the pepper; if you don't, opt for a deseeded jalapeño or omit it.

To safely remove the seeds, cut the chili in half and scrape them out, along with the pithy veins, using a small spoon. Never use your fingers: the oil lingers and can burn your eyes and mouth.

8 ounces whole-wheat spaghetti or angel-hair pasta

Sauce

4 tablespoons natural unsalted peanut butter

4 cloves garlic, smashed and chopped

1 serrano chili, deseeded and chopped

2 packed tablespoons brown sugar

Zest and juice of 2 limes (about ¼ cup juice)

2 teaspoons low-sodium soy sauce

1 teaspoon yellow curry powder

½ head bok choy

1 medium white or yellow onion, sliced into strips (about ½ cup)

1 cup grated carrots

1 bell pepper, sliced into strips (about 1 cup)

2 tablespoons chopped dry-roasted unsalted peanuts

Chopped fresh cilantro or basil (optional)

Bring a large saucepan of water to a boil, break the pasta in half, and cook according to package directions. Drain when ready, but reserve ¼ cup of the pasta cooking water. Set aside.

Meanwhile, prepare the sauce. Using a fork, in a medium bowl whisk together the peanut butter with ⅓ cup of hot tap water until smooth, then add the remaining sauce ingredients to the bowl—the garlic, serrano chili, brown sugar, lime zest, lime juice, soy sauce, and curry powder—and stir to combine. Set aside.

Cut the bottom 2 inches off the head of bok choy. Finely chop the green tops and slice the stalks into bite-size pieces.

Coat a wok or your largest skillet with cooking spray and place it over high heat. Sauté the onion and carrots for 2 minutes, then add the tops and stalks

of the bok choy and the bell pepper and sauté for 3 more minutes. Add the reserved ¼ cup of pasta water to the vegetables.

Add the drained pasta along with the sauce to the skillet. Stir to combine and cook until the sauce is heated through, about 2 minutes.

Divide the mixture between four serving plates and sprinkle with the peanuts and optional chopped herbs.

This dish can also be prepared a day in advance and stored in the refrigerator. If you're serving this dish cold, reserve half of the sauce and dress it just before eating.

Nutrition Information per Serving

Calories: 391.5	Sodium: 90.3 mg	Fiber: 10.0 g
Fat: 11.8 g	Carbs: 63.3 g	Protein: 15.4 g
Cholesterol: 0.0 mg		

Twenty-Minute Fish Tacos with Homemade Pico de Gallo

Give ground beef the night off, and lighten up your tacos. Choose any white-fleshed fish for this recipe. I like cod but pollock, flounder, or tilapia are good too. Served with a fresh tomato salsa and creamy avocado, these tacos are ready in twenty minutes.

Prep Time: 10 minutes
Cooking Time: 10 minutes
Yield: serves 4
Serving Size: 2 tortillas, ¼ cup pico de gallo, and 1½ ounces fish

> SPARK SWAPS TIPS

The pico de gallo can be made ahead of time, and it will keep up to four days in the fridge.

If tomatoes are out of season, use canned petite diced tomatoes (no salt added, of course). Drain them to avoid soggy salsa.

You can also turn this recipe into a taco salad.

Fish and seafood, unlike meat, can only be marinated for a short time—never more than 20 minutes. Due to the lack of connective tissue in the flesh, fish and seafood can actually cook in acidic marinades if left for too long (e.g., ceviche).

Marinade
> 2 teaspoons olive oil
> ½ teaspoon dark chili powder
> Zest and juice of 2 limes

> 1 pound cod, cut into four equal portions

Pico de Gallo
> 1 large white or yellow onion, finely chopped (about ¾ cup)
> 1 tablespoon red wine vinegar
> ½ teaspoon sugar
> 2 pounds tomatoes, chopped with juice and seeds (about 3 cups)
> ¼ cup chopped fresh cilantro, leaves only
> 1 banana pepper, deseeded and chopped
> ¼ teaspoon black pepper
> ⅛ teaspoon salt

> 8 6-inch corn tortillas
> 1 avocado, diced

Prepare the marinade in a pie plate or flat dish, whisking together the olive oil, chili powder, lime zest, and lime juice. Set the fish in the marinade, flipping to coat both sides. Cover and refrigerate.

Meanwhile, make the pico de gallo. In a medium bowl, combine the onion, vinegar, and sugar, stirring well, then add the tomatoes, cilantro, and banana pepper. Season with salt and pepper.

Place a nonstick skillet over medium heat. Coat both sides of each tortilla with cooking spray. Heat each one for 30 seconds until slightly toasted, flip, and cook another 30 seconds. Set all of them aside on a plate or serving platter.

Remove the pan from heat, generously coat it with more cooking spray, and return it to medium heat. Remove the fish from the refrigerator, and cook each piece of the fish for 4 minutes, then flip and cook an additional 2 minutes, until the flesh is opaque and easily flakes. Remove from heat, and flake the fish with a fork.

Fill each tortilla with ¼ cup pico de gallo and 2 ounces of fish. Top with the avocado, and serve with additional pico de gallo.

For Chicken Tacos: Marinate 1 pound boneless, skinless chicken breasts up to overnight.

For Bean Tacos: Mix 2 14.5-ounce cans drained and rinsed black or pinto beans with the marinade and heat in a small skillet or in a microwave-safe bowl. Mash half of the beans and mix, for a chunky texture.

Nutrition Information per Serving

Calories: 346.0	*Sodium: 179.6 mg*	*Fiber: 8.6 g*
Fat: 12.3 g	*Carbs: 37.2 g*	*Protein: 25.6 g*
Cholesterol: 49.3 mg		

Splendid Sides

Baked Garlic-Herb Fries

Fingerling potatoes are perfect for oven fries. They cook up quickly and get a nice brown color in the oven. You can alternately use any waxy variety of potato, such as red-skin, Yukon Gold, or new potatoes.

Prep Time: *3 minutes*
Cooking Time: *20 minutes*
Yield: *serves 4*
Serving Size: *½ cup*

> SPARK SWAPS TIPS

To strip herbs from their stems, hold the bottom of the stem and pull your fingers firmly upward. The leaves will come off easily.

Don't throw away the herb stems. Place them in the dish to impart extra flavor.

1 pound fingerling potatoes (about 12), thinly sliced
2 cloves garlic, sliced
1 teaspoon minced fresh rosemary
1 teaspoon fresh thyme leaves

Preheat the oven to 400°F. Coat a 9 × 13-inch glass baking dish with cooking spray.

Toss all the ingredients together in the dish and spread the potatoes in a single layer. Coat the tops of the potatoes with a layer of cooking spray and bake for 20 minutes.

Nutrition Information per Serving

Calories: 112.7	*Sodium: 0.3 mg*	*Fiber: 2.1 g*
Fat: 0.5 g	*Carbs: 26.6 g*	*Protein: 3.1 g*
Cholesterol: 0.0 mg		

Better "Buttermilk" Biscuits

Okay, you caught me. There's no actual buttermilk in this recipe. That's because I knew that most of you wouldn't have any on hand. You can make a buttermilk substitute by combining skim milk and lemon juice or white vinegar, items you're more likely to have and use regularly.

This Southern staple gets a dose of fiber, and has half the fat of the original. Make a double batch over a weekend and freeze for the busy weekday mornings. We used them with Slim Sausage Gravy (page 166) and Meg's Pan-Fried Chicken (page 200).

Prep Time: *15 minutes*
Cooking Time: *15 minutes*
Yield: *serves 6*
Serving Size: *1 biscuit*

> SPARK SWAPS TIPS
For a shiny top, brush the muffins with milk before baking.

½ **cup skim milk**
1½ **teaspoons lemon juice or white vinegar**
1 **cup whole-wheat flour**
½ **teaspoon sugar**
1 **teaspoon baking powder**
¼ **teaspoon baking soda**

Pinch of salt
2 tablespoons cold unsalted butter, diced

Mix the milk with the lemon juice or vinegar. Set aside for 5 to 10 minutes.

Preheat the oven to 400°F. Coat a baking sheet with cooking spray or line it with a silicone baking mat.

In a large mixing bowl, combine the flour, sugar, baking powder, baking soda, and salt. Work the butter into the dry ingredients using a pastry cutter or two forks. Add the milk mixture and stir until just combined.

On a lightly floured cutting board, roll out the dough, gently patting it into a flat 4-inch circle, 1 inch thick. Using a 2-inch circle cookie cutter, or the rim of a glass, cut the dough into four circles. Gather and roll out the remaining dough, and cut out two final biscuits.

Bake the biscuits on the prepared baking sheet for 14 to 15 minutes, or until lightly browned on the bottom. Serve warm, or allow to cool before freezing and reheat in a toaster oven until just warmed.

Nutrition Information per Serving

Calories: 108.0	*Sodium: 67.7 mg*	*Fiber: 2.4 g*
Fat: 4.2 g	*Carbs: 15.8 g*	*Protein: 3.2 g*
Cholesterol: 10.6 mg		

Creamy Herb Pesto

Traditional pesto contains loads of oil and nuts to bind the herbs and cheese; this one uses Greek yogurt instead, with a bit of olive oil and toasted almonds for flavor. Ready in ten minutes, with no cooking required, this fresh take on pesto is perfect over angel-hair pasta, grilled fish, or simple steamed or grilled vegetables. You can also spread it on a sandwich or use it as a dip for crudités.

Prep Time: *10 minutes*
Yield: *serves 4*
Serving Size: *¼ cup*

> SPARK SWAPS TIPS

You can use a blender, but start by adding the wet ingredients, plus add a couple tablespoons of water to loosen the mixture, if needed.

2 cups fresh parsley or basil, leaves only (about 2 ounces)
1 cup (about 3 ounces) fresh arugula or spinach
2 tablespoons fresh thyme, or 1 tablespoon dried thyme
4 green onions, chopped
2 cloves garlic
2 tablespoons sliced almonds, toasted in a dry pan until just fragrant
2 teaspoons tomato paste*
2 tablespoons fat-free plain Greek yogurt
1 tablespoon olive oil
1 tablespoon shredded Parmesan cheese

Or 2 sun-dried tomatoes, soaked in hot water for 5 minutes

In a food processor, pulse all the ingredients several times to combine, then purée until smooth. Cover and refrigerate until ready to eat. The pesto will keep in the fridge up to two days or frozen for up to three months.

Nutrition Information per Serving

Calories: 100.8	Sodium: 60.4 mg	Fiber: 2.4 g
Fat: 6.4 g	Carbs: 6.1 g	Protein: 4.6 g
Cholesterol: 0.8 mg		

Creamy Roasted Red Pepper Pasta Sauce

Pair pantry staples with fresh herbs and garlic for a sauce that's rich yet low in fat. Serve this sauce over grilled fish, green salads topped with chicken, cheese ravioli, or even scrambled eggs.

Prep Time: *5 minutes*
Cooking Time: *5 minutes*
Yield: *serves 4*
Serving Size: *¼ cup*

> SPARK SWAPS TIPS

Roasted red peppers add a sweet, smoky flavor to any dish. Roast your own or use the jarred variety. Drain and rinse them to remove as much salt as possible.

Never skip the step of rinsing canned beans. Not only does it remove up to 40 percent of the sodium, but it also eliminates the starches that can cause stomach discomfort.

4 ounces roasted red peppers, drained and rinsed (2 peppers)
1 cup canned cannellini (white kidney) beans, drained and rinsed*
1 cup fresh parsley, leaves only (about ½ bunch)
1 clove garlic
2 tablespoons red wine vinegar
½ teaspoon paprika
¼ teaspoon cayenne pepper

* If you can't find cannellini beans, use Great Northern or navy beans.

In a food processor or blender, purée all ingredients until smooth. Transfer to a saucepan and cook over medium heat until warm, about 3 minutes.

If you prefer a thinner sauce, add water until you reach the desired consistency.

Nutrition Information per Serving

Calories: 74.8	*Sodium: 91.3 mg*	*Fiber: 5.1 g*
Fat: 0.3 g	*Carbs: 16.2 g*	*Protein: 4.8 g*
Cholesterol: 0.0 mg		

Hot-and-Sweet Rainbow Slaw

Creamy coleslaw pairs well with fried chicken, but who needs all that mayonnaise? This one uses—you guessed it—plain Greek yogurt and a healthier mayonnaise, plus a few other special ingredients. We used a packaged slaw mix from the supermarket to save time.

Prep Time: *5 minutes*
Yield: *serves 4*
Serving Size: *½ cup*

> SPARK SWAPS TIPS

This dish tastes better the longer it sits, so make it up to a couple of days ahead.
Use any leftovers on a Sandwich Thin with pork tenderloin or chicken topped with barbecue
sauce.

Dressing

½ teaspoon Dijon mustard
1½ teaspoons olive-oil or canola-oil mayonnaise
1½ tablespoons fat-free plain Greek yogurt
Dash of hot sauce
1½ teaspoons lemon juice

6 ounces rainbow slaw*
1 Granny Smith apple, sliced into matchsticks or grated

This variety has broccoli, cauliflower, carrots, and red cabbage.

In a large bowl, whisk together all the dressing ingredients—the mustard, oil mayonnaise, yogurt, hot sauce, and lemon juice—then toss with the slaw and apple, coating thoroughly. Serve immediately or refrigerate.

Nutrition Information per Serving

Calories: 41.9	Sodium: 44.4 mg	Fiber: 2.0 g
Fat: 0.9 g	Carbs: 8.2 g	Protein: 1.5 g
Cholesterol: 0.6 mg		

Kale Pesto

This thick, creamy pesto will melt into a thick, flavorful sauce when used on pasta or grilled vegetables. But there are two tricks to this recipe: we swapped kale for the herbs and swapped white beans for the oil.

Prep Time: *5 minutes*
Cooking Time: *1 minute*
Yield: *serves 4 as a pasta sauce or serves 8 as a veggie topping*
Serving Size: *¼ cup pasta sauce or 2 tablespoons veggie topping*

> SPARK SWAPS TIPS

To separate kale leaves from their stems, hold each leaf upside down and pull down forcefully along the stem. The leaves will easily come off. Discard the tough stems and chop or tear the leaves.

½ bunch kale, tough stems removed, leaves chopped (about 1½ cups)

2 tablespoons shelled, unsalted pistachios*

½ cup canned cannellini (white kidney) beans, drained and rinsed**

½ teaspoon black pepper

1 tablespoon lemon juice

¼ cup shredded Parmesan cheese

Toasted, unsalted almonds or hazelnuts could be substituted.

*** If you can't find cannellini beans, use Great Northern or navy beans.*

Place the kale in a microwave-safe dish with 1 tablespoon water. Cover with plastic wrap and cook on high for 1 minute, until brighter in color and slightly wilted.

Transfer the kale and any water in the dish to a food processor. Add the nuts, beans, pepper, and lemon juice. Pulse several times to combine, then purée until smooth. Transfer to a small bowl and stir in the cheese. Cover and refrigerate for up to four days or freeze for up to three months.

Nutrition Information per Serving

Calories: 80.9	*Sodium: 118.2 mg*	*Fiber: 3.0 g*
Fat: 3.3 g	*Carbs: 9.1 g*	*Protein: 5.4 g*
Cholesterol: 3.8 mg		

Lemon Roasted Cauliflower

Roasted cauliflower is a simple side dish that will convert any veggie hater. The trick is in the smash. To use less oil and still achieve the texture and color you want, place the cauliflower and oil in a large, sealable plastic bag and smash the florets with the heel of your hand.

Prep Time: *5 minutes*
Cooking Time: *30 minutes*
Yield: *serves 4*
Serving Size: *¾ cup*

> SPARK SWAPS TIPS

This same roasting technique can be used for almost any vegetable; try parsnips, fennel, or broccoli.

**1 small head cauliflower, core removed, chopped (about
    3 cups florets)
1 tablespoon olive oil
3 cloves garlic, sliced
½ teaspoon dried thyme
½ teaspoon black pepper
½ lemon, cut into 4 pieces**

Preheat the oven to 400°F. Line a baking sheet with foil, then coat the foil with cooking spray.

Put the cauliflower florets, oil, garlic, thyme, and pepper in a large ziplock bag, close the bag, and use the heel of your hand to smash the cauliflower into equal size pieces and distribute the oil. Add the lemon, shake, and pour onto the baking sheet. Roast for 15 minutes, stir, and roast another 10 minutes, until the cauliflower is soft and golden brown in places.

Squeeze the roasted lemon wedges over the cauliflower, then discard them. Serve immediately and refrigerate any leftovers.

Nutrition Information per Serving

Calories: 89.2   *Sodium: 63.9 mg*   *Fiber: 6.0 g*
Fat: 3.9 g   *Carbs: 13.3 g*   *Protein: 4.5 g*
Cholesterol: 0.0 mg

Microwave Pasta Sauce

Take one jar basic tomato sauce and add half a bag of frozen spinach. Purée and voilà: a serving of veggies in your pasta. Top whole-wheat penne with the sauce and a slice of provolone, and dinner is ready in no time.

Prep Time: *1 minute*
Cooking Time: *2 minutes*
Yield: *serves 4*
Serving Size: *½ cup*

> SPARK SWAPS TIPS

Pasta aside, use this sauce on grilled flatbreads or as a dipping sauce for steamed or grilled vegetables.

2 cups no-salt-added tomato-based pasta sauce
5 ounces fresh or frozen spinach

Place the spinach in a large microwave-safe bowl. If using fresh spinach, add 1 tablespoon water. Microwave on high for 1 minute for fresh spinach, up to 5 minutes for frozen. Remove from the microwave and drain any excess water.

In a food processor or blender, purée the spinach and tomato sauce until smooth. Return to the bowl and microwave for 1 minute, until the sauce is hot.

Nutrition Information per Serving

Calories: 78.2	*Sodium: 68.0 mg*	*Fiber: 2.8 g*
Fat: 2.6 g	*Carbs: 13.3 g*	*Protein: 3.0 g*
Cholesterol: 0.0 mg		

Perfect Mashed Potatoes

Warm, creamy, and rich, mashed potatoes are the ultimate comfort food. While this supper staple is easy to make, most iterations rely solely on cream and butter for flavor. Not this one. We've added some surprising sweetness with

parsnips, helped by a few herbs and spices. We used just 1 tablespoon of light sour cream for creaminess, and we kept the skins on the potatoes for fiber and texture.

Prep Time: *3 minutes*
Cooking Time: *20 minutes*
Yield: *serves 4*
Serving Size: *½ cup*

> SPARK SWAPS TIPS

If you don't dry out the potatoes, they will not get fluffy.

3 medium red potatoes, quartered (about 12 ounces)
2 small parsnips, peeled and chopped (about ¾ cup)
1 clove garlic
¼ teaspoon black pepper
1 teaspoon chopped fresh thyme
1 tablespoon low-fat sour cream or fat-free plain Greek
    yogurt

Place the potatoes, parsnips, and garlic in a large saucepan and fill with cool water. Cover, bring to a boil, then simmer for 20 minutes, until the vegetables can be easily poked with a fork. Turn off the heat and carefully drain the vegetables using a colander. Return them to the pan and turn the heat to medium. Allow the vegetables to dry out, which should take about a minute.

Remove from the heat and stir in the pepper, thyme, and sour cream. Mash the mixture using a fork or potato masher to your desired consistency. Serve warm.

Nutrition Information per Serving

Calories: 88.9
Fat: 0.7 g
Cholesterol: 1.5 mg

Sodium: 9.8 mg
Carbs: 19.1 g

Fiber: 2.6 g
Protein: 2.2 g

Ten-Minute Garden Harvest Pasta Sauce

Your family will think you had this sauce on the stove for hours. Only you will know that it took a mere ten minutes. Try it on grilled pork, grilled eggplant, or whole-wheat pasta.

> **Prep Time:** *5 minutes*
> **Cooking Time:** *7 minutes*
> **Yield:** *serves 4*
> **Serving Size:** *¾ cup*

> SPARK SWAPS TIPS

To add fiber and texture, we didn't peel the eggplant or zucchini.

Change up the veggies: try carrots, bell peppers, summer squash, or mushrooms.

> **1 small white or yellow onion, chopped (about ½ cup)**
> **1 clove garlic, chopped**
> **1 small eggplant, chopped (about 1 cup)**
> **1 small zucchini, chopped (about 1 cup)**
> **1 teaspoon dried thyme or oregano**
> **2 cups basic tomato-based pasta sauce***

* Choose a low-sodium sauce, if possible, and avoid sauces with added cheese or meat. For this recipe, a basic marinara or tomato-basil works well.

Place a large skillet over medium-high heat. When the skillet is hot, remove it from heat, coat it with cooking spray, and return it to the heat. Sauté the onion, garlic, eggplant, and zucchini for 3 or 4 minutes, until soft. Stir in the thyme or oregano and ¼ cup water, and cook for another minute. Then stir in the pasta sauce, combining well.

For a chunky sauce, heat thoroughly and serve. For a smooth sauce, remove the skillet from the heat, transfer the sauce to a food processor or blender, and purée until smooth. Return to the pan and heat thoroughly.

> **Nutrition Information per Serving**
>
> | | | |
> |---|---|---|
> | *Calories: 94.6* | *Sodium: 101.3 mg* | *Fiber: 3.7 g* |
> | *Fat: 2.6 g* | *Carbs: 17.9 g* | *Protein: 2.8 g* |
> | *Cholesterol: 0.0 mg* | | |

Tomato-Basil Aioli

Traditionally, aioli is a garlicky sauce made with olive oil and egg yolks—a fancy mayonnaise. Outside of French or Spanish cooking, the definition has loosened, and it has come to refer to any souped-up mayonnaise. Our aioli contains no mayonnaise, egg yolks, or oil; instead, its creaminess comes from Greek yogurt.

Prep Time: *5 minutes*
Yield: *serves 1*

> SPARK SWAPS TIPS

Use this recipe as a template. Swap the herbs, add garlic, or use vinegar in place of the lemon juice.

1 sun-dried tomato* or 1 tablespoon chopped roasted red pepper
1 tablespoon fat-free plain Greek yogurt
1 tablespoon chopped fresh chives
1 tablespoon chopped fresh basil
1 teaspoon lemon juice

* If using jarred sun-dried tomatoes, opt for those packed in water. You could also use 1 teaspoon sun-dried tomato paste.

Place the sun-dried tomato in a small dish and cover it with hot water. Steep it for 3 minutes, then drain and chop. Combine the chopped tomato with the remaining ingredients—the yogurt, chives, basil, and lemon juice—by stirring, and refrigerate or use immediately.

Nutrition Information per Serving

Calories: 20.1	*Sodium: 52.1 mg*	*Fiber: 0.4 g*
Fat: 0.1 g	*Carbs: 2.4 g*	*Protein: 2.9 g*
Cholesterol: 0.0 mg		

Super Snacks and Sweets

Banana Chocolate Muffins

One recipe, two treats. The banana you had for breakfast turns into a healthy treat with the simple addition of chocolate chips. This recipe makes a dozen, so freeze some for later, share a few with your coworkers, or put them in your kids' lunchboxes.

Prep Time: *5 minutes*
Cooking Time: *15 minutes*
Yield: *serves 12*
Serving Size: *1 muffin*

> SPARK SWAPS TIPS

To freeze, place cooled muffins in ziplock bags. Thaw overnight at room temperature or microwave for 30 seconds.

Prepared batter of 1 recipe Better Banana Bread (page 230)
½ cup semisweet or dark chocolate chips

Preheat the oven to 350°F. Grease a muffin tin with cooking spray or line with paper baking cups.

Place 1 tablespoon of the batter in the bottom of each well of the muffin tin, then fill with 2 teaspoons chocolate. Top with another tablespoon of batter. Divide any remaining batter equally among the wells.

Bake 13 to 14 minutes, until the tops are firm and the muffins are golden brown. Cool slightly in the muffin tin before eating. Let cool completely before freezing. Thaw overnight at room temperature or in the microwave for 30 to 40 seconds on high.

Nutrition Information per Serving

Calories: 121.0	*Sodium: 67.7 mg*	*Fiber: 2.9 g*
Fat: 3.3 g	*Carbs: 23.3 g*	*Protein: 3.5 g*
Cholesterol: 0.0 mg		

Berry Cobbler Cup

Not only is this cobbler ready in under five minutes, but it's the perfect portion too. No leftovers means no temptation.

Prep Time: *2 minutes*
Cooking Time: *2 minutes*
Yield: *serves 1*

> SPARK SWAPS TIPS

As an alternative, substitute canned chopped peaches for the berries and add a pinch of cinnamon.

1½ tablespoons skim milk
1½ tablespoons whole-wheat flour
2 teaspoons sugar
¼ teaspoon baking powder
⅓ cup fresh or frozen berries (blueberries, blackberries, raspberries)

Coat a coffee mug with cooking spray. Add the milk, flour, sugar, and baking powder, and stir with a fork until well combined. Stir in half of the berries, then pour the remaining berries on top. Microwave on high for 2 minutes. Cool slightly before eating.

Nutrition Information per Serving

Calories: 104.2	*Sodium: 136.2 mg*	*Fiber: 2.6 g*
Fat: 0.2 g	*Carbs: 24.5 g*	*Protein: 2.5 g*
Cholesterol: 0.4 mg		

Better Banana Bread

With most produce, you're out of luck if you let it go past its peak ripeness. Not with bananas. The longer they sit on the counter, the better they are—for banana bread. The natural sweetness of the fruit means you need little added sugar, despite what some recipes call for. Ours has no oil and gets a burst of bright orange flavor.

Prep Time: *5 minutes*
Cooking Time: *25 minutes*
Yield: *serves 6*
Serving Size: *1 slice*

> SPARK SWAPS TIPS

To change up the flavor, swap the orange juice for milk and add almond extract.

2 tablespoons ground flaxseeds
2 medium ripe bananas, mashed (about 1 cup)
1 large egg
¼ cup fat-free plain Greek yogurt
¼ cup packed brown sugar
Zest and juice of 1 medium orange
1¼ cups whole-wheat flour
½ teaspoon baking soda
¼ teaspoon salt
2 tablespoons sliced almonds
½ teaspoon cinnamon

Preheat the oven to 350°F. Grease a 5 × 9-inch loaf pan with cooking spray.

In a small dish, soak the ground flax in 3 tablespoons of water for 3 minutes, until a thick paste forms. In a large mixing bowl, combine the flax mixture, bananas, egg, yogurt, sugar, orange zest, and 1 tablespoon of the orange juice, stirring with a rubber spatula until somewhat smooth. Add the flour, baking soda, salt, almonds, and cinnamon, and mix until just combined.

Pour into the prepared pan. Bake 25 to 27 minutes, until the bread is golden brown and firm to the touch. Allow to cool for 10 minutes before turning the loaf onto a plate or wire rack. Allow to cool completely before storing in a plastic bag. The bread will keep for up to four days on the counter. You can also freeze individual slices and thaw as needed.

Nutrition Information per Serving

Calories: 186.6	*Sodium: 145.5 mg*	*Fiber: 5.0 g*
Fat: 3.2 g	*Carbs: 37.7 g*	*Protein: 7.4 g*
Cholesterol: 30.8 mg		

Cherry Fro-Yo Sandwich

Satisfy cravings in no time. These frozen-yogurt sandwiches are ready quickly and easily customized: chocolate graham crackers with chocolate frozen yogurt and strawberries; cinnamon ones with vanilla and raisins; honey graham crackers with cinnamon, vanilla yogurt, and banana slices.

Prep Time: *5 minutes*
Yield: *serves 1*

> SPARK SWAPS TIPS

If fresh cherries are out of season, use thawed frozen ones. They're already pitted!

1 sheet low-fat graham cracker, broken in half
2 tablespoons slow-churned vanilla frozen yogurt
3 cherries, pitted and chopped

Sandwich the frozen yogurt and chopped cherries between the two graham cracker halves.

Nutrition Information per Serving

Calories: 98.9	*Sodium: 94.1 mg*	*Fiber: 0.9 g*
Fat: 1.6 g	*Carbs: 20.7 g*	*Protein: 1.7 g*
Cholesterol: 2.6 mg		

Cherry-Pistachio Yogurt Sundae

This combination is so simple but so good. Swap in your favorite fruit and nuts.

Prep Time: *5 minutes*
Yield: *serves 1*

> SPARK SWAPS TIPS

To pit fresh cherries without a cherry or olive pitter, gently press down on them with the flat side of your knife as you would a garlic clove.

¼ cup cherries, pitted and sliced (about 6 to 7 cherries)
1 tablespoon chopped unsalted pistachios
¼ cup fat-free vanilla Greek yogurt

In a small dish, combine the chopped cherries and pistachios, then stir in the yogurt. Serve immediately or refrigerate until you're ready to eat.

Nutrition Information per Serving

Calories: 103.9   *Sodium: 25.1 mg*   *Fiber: 1.5 g*

Fat: 3.3 g   *Carbs: 12.2 g*   *Protein: 7.2 g*

Cholesterol: 0.0 mg

Chocolate Fondue

Fondue is a favorite dessert, but staying in control when faced with a giant vat of bubbling chocolate can be difficult. Plus, who's measuring the amount of chocolate consumed with each dunk of the fondue fork? This recipe solves that problem. It makes just enough for one, and it's under 100 calories.

Prep Time: *3 minutes*
Cooking Time: *1 minute*
Yield: *serves 1*

> SPARK SWAPS TIPS

Keeping the greens on the strawberries makes for easier dipping.

To ensure the chocolate clings to the berries, pat the berries dry after rinsing them.

If having an entire bag of chocolate chips in the house is too tempting for you, use a single chopped square of dark chocolate instead.

1½ teaspoons fat-free evaporated milk
1 tablespoon semisweet chocolate chips
½ teaspoon vanilla extract
½ cup fresh strawberries (6 medium or 3 large)

In a small microwave-safe dish, combine the milk, chocolate, and vanilla and microwave on high for 30 seconds, checking and stirring every 10 seconds. When the chocolate is 75 percent melted, remove the dish from the microwave (the residual heat will melt it completely). Serve immediately with the berries.

Nutrition Information per Serving

Calories: 79.9	*Sodium: 10.7 mg*	*Fiber: 2.3 g*
Fat: 3.3 g	*Carbs: 13.3 g*	*Protein: 1.5 g*
Cholesterol: 0.3 mg		

Chocolate Fro-Yo Sandwich

These freeze well, so go ahead and make several while you have the ingredients out and handy. Wrap each in parchment paper for a no-mess handheld treat.

Prep Time: *3 minutes*
Yield: *serves 1*

1 chocolate graham cracker, broken in half
2 tablespoons slow-churned vanilla frozen yogurt
½ tablespoon ice cream sprinkles

Sandwich the frozen yogurt between the two graham cracker halves. Press the sprinkles into the yogurt along the sides. Serve immediately or freeze.

Nutrition Information per Serving

Calories: 99.0	*Sodium: 64.4 mg*	*Fiber: 0.0 g*
Fat: 3.4 g	*Carbs: 15.8 g*	*Protein: 1.6 g*
Cholesterol: 2.6 mg		

Creamy Orange Soft-Serve

While this treat does take a bit of time (and patience) to freeze, it takes no time to prep. If you're in the mood for something sweet yet light, this is a tasty treat. Even unfrozen, this is a fun way to eat your yogurt.

Prep Time: *5 minutes*
Yield: *serves 1*

½ orange
¼ cup fat-free vanilla Greek yogurt

Cut a small slice from one end of the orange to create a flat surface. Remove the flesh from the orange by running a small knife around the inside of the fruit, between the pith (the white part) and the flesh. Pull away the white membrane from the inner sections and chop the orange segments. Set the leftover peel cup aside.

In a small dish, mix the orange segments and any juice from the orange with the yogurt, then spoon the mixture into the orange-peel cup. Place on a small plate and freeze for 1 hour for soft-serve or 3 hours for a completely frozen treat.

Nutrition Information per Serving

Calories: 79.2	*Sodium: 33.3 mg*	*Fiber: 1.1 g*
Fat: 2.1 g	*Carbs: 13.7 g*	*Protein: 2.8 g*
Cholesterol: 8.3 mg		

Fruit-Stuffed Ice Cream Cone

The fruit fills the cone and gives you two treats in one. This is like a healthy shortcake and ice cream treat rolled—stuffed!—into just 87 calories.

Prep Time: *3 minutes*
Yield: *serves 1*

> SPARK SWAPS TIPS

Substitute any fruit that's on sale or in season. Try sliced bananas, chopped fresh peaches and plums, canned pineapple, blueberries, or raspberries.

1 ice cream cone*
2 tablespoons chopped blackberries
2 strawberries, chopped
¼ cup slow-churned vanilla frozen yogurt

* We use the sugar variety.

Fill the cone with chopped fruit, then top with frozen yogurt. Serve immediately.

Nutrition Information per Serving

Calories: 86.9	Sodium: 32.7 mg	Fiber: 1.5 g
Fat: 1.7 g	Carbs: 16.6 g	Protein: 2.3 g
Cholesterol: 5.0 mg		

Grilled Pineapple with Toasted Coconut

If you like piña coladas, you'll love this sweet snack. Pineapple gets sweet and caramelized in a hot skillet, then rich, creamy coconut milk and toasted coconut transform it from fruit to dessert.

Prep Time: *2 minutes*
Cooking Time: *4 minutes*
Yield: *serves 1*

> SPARK SWAPS TIPS

If you don't have coconut milk on hand, you can omit it.

Freeze leftover coconut milk in ice cube trays, then transfer the cubes to a plastic freezer bag for storage. They'll keep for six months. They add tropical flair to smoothies, and when thawed, they're great in pancake or muffin batter.

2 teaspoons unsweetened shredded coconut
2 slices pineapple, fresh or canned in natural juice
2 tablespoons light coconut milk

Heat a small skillet over medium heat. Add the coconut to the dry pan and toast lightly, about 2 minutes. Set aside.

Heat the same small skillet over high heat. Sauté the pineapple 2 minutes per side, then transfer to a small serving plate, top with the toasted coconut, and drizzle with the coconut milk. Serve immediately.

Nutrition Information per Serving

Calories: 114.5   Sodium: 2.4 mg   Fiber: 2.3 g

Fat: 3.7 g   Carbs: 21.8 g   Protein: 0.8 g

Cholesterol: 0.0 mg

Hot Apple Tart

There's no dessert more comforting on a cool fall night than a slice of home-made apple pie. There are also few desserts more tempting. Save time and calories with a version that's ready in three minutes flat.

Keep the peel on the apple for fiber and texture.

Prep Time: 3 minutes
Cooking Time: 3 minutes
Yield: serves 1

> SPARK SWAPS TIPS

You can also make this recipe in the microwave. Heat on high for 90 seconds.

½ Granny Smith apple, diced
¼ teaspoon cinnamon
1 packed teaspoon brown sugar
½ low-fat honey or cinnamon graham cracker, crumbled
1 tablespoon light whipped topping

In a small skillet set over medium-high heat, combine the apples, cinnamon, and brown sugar. Stir constantly for 3 minutes, until the apples start to brown.

Transfer to a small serving dish, sprinkle with the graham cracker crumbles, and finish with the whipped topping. Eat immediately.

Nutrition Information per Serving

Calories: 124.5   Sodium: 86.3 mg   Fiber: 2.8 g

Fat: 1.9 g   Carbs: 29.8 g   Protein: 1.1 g

Cholesterol: 0.0 mg

Strawberry Crunch Sundae

Call it a parfait. Call it a sundae. Call it anything you want. Just call on it at snack time.

Prep Time: *5 minutes*
Yield: *serves 1*

> SPARK SWAPS TIPS

Other fruit options: canned peaches or pineapple, blueberries, blackberries, raspberries, sliced banana, or halved grapes.

Desktop Dining. To keep the granola crunchy, store it separately from the yogurt and berries until you're ready to eat.

¼ cup fresh strawberries, sliced
¼ cup fat-free vanilla Greek yogurt
1 tablespoon Quick and Easy Granola (page 165)

In a small bowl, mash the strawberries with a fork, then top with the yogurt and the granola. Serve immediately.

Nutrition Information per Serving

Calories: 101.6   *Sodium: 23.1 mg*   *Fiber: 2.1 g*
Fat: 1.8 g   *Carbs: 14.7 g*   *Protein: 6.9 g*
Cholesterol: 0.0 mg

Tiramisu Sandwiches

We downsized tiramisu. Vanilla wafer cookies stand in for ladyfingers and ricotta cheese for mascarpone, but all the flavors and textures you crave remain.

Prep Time: *3 minutes*
Yield: *serves 1*

1 ground coffee bean or ¼ teaspoon instant coffee
2 tablespoons low-fat ricotta cheese

¼ teaspoon vanilla extract
4 low-fat vanilla wafer cookies
¼ teaspoon unsweetened cocoa powder

In a small cup or bowl, combine the coffee, cheese, and vanilla. Spread the mixture on two cookies and sandwich them with the remaining two cookies. Dust both with cocoa powder and eat immediately.

Nutrition Information per Serving

Calories: 102.9	*Sodium: 95.0 mg*	*Fiber: 0.1 g*
Fat: 3.6 g	*Carbs: 13.9 g*	*Protein: 4.2 g*
Cholesterol: 9.9 mg		

Spark Solution Fitness Plan

The Spark Solution incorporates a six-day workout program, alternating days of cardio and strength training, plus one rest day. Here's a refresher on the basics that we introduced in "The Spark Solution Metabolic Makeover" in Part 1:

Cardio (cardiovascular exercise) elevates your heart rate and keeps it pumping faster for at least ten consecutive minutes. You can split your cardio sessions into smaller intervals, but they must be at least ten minutes each for them to count.

Cardio burns fat while strengthening your heart and lungs. You'll do cardio workouts three times a week, of twenty to thirty minutes' duration in the first week and thirty to forty-five minutes' duration in the second. You'll also change up your intensity and your activity.

You get to choose which type of cardio you do. If you don't like running, you don't have to run. If you love to use the elliptical while catching up on your favorite TV shows, go for it. We encourage you to do at least two different forms of cardio and change them up regularly to avoid overuse injuries, to work your muscles in different ways, and to ward off boredom.

Strength training entails exercises performed against resistance—from a machine, a weight, or even your body's weight. Not only does this type of exercise build muscles, it also strengthens bones, tendons, and ligaments.

You'll strength train three days a week, but not on the same days you'll do cardio. Each day will vary in intensity and length.

We offer step-by-step photos and instructions for each move, along with modifications to make each exercise appropriate for your fitness level.

Flexibility (stretching) exercises lengthen your muscles and develop or maintain range of motion. Stretch after both cardio and strength workouts

241

to reduce injuries. Increased flexibility may also help you with coordination. You'll stretch for a few minutes after every workout.

Lifestyle Activities: NEAT

Cardio, strength, and flexibility are the standard forms of exercise with which you're probably somewhat familiar. You may have noticed how specific they are in their parameters and descriptions: how cardio *has* to last for ten minutes and be at a somewhat challenging intensity to really "count," or how strength training *must* work certain muscles in a certain number of repetitions. It's true that for planned exercise to really count— meaning that it gives you the health, fitness, and weight-loss benefits you're aiming for—you have to follow these guidelines. But what about all the other movement in your life? Taking the stairs at work might not be intense enough or last long enough to count as a cardio workout, but does that mean it's pointless?

Far from it. These are what we call lifestyle activities, or NEAT (non-exercise activity thermogenesis), and they benefit both your health and your waistline. In fact, many studies show that this type of movement is just as important as planned exercise. NEAT includes all activities that aren't exercise, sleeping, or eating—everything from carrying the laundry to the basement and back to playing with your kids to pushing a grocery cart around the supermarket. When you think about it, even when following a consistent and intense exercise program—say, working out an hour a day—your body is mostly sedentary for the remaining twenty-three hours. Those long stretches of inactivity can wreak havoc on your metabolism, blood sugar, posture, and more, but by incorporating more quick-and-easy lifestyle activity into your days, you're upping your overall calorie burn and boosting your health.

- *How Much.* While there has been far less research conducted on the amount of lifestyle activity a person needs for ideal health, most experts agree the more the better. Even on days that you do cardio and/or strength training, you should still aim to be as active as possible throughout the day. Try to accumulate up to one to two hours of NEAT per day.

- *How Often.* NEAT is something you accumulate a few minutes at a time here and there throughout the day, but it should be a part of your daily routine.

- *How Long.* Unlike other types of exercise, NEAT doesn't have to last any particular length of time to be effective. It could last as little as five seconds (standing up to grab the phone) or for several hours (bowling, yard work, etc.).

- *What Counts.* Anything that gets you on your feet counts as NEAT. Even standing counts—but you have to stand, not sit. Little activities like walking from your desk to talk to a coworker, taking the stairs, parking farther from the door, pacing while you talk on the phone, or standing up in a waiting room all add up.

Your Two-Week Spark Solution Fitness Plan

You will want to spend a few minutes warming up before each workout. After each session, spend a few minutes cooling down, and then stretch all your major muscle groups.

Day	Workout	Instructions	Daily NEAT Minute Goal
1	Cardio: 20 minutes	Choose any activity and accumulate minutes in two 10-minute chunks or all at once. Work "somewhat hard" (8 out of 10) so you are slightly breathless the entire time. Need help deciding what to do? Check out the appendix for a list of workouts.	30 minutes
2	Strength training: two sets of ten reps	Perform the exercises in the Spark Swaps Strength Workout (page 247) in the order listed, moving quickly from one exercise to the next for one set, then repeat for a second set. For exercises performed on one side at a time, perform all reps on each side before switching. Then move on to the next exercise.	45 minutes
3	Cardio intervals: 30 minutes	Choose any form of cardio and alternate between high intensity and low intensity using this guide: 1 minute of "all out" (9 out of 10) followed by 3 minutes of "moderate" (6 out of 10). Repeat this sequence of intervals 6 times (24 total minutes). Warm up before and cool down after for 3 minutes each.	30 minutes

Day	Workout	Instructions	Daily NEAT Minute Goal
4	Strength training: AMRAP	Perform the exercises in the Spark Swaps Strength Workout (page 247) in the order listed, this time doing as many reps as possible (AMRAP) and every exercise for 1 full minute, fitting in as many controlled, good reps as you can. Move quickly to the next exercise (with little or no rest) until you've done them all. For exercises performed on one side at a time, perform 1 full minute on each side before switching. Then move on to the next exercise. Record your score (reps) for each move for later reference.	45 minutes
5	Cardio: 20 minutes	Choose a different activity than Day 1 and accumulate minutes in two 10-minute chunks or all at once. Work "somewhat hard" (8 out of 10) so you are slightly breathless the entire time.	30 minutes
6	Strength training: two sets of twelve reps	Perform the exercises in the Spark Swaps Strength Workout (page 247) in reverse order, moving quickly from one exercise to the next for one set, then repeat for a second set. For exercises performed on one side at a time, perform all reps on each side before switching. Then move on to the next exercise.	45 minutes
7	Rest day	No cardio or strength today. Rest up, rebuild, and recover.	75 minutes
8	Cardio: 30 minutes	Choose any activity and accumulate minutes in three 10-minute chunks, two 15-minute chunks, or all at once. Work "somewhat hard" (8 out of 10) so you are slightly breathless the entire time.	45 minutes
9	Strength training: two sets of fifteen reps	Perform the exercises in the Spark Swaps Strength Workout (page 247) in the order listed, moving quickly from one exercise to the next for one set, then repeat for a second set. For exercises performed on one side at a time, perform all reps on each side before switching. Then move on to the next exercise.	60 minutes
10	Cardio intervals: 45 minutes	Choose any form of cardio and alternate between high intensity and low intensity using this guide: 3 minutes of "moderate" intensity (6 out of 10) followed by 2 minutes of "somewhat hard" intensity (8 out of 10), then 1 minute of "all-out" intensity (9 out of 10). Repeat this sequence of intervals 7 times (42 total minutes). Warm up before and cool down after for 3 minutes each.	30 minutes

Day	Workout	Instructions	Daily NEAT Minute Goal
11	Strength training: AMRAP	Perform the exercises in the Spark Swaps Strength Workout (page 247) in the order listed, doing as many reps as possible (AMRAP) and every exercise for 1 full minute, fitting in as many controlled, good reps as you can. Move quickly to the next exercise (with little or no rest) until you've done them all. For exercises performed on one side at a time, perform 1 full minute on each side before switching. Then move on to the next exercise. Your goal today is to beat last week's score for each exercise.	60 minutes
12	Cardio: 30 minutes	Choose a different activity than Day 8 and accumulate minutes in three 10-minute chunks, two 15-minute chunks, or all at once. Work "somewhat hard" (8 out of 10) so you are slightly breathless the entire time.	45 minutes
13	Strength training: three sets of ten reps	Perform the exercises in the Spark Swaps Strength Workout (page 247) in reverse order, moving quickly from one exercise to the next for one set, then repeat for a second set. For exercises performed on one side at a time, perform all reps on each side before switching. Then move on to the next exercise.	60 minutes
14	Rest day	No cardio or strength today. Rest up, rebuild, and recover.	90 minutes

Rate of Perceived Exertion

Rate of perceived exertion (RPE) may be the most versatile method to measure exercise intensity for all age groups. Using this method is simple,

10	Maximal exertion
9	Very hard
8	Extremely hard
7	Hard (heavy)
6	Moderately hard
5	Somewhat hard
4	Fairly light
3	Light
2	Very light
1	Rest

because all you have to do is estimate how hard *you feel* like you're exerting yourself during exercise. RPE is a good measure of intensity because it is individualized—it's based on your current fitness level and overall perception of exercise. The scale ranges from 1 to 10, allowing you to rate how you feel physically and mentally at a given intensity level.

An RPE between 5 and 7 is recommended for most adults. This means that at the height of your workout, you should feel you are working "somewhat hard" to "hard."

The Talk Test

The final method for measuring exercise intensity is the talk test. Like the RPE, the talk test is subjective and quite useful in determining your aerobic intensity, especially if you are just beginning an exercise program.

Using this method, you aim to work at a level where you can answer a question but not comfortably carry on a conversation. In simple terms, you're working out too hard if you have to take a breath between every word you say. Conversely, you would be exercising too easily if you could sing the chorus of a song without breathing hard.

Work at an intensity that allows you to breathe comfortably and rhythmically throughout all phases of your workout. This will ensure a safe and comfortable level of exercise.

Spark Swaps Strength Workout

Squat and Reach

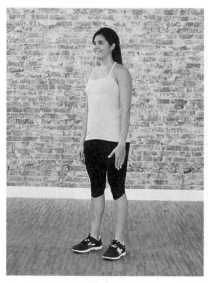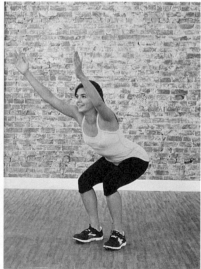

Stand with your feet hip-width apart, your arms at your sides (above left). *Squat (bending your knees and hips) as you lift your arms straight up next to your ears* (above right). *Return to the starting position to complete one rep.*

Tip: Throughout the movement, keep your abs (abdominal muscles) tight, your back straight, and your chest lifted. Only raise your arms up as high as you can while maintaining balance and good form.

Curtsey Lunge

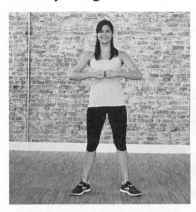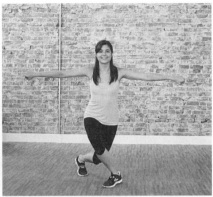

Stand with your feet turned slightly outward and wider than your hips. Bend your elbows and place your arms in front of your chest, with your palms facing your body (above left). Step your right leg diagonally behind your left leg, then bend both knees into a lunge position while simultaneously extending your arms out, reaching your pinkies toward the ceiling (above right). Step back to the starting position (above left) to complete one rep. Perform all the intended reps on one side before switching legs. Be careful that your knees always point in the same direction as your toes throughout this movement.

Lunge with Rotation

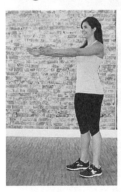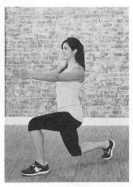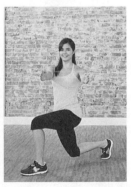

Stand with your feet hip-width apart and your arms extended out in front of your shoulders (above left). Step forward with your right leg and lower down into a lunge, keeping both knees bent around ninety degrees (above middle). Hold the lunge position and rotate your torso to the right (above right). Rotate back to center (above middle), then step back to the starting position (above left) to complete one rep. Repeat all the intended reps on one side before switching sides.

Kneeling Leg Lifts

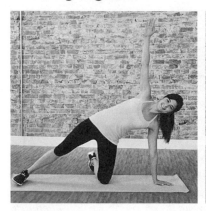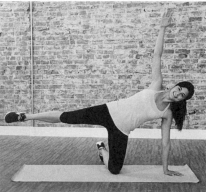

Begin by kneeling, setting both your knees on the floor. Extend your left leg out and carefully reach out with your right arm until your hand touches the floor and your opposite arm extends overhead. This is the starting position (above left). Make sure your hips and shoulders are square toward the front (not rotated at all). Slowly lift your extended leg as high as possible (above right), then return to the starting position (above left) to complete one rep. Repeat all the intended reps on one side before switching sides.

Triple Toner

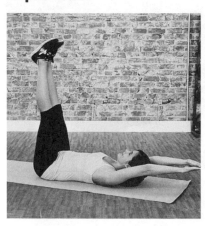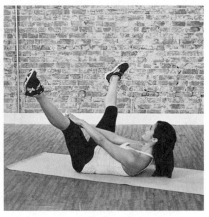

Lie flat on your back with your legs straight up (in line with your hips) and your arms extended in line with your shoulders, one hand stacked on top of the other (above left). Crunch up (lift your head, neck, and the tips of your shoulder blades off the floor) as you open your legs wider than your hips and bring your hands between your thighs (above right). Slowly lower back to the starting position to complete one rep.

Swim Triceps Trim

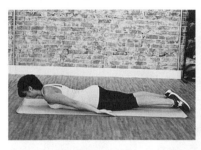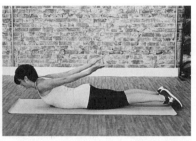

Lie flat on the floor, chest down, with your arms extended next to your hips, your spine neutral, and your legs as close together as is comfortable (above left). Lift your head, neck, and chest up from the floor (keeping your legs on the floor) as you hinge from the shoulder to lift your arms higher toward the ceiling (above right). Return to the starting position to complete one rep.

Pushup to Side Plank

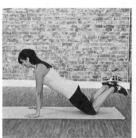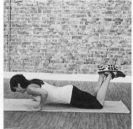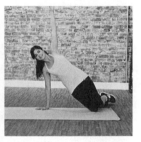

Begin in a modified (kneeling) plank position with your wrists under your shoulders, your arms straight, your legs together, and your body forming a continuous straight line from shoulder to hip to knee (above left). Keeping your body straight, bend your elbows to lower into a pushup (above middle). Straighten your arms to push back up to the starting position (above left). Lift your right hand off the floor and rotate to a modified (kneeling) side plank position, keeping your legs stacked (above right). Rotate back to the starting position (above left) to complete one rep. Alternate sides after each pushup.

If your strength allows, do these pushups and side planks with straight legs instead of with your knees bent.

Plank to Pike

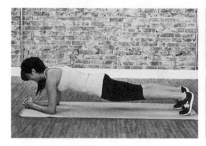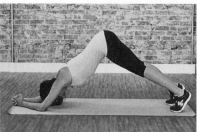

Come to a modified (elbows bent) plank position, with your elbows directly under your shoulders, your feet hip-width apart, your legs straight, and your body in a continuous straight line from shoulder to heel (above left). Engage your abs and slowly lift or "pike" your hips toward the ceiling as high as you can while keeping your legs straight and your back straight (above right). Return to the starting position to complete one rep.

For an added challenge or variety, try this move with straight arms instead of bent elbows.

Stable Table

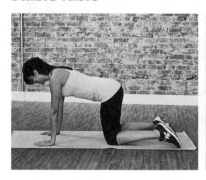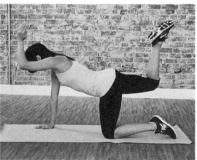

Kneel on all fours, placing your wrists directly under your shoulders and your knees directly under your hips (above left). Engage your abs and keep your back straight. Imagine your back, hips, and shoulders are flat like a tabletop. Maintain that flat surface as you lift a hand and an opposite leg up (don't tip!), keeping your joints bent at ninety degrees (above right). Return to the starting position (above left) and repeat on the other side to complete one rep. Continue alternating sides to complete all reps.

For an added challenge, throughout the exercise try this move with your knees hovering just a couple inches off the floor.

What Comes Next

The Next Two Weeks

When you trade the Standard American Diet for the Spark Solution's Spark Swaps, you can shed almost 5 pounds in two weeks, and 9.3 pounds in a month. Keep up the plan for three months and you can lose almost 28 pounds. After six months with the Spark Solution, 55.8 pounds down. Nine months, 84 pounds lost. And after a year, you will have lost 112 pounds!

Think about that for a moment. Whether you have 20, 50, or 100 pounds or more to lose, you can suddenly see that it's possible to reach your goal weight and achieve a healthier, happier you.

With that image in mind, you're ready to conquer the rest of your life. But first, let's start with the next two weeks. We're not taking the training wheels off just yet, but we are going to build in new healthy habits on top of the ones you've committed to during the first fourteen days.

We understand that life happens. Maybe you had a few late nights at the office, your child was ill, or you just couldn't find the time to fit in a workout one day. That's okay. No matter how much you accomplished, you're still on your way to a healthier you. Success is measured in myriad ways. If you're feeling better about yourself in any way, shape, or form, count it.

For the next two weeks, you'll start to gain independence in the kitchen and during your workouts. This is not a race, so if you want to take things slow and repeat a week, go for it. You'll continue to see results, and you'll reinforce all the lessons and habits you've committed to thus far.

We brought back those Spark It Up and Make It Work tips, which will differentiate the two plans for Week 3 and Week 4.

Setting Fitness Goals and Changing Your Routine

Every six to eight weeks vary your exercise program to avoid boredom and plateaus. This is crucial to keep your body's muscles surprised and constantly adapting. They'll have to work harder, you'll be challenged, and you'll burn more calories and build more lean muscle in the process.

CONTINUED ON PAGE 256

Cardio

Gradually work up to about sixty minutes over time, adding 10 percent more minutes each week, and vary between shorter and longer sessions. If you run or walk, increase your mileage by no more than 10 percent each week. The longer you work out and the farther you walk or run, the more calories you'll burn and the more endurance you'll build. Time can be cumulative. You don't have to do sixty minutes all at once. You can do several ten-minute mini workouts each day and add them up for pretty much the same benefits. Listen to your body and go at a pace that feels good to you. Plus, always warm up before each session, and cool down and stretch after. Continue to vary your workouts by including two or more cardio activities per week and alternating steady-state and interval workouts to keep that metabolism tuned up.

Strength Training

As you lose weight, continue to strength train to tighten your body and replace that lost fat with muscle. Start with light weights, as you perfect your form and get accustomed to strength training. Over time, gradually increase the amount of weight you lift, but by no more than 10 percent each week. If you're using your body weight for resistance, add another set each week and continue to alternate your speed and intensity.

When you're ready to try something new, start with strength-training DVDs, the free videos on SparkPeople.com, or gym machines. The machines usually have detailed instructions and a picture on them, plus they show which muscles you are working. They are set up to put your body in proper form and isolate the right muscles. In a typical weight room, the machines are often grouped together depending on their muscle focus (upper body, chest, arms, legs, etc.), so you can easily move through them and target every major muscle group.

Don't hold your breath, which can be dangerous. (It increases blood pressure and can cause lightheadedness, for example.) Exhale fully and forcefully on the exertion phase—usually the phase when you're lifting the weight. Inhale deeply on the easier phase—usually when you're returning to the starting position. Try to keep this rhythm throughout every set. In the beginning, it will take some concentration, but after a while, it will become habit.

Week 3

Eating

SPARK IT UP: SHAKE IT UP IN THE KITCHEN

Stick with the 1,500-calorie-per-day meal plan you've been following for the past two weeks, but mix it up. You have the freedom to choose any of our recipes, in any order. We included plenty of extra recipes in Part 3, so you'll find new dishes to try. We also added variations and alternative serving suggestions, so you can give the meals you've already tried a new twist.

If you want to have Better Banana Bread for breakfast three days in a row, go for it, as long as it fits into your meal plan. If you want to eat breakfast for dinner or a dinner meal for lunch, do it. What's important is that you continue to track everything you eat, measure your portions, and enjoy what you're eating. After all, healthy living should be fun!

MAKE IT WORK: STICK WITH WHAT WORKS

If you don't want to start choosing meals on your own, return to Week 1 and follow that week's meal plan again. Feel free to swap out the fruit and vegetable choices based on your preferences and what's in your kitchen, but stick to 1,500 calories a day.

Exercise

SPARK IT UP: THE POWER OF TEN

If you felt strong during last week's workouts and you're ready to do more, you'll start to lengthen and intensify your workouts. Follow the rule of ten: add no more than ten additional minutes to each workout, or if you measure fitness in miles, add no more than 10 percent more distance each week. So, if your cardio workouts lasted for twenty, thirty, and forty-five

minutes last week, change them in Week 3 to thirty, forty, and fifty-five minutes, respectively. If you usually walk four miles three times a week (a total of twelve miles a week), add no more than 1.2 extra miles (to total 13.2 miles) this week.

For your strength workouts, add an extra set, or tack another ten seconds on your one-minute AMRAP sessions. So rather than doing two sets of fifteen, you'll do three. And instead of doing one-minute intervals of your strength exercises, you'll do seventy seconds.

Please note that you do not have to add more time or intensity to every workout. Adding an extra ten minutes for just one day is a great place to start. Listen to your body and don't push yourself too hard.

You can also aim for an extra ten minutes of NEAT each day. And keep that rest day. You've earned it!

MAKE IT WORK: HOLD TIGHT

If last week's workouts were a challenge, repeat them again this week. Choose two different cardio workouts, and keep doing your strength-training exercises as laid out in the plan.

Week 4

Eating

SPARK IT UP: CHOOSE YOUR OWN ADVENTURE

Last week you practiced swapping in different recipes for your 1,500-calorie plan. This week you'll take it one step farther: work in some recipes that aren't included in this book. Use SparkRecipes.com to calculate the nutrition information in your favorite recipes, or choose from websites or cookbooks that provide that data for you. Follow the same guidelines, choosing recipes that fit within the nutrition criteria you've been using since Day 1. Of course, you can always use our recipes if you prefer.

You can even dine out once this week, using the principles you've learned. Check out menus ahead of time, visually portion your food, and make Spark Swaps. You can do this! Remember to track your food, even if you didn't cook it yourself.

MAKE IT WORK: TACKLE WEEK 2

If you returned to the beginning of Week 1 last week, continue with the plan, following Week 2's meal plan this week.

Exercise

SPARK IT UP: KEEP IT MOVING

Keep following the rule of ten. Add ten minutes to a workout or two, or increase your intensity with your strength training. Squeeze in another ten minutes of NEAT, and enjoy your rest day.

MAKE IT WORK: START SMALL

Are you ready to add to your workouts? You'll again follow the rule of ten we explained in Week 3.

Take it slow, listen to your body, and feel free to drop back to the Week 2 plan if needed.

The Rest of Your Life

It's been a month since you started this journey, and the detailed meal plans are complete. You've learned so much about healthy eating, and you've proved to yourself—and the world—that you could do it. We believed in you all along. We're so proud of you!

At SparkPeople, when we celebrate a goal, we shout "woohoo!" Today is definitely an occasion to yell "woohoo!" This leg of your journey is ending, but the road is long and you are strong. As you continue to build on your healthy habits, we encourage you to hold on to some lessons:

- Keep the Eight Habits of Super Successful Dieters in mind (see page 25 for a refresher).
- Follow the guidelines of the Spark Solution's Metabolic Makeover whether you're dining out or cooking at home (see page 31 any time you need a reminder).
- Continue to move your body, building strength as you shed weight (refer to the Spark Solution Fitness Plan on page 241 as you build your own workout schedule).
- Track your food, measure it, keep your plate filled with calorie-burning whole foods, and enjoy what you eat.

Throughout the rest of this section, you'll find resources to help you overcome hurdles you might encounter as you continue to lose weight. You'll learn how to:

- overcome plateaus
- identify and deal with diet saboteurs

- determine whether your brain or your belly is hungry
- avoid eating when you're not hungry
- reward yourself, and why that's so important

If at any time in your life you feel like you need a "refresher course," return to Week 1 of the Spark Solution and give yourself a two-week jolt of enthusiasm and motivation. You can do this!

What's the Difference Between Hunger and Cravings?

It's an hour after dinner, and you're relaxing in front of the TV. Suddenly the image of a juicy burger topped with sizzling bacon and melted cheese on a fresh sesame seed bun appears on the screen. *I'm hungry,* you immediately think. Are you sure you're hungry—as in, true grumbling-belly hungry? Maybe, maybe not.

There are two types of hunger: stomach hunger and mouth hunger. Stomach hunger can be identified by the stomach rumbling or growling or an empty ache in your belly area. You may feel a little cranky, faint, dizzy, or lightheaded. Mouth hunger is simply the desire for the taste of a certain food right at that moment. It has nothing to do with the body's need for calories or energy from food.

While neither type of hunger is good or bad, it's important to learn to identify both types of hunger so you can deal accordingly.

You should eat when you feel stomach hunger. This is your body's way of telling you it needs fuel. If your hunger is indeed stomach hunger, rate your hunger on a scale of 0 to 5.

Hunger Scale

0 = starving—feeling sick, dizzy, or cranky
1 = very, very hungry
2 = hungry with strong urge to eat
3 = neither hungry nor full; comfortable
4 = comfortably full
5 = overly stuffed and uncomfortable

The goal is to start eating when you're at level 2 and stop eating when you reach level 4, comfortably full. If you wait for your hunger to be at a level 0 or 1, you're more likely to grab any food in sight, quickly devouring the contents with little control. Eating meals and snacks at a table—away from distractions—can help you tune in to your levels of hunger and fullness so you don't overeat.

If your hunger is mouth hunger, ask yourself, *What food am I hungry for?*

Sometimes ignoring mouth hunger isn't the best call if you're craving something sweet and eat carrots instead. The craving doesn't go away, and you consume more calories as you eat the carrots, an apple, and *then* a bag of chocolate. Instead, eat a small amount of what you're craving while sitting at the dinner table, and focus on enjoying the food. Satisfy your mouth hunger and then move on.

If your mouth hunger never goes away, is there something else going on? Are there feelings or emotions triggering the mouth hunger? Are you feeling afraid, angry, anxious, awkward, bored, embarrassed, excited, guilty, happy, lonely, overwhelmed, irritated, sad, shy, stressed, or upset?

Think of other activities to do besides eating. Our members fight mouth hunger by journaling, talking, exercising, reading a book, listening to music, meditating, going to the movies, doing a craft or hobby, or writing a letter to a friend. Sometimes talking to a counselor can help when emotions are closely tied to the desire to eat.

You're born with natural hunger signals that tell you when to start eating and fullness signals that tell you when to stop, based on your body's caloric needs. Unfortunately, too many external signals and a limitless amount of food have made it difficult to tune in to your hunger level. By assessing your hunger before eating, you can learn how to regulate the amount of food you eat every day.

Why Do You Eat When You're Not Actually Hungry?

You're using food to cope with stress. You know the scenario. A big project is due at work, the pressure is building, and you reach for a bag of chips to cope. Stress can influence your eating. It's almost as if the stress pulls

you toward food; your body craves food to feel better and forces you to eat more.

Spark Solution: Soothe yourself with other activities—listen to music, read a good book, go for a walk, do a craft, go fishing, meditate, or connect with a friend. Another way to cope is to reduce the stressful situation. Think about ways to change the event or lessen your response. Don't procrastinate on responsibilities, but limit your exposure to people who create stress in your life, change your thoughts regarding events that cause stress, and practice relaxation techniques.

You suffer from clean-plate syndrome. Does your mom's voice resonate in your head with phrases from your childhood, such as "No dessert, young lady, unless you eat everything on your plate"? The good old clean-plate club can have devastating effects on your eating habits. Remember, only you can assess your hunger and fullness level; neither other people nor the sight of food on a plate should cause you to keep eating.

Spark Solution: For the next two weeks, leave on your plate at least one bite of every food you were consuming. Let your brain and belly reconnect as you eat based on your hunger level, not the fact that food is still on your plate.

You can't resist free (or cheap) food. The family-size bags of chips are on sale this week. For just another dollar, you can add a side to your meal. Supersize those fries for a mere twenty-five cents. Talk about temptations at every turn. Who doesn't want the best deal on food? However, the food that's cheap is seldom the food we should be eating regularly.

Spark Solution: Resist cheap food in three steps. First, shop with a list and only buy foods on sale if they also benefit your health. Second, before going out to eat, read the menu online or create a mental plan of what you want to eat to avoid impulsive ordering. Third, when free food is offered, just say no or stick to a single bite. Enjoy the bite, then decide if having a larger portion is worth the extra calories.

You eat by the clock. It's lunchtime, but you're not hungry. Should you eat anyway? You know it's important to assess your hunger and eat according to how you feel. You also know that skipping a meal can bring about excessive hunger in the afternoon and result in a bingeing frenzy.

Spark Solution: Don't indulge in a complete meal when you really aren't that hungry. Instead, have a sensible snack to tide you over. If you're hun-

gry later, you can always finish the food you had planned to eat for lunch and still keep the bingeing at bay.

You can't say no to food pushers. At the office you hear, "Come on. It's Sandy's birthday. You must have a piece of cake." At the neighborhood party you're told, "It's a family recipe. Let me know what you think." At home, work, and social gatherings, are you surrounded by people pushing food? While some may be unaware of your weight-loss commitment, others may be trying to comfort you with foods. Still others may be jealous of your success, not wanting you to succeed or testing your determination.

Spark Solution: Be polite yet firm with people. Stand up for yourself and refuse the foods offered. Be upfront with folks. Let them know you're trying to lose weight or tell them your doctor has you on a special diet. After a few polite refusals, most people will get the message and quit pestering you. Above all, ask for their support and continued encouragement, which may give them ideas about how they can truly help you in your effort.

You eat when you're bored. Have you wired your brain to use food as a coping method for boredom? Many adults report reaching for food when they're bored and have nothing to do.

Spark Solution: Keep your brain entertained by rediscovering the simple pleasures in life or taking time to explore a new opportunity—a skill, craft, or hobby. Go fishing; shoot hoops; practice putting or chipping; learn to play the keyboard; take up knitting, crocheting, scrapbooking, or photography; visit a museum; or study a new language.

You eat because you're tired. Inadequate sleep alters the levels of the hormones that regulate hunger and satiety. Therefore, being sleep deprived results in increased food cravings, especially for foods high in sugar, fat, and carbohydrates, such as doughnuts and pastries.

Spark Solution: Aim for at least seven to eight hours of sleep nightly. Even if you get that much sleep, do you still notice feeling tired and lethargic during the day? Does your sleep partner report that you snore heavily or sound as if you're gasping for breath? If so, make an appointment with your doctor and discuss the need for a sleep assessment.

You eat on special occasions. Nowadays food is served everywhere—sporting events, weddings, parties, church socials, and more. Those innocent little nibbles and tastes from the buffet line and bar can tally up to hundreds, even thousands, of unplanned calories.

Spark Solution: Rely on calorie banking to get you through. "Save" a few calories from other meals during the day, or even earlier in the week, to "spend" at the special occasion. If you usually plan on about 500 calories for an evening meal, and you skip your snacks and eat at the low end of your calorie range for a few days, your calorie bank may amount to 1,000. Plan how you're going to spend those calories throughout the occasion. Though you may end up over for that day, your weekly average will be right on target for your weight-loss plan.

You eat because you're staring at a screen. Here is the equation, plain and simple: TV or computer screen plus food or caloric beverage equals unconscious and uncontrolled eating. It happens with every type of screen and can occur for hours throughout the day. Think of the amount of minutes or hours you spend eating or drinking while watching TV, tied to your computer, or using your tablet or smartphone, playing, typing, and texting.

Spark Solution: Establish two rules. First, no food or caloric beverage is allowed while using any device with a screen. If this brings about the shakes from withdrawal, formulate a plan to wean yourself off the habit over the next several weeks. Second, no more than two hours of pleasure (non-work-related) screen time daily. Think about it. When you're sitting at a screen, the rest of your body is inactive. No NEAT minutes here!

You eat out of habit. Does your morning drive to the office have you stopping at the doughnut shop and picking up a cream-filled goodie or two? Does your afternoon walk take you past the vending machine for a chocolate bar? If your day is filled with these types of habitual food adventures, it's time to reroute your routine.

Spark Solution: By reshaping your environment and making gradual step-by-step changes in your behavior, you can completely avoid some of the food distractions that derail and destroy your diet. You may need to restructure your drive to work, take a different walking path, reorganize your kitchen, or alter your desk area. The less contact you have with food during the day, the more successful you'll be.

The path to healthy living is different for all of us. The key to success is to not let bumps in the road slow you down for long. Let's examine some of the most common setbacks and how to move past them.

Defend Yourself Against Diet Saboteurs

One of the reasons SparkPeople relies so heavily on community support for weight-loss success is that, in addition to being a fun way to stay motivated, losing weight and getting healthy can be very isolating experiences for many people. Often, you're the only person in your family or social circle who needs to or, more likely, wants to improve your health. While you—and we—know what you're doing is a great thing, others in your life might not be so excited.

Perhaps you're gung ho about these healthier recipes from Chef Meg, but your husband is bringing home greasy barbecue ribs, fried potatoes, and corn dripping in butter. We hear this often on the SparkPeople message boards. Members are desperately searching for ways to get their significant others, families, and close friends on board.

Why do people around you challenge you when you're trying to get healthy? We're creatures of habit. You're trying to change and build lifelong healthy habits; those around you want to stay in their comfort zone. It usually elicits one of three responses:

They feel guilty. You're shaping up and your partner or best friend is not. If you return to the status quo, they don't have to worry about their own weight or health.

They miss the old you. Food has a way of uniting us. If you're blowing off happy hour for the gym or skipping pizza and getting a salad at the monthly meet-up, your loved one might worry that he or she is losing you.

They don't get it. Say your sister has been thin all her life. She likely has no idea what you're going through. She doesn't understand what it's like to be mindful of your eating and exercise.

So how do you deal?

Don't assume the worst. Unless you're surrounded by mean-spirited personalities or frenemies, most people aren't out to get you. Sharing unhealthy food with you or encouraging you to skip the gym to go to the movies is likely a way to spend more time with you, not to get you to gain weight.

Also, start by talking. Have a heart-to-heart talk about why these new habits are important to you. Discuss how these actions can improve every-

one's health, weight, and energy level. Showing concern for your loved one's health can help break down the barriers and get everyone in the household on the road to better health. Discussing ways to include favorite family recipes along with the new recipes can also help you get an unwilling spouse on board.

Sometimes your partner just refuses to be supportive and wants no part of the program. This is your partner's right, and you need to show respect, but it doesn't mean you need to give in and become a short-order cook, preparing two separate meals night after night. Plan the healthier meals most nights and include your partner's old favorites from time to time. Cook the food, serve the food, smile, and enjoy the food. If the other adults in the family are not happy with the food served, they can make their own food. Yes, this sounds harsh, but your first job is to take care of yourself, your body, and your health.

Find Support Elsewhere

Most people do better when there is someone they can turn to when the going gets rough or they just need that little inspiring boost. One-third of our success stories found someone they could talk to about their new habits during the first two weeks. While you may assume your significant other or spouse will naturally become your weight-loss support person, it doesn't necessarily have to be this way.

Think about the people with whom you have daily or weekly contact: your best friend, your yoga teacher, your mother, or your brother. Ask yourself these questions to determine if the person you have in mind would make a good cheerleader, so to speak:

- Will it be easy for me to talk to this person about my weight?
- Is this person truly interested in helping me improve my health?
- Will this person understand the struggle of losing weight?
- Will this person become jealous if I lose weight?
- Does this person ever try to force me to eat foods I don't want?
- Can I talk to this person about my weight even during difficult times?

Once you have identified your cheerleader, talk to that person. Be as specific as possible regarding how he or she can help. Do you want to be praised? Do you want to be scolded? Do you want the partner to assist you with your weekly weigh-in? Would you like someone to exercise with you? You might want to find a cheerleader who's also actively losing weight. This can work well, as long as it's a supportive environment for both of you and not a competition.

Erin encountered diet saboteurs after she reached her initial goal weight, after she had lost the 100 pounds she'd aimed to lose. It had seemed like such a lofty goal, that 100 pounds, but she reached it. Then she decided to lose a bit more, and that's when people started offering her treats, criticizing her decisions, and telling her to stop losing weight.

"Everyone around me is telling me that I should stop losing weight now, but I disagree," she wrote in 2010. "I do have some areas that I would like to improve, but the problem is that when I tell people, they roll their eyes."

Though her weight was well within the healthy range, loved ones accused her of starving herself, which hurt her to hear after she had spent so much time overcoming binge eating. Eventually, she was able to convey her feelings about her body and her weight loss, and today she is at peace with her body and those around her.

Pop Quiz: A Pound of Fat Versus Muscle

True or false? A pound of fat weighs more than a pound of muscle.

False. A pound of fat, a pound of feathers, a pound of lead, a pound of muscle—they all weigh the same amount. Sixteen ounces equals a pound.

The volume is what's different. A pound of fat takes up more space in the body than a pound of muscle. Picture the fat on a piece of chicken. It doesn't really have a defined shape, and it's tucked into nooks and crannies all over the surface. Compare that to muscle tissue, which is dense and compact.

So, while a pound of fat weighs the same as a pound of muscle, the fat takes up more space in your body while the muscle is compact and tight, taking up less space.

This explains why your scale hasn't budged but your jeans feel looser. You are burning fat and gaining muscle, so don't feel discouraged.

No More "Bad" Foods, No More Cheating

If you feel the desire to cheat on your diet, it may not be your fault. Your view of how you "should" or "need to" eat to lose weight or be healthier is the real culprit. We hope that in the last two weeks we've helped you realize that there is no such thing as a bad or a good food.

Try these strategies to bring your eating habits back to normal. First, remember that all foods can fit. No single food causes weight gain. There is no such thing as good food or bad food. Your weight loss is based on your total calorie intake, not the severe restriction of certain ingredients, foods, or food groups. All foods can fit into a healthy eating plan. Instead of thinking about foods as being good or bad, change your food vocabulary.

Don't say, "This is a bad food." Say, "Wow! This food has lots of calories; therefore, I'll have a small piece."

Don't say, "I cheated." Say, "I ate more than I planned to eat today, but by saving some calories during the next few days, my weekly average intake will still be within my calorie range."

Also, start to incorporate small portions of foods you feel are bad (think potato chips, cake, or soda). Measure the food, then sit down, take your time, and savor every bite while eating. There should be no guilt. You are in control of the food; the food is not controlling you. Studies, including one in 2004 and another in 2005 in the *International Journal of Eating Disorders,* have found that restricting foods ultimately backfires and leads to overeating. Researchers have also found that creating arbitrary food restrictions and rules can increase feelings of guilt, anxiety, and depression, and according to a 2007 study in the journal *Appetite* it can negatively impact body image.

The Importance of Rewarding Yourself

The Spark Solution takes a positive approach to weight loss and healthy living. As part of that can-do attitude, we encourage people to focus on what they can do and what they've done, not how far they have to go or what they can't do. Beating yourself up only leads to more self-loathing

and unhealthy choices, so that's why we're doing things differently this time. We're setting goals and keeping our eyes on the prize: a healthier weight, a stronger body, and a happier you.

We approach goals from a position of possibility. Find ways to use regular rewards to pat yourself on the back and give a word of encouragement. Instead of focusing on what you do wrong, try paying more attention to what you do right. While straight talk and brutal honesty are often good for getting your butt moving, for sustained motivation a more positive approach will keep you from burning out.

Rewards create a feeling of doing something you want to do, not just what you're forcing yourself to do. Even the smallest of rewards can work wonders as you travel from milestone to milestone, pound to pound, and goal to goal. Stacey from Arizona has rewarded herself throughout her 97-pound weight loss. To her, rewards "help you see that hard work is worth the effort." She gave herself a heart-rate monitor to keep tabs on her workouts and new exercise clothes to help her feel more confident. She also gave herself a more permanent reward, a tattoo written in Latin that translates as "she flies with her own wings."

"It was a meaningful saying to me after I achieved several of my weight-loss and fitness goals, because I felt as though I could do anything and I could do it all by myself," she says. "Seeing the tattoo on a daily basis is a constant reminder to me that I am powerful and can do anything I set my mind to, and nothing will stand in my way."

Here's how to set up your own rewards system:

- Decide how often you'll reward yourself and with what. Some people reward themselves for every 10 or 20 pounds lost, while others count the weeks or months they've stuck with the program. You can also reward yourself for non-weight-related achievements, such as drinking eight 8-ounce glasses of water a day, going a certain amount of time without smoking, or not bingeing for a set period.

- Choose rewards that matter and are useful. Sometimes the best rewards are those you can't buy. Consider a hot bath, a new book from the library, or a night to relax on the couch and do nothing, as well as tangible rewards like new clothes, shoes, and jewelry. Pick rewards that matter to you and fit within your budget.

- Set small and big rewards. A lot of small rewards, used for meeting smaller goals, are more effective than relying solely on the bigger rewards that require more work and more time.

- Don't use food as a reward, even if it's nutritious food. It's too much of a slippery slope and reinforces negative behavior and that good-food-versus-bad-food mentality.

- Plan to celebrate. Figure out now how you're going to celebrate reaching your ultimate health, fitness, or nutrition goal. Involve other people. Tell them about it. Create a celebration you can anticipate and then keep it within sight all the time.

- Be honest with yourself. Over- or underestimating the numbers or "borrowing" against the next reward hurts the ultimate goal of building a new life habit. Remember to keep your focus on building a habit, not just figuring out how to get the reward.

We asked our success stories how they rewarded themselves. Almost 40 percent rewarded themselves within the first two weeks, and most of them continue to reward themselves today. What was interesting to note was that the rewards themselves actually feed into the virtuous cycle. Rather than reward themselves with a cheat day or a binge (two tactics that backfire and should be avoided), they reward themselves with things that make healthy living easier and fun:

- "A massage. I used to be too embarrassed by my body to get one."

- "I don't really reward as much as I contribute to my own success. I allow myself to spend money on good workout clothes, shoes, and music for my iPod. I think it's important because it reinforces that your habits and hobbies are good ones."

- "Wearing tighter clothes and makeup and allowing myself to feel confident."

- "I like to buy new workout equipment or DVDs, not only as a reward but as a way to stay focused on fitness and staying healthy. I think rewarding yourself is important because it helps you to acknowledge the hard work you have done, as well as creating a goal and reward system so that you are more likely to stay on track. "

- "My most memorable reward was our trip to Key West. I wore a bikini!"
- "Now that I've had to work hard to get my body back, it's so much more rewarding to see what I've done. Purchased rewards really pale in comparison to seeing my hard work pay off."
- "New jeans!"
- "I reward myself every 10 pounds with new clothes or workout gear."

> The best advice: "Don't reward yourself with food. You're not a dog. Exercise isn't the trick for a reward. It's the life source for energy!"
>
> —Shelly, 30 pounds lost

Here are some other good rewards to get you started:

- Compliment yourself. Write down what you would say to anyone else who accomplished what you did.
- Take a vacation or weekend getaway.
- Put one dollar in a jar every time you meet a goal. Use the money for something fun when you reach your ultimate goal.
- Create a scrapbook with mementos from your accomplishments.
- See a movie.
- Make a grab bag of little prizes—bottles of nail polish, gift cards, new pens. When you reach a significant goal, reach in and get your reward.
- Go for a spa treatment or massage.
- Buy yourself a gift certificate.
- Subscribe to a magazine you always wanted.
- Go canoeing or do something in nature.
- Watch your favorite TV show.
- Buy something for your hobby.
- Read a funny book.

- Find time to be by yourself.
- Pay someone to do the yard work or house cleaning this week.
- Fly a kite.

Dealing with the Dreaded Plateaus

If you've been exercising and cutting calories for several weeks, and you're no longer seeing the same results you experienced in the beginning, then you've probably hit a plateau. This occurs when your progress comes to a standstill and can be described as not making any gains (such as improving your fitness level or losing weight) but not necessarily moving backwards (losing endurance or gaining weight).

While a rare few of our success stories hit plateaus early on, 72 percent lost steadily for at least two months. Another 11 percent didn't hit a plateau for at least six weeks.

And how did they bust through it and still remain positive?

- "Switch up your workouts: the type of workout, intensity, and duration. You will be back to losing weight in no time!" —Marie, 80 pounds lost

Ten Steps to Meeting Your Goals

1. Start small.
2. Get it on paper.
3. Focus on everyday habits.
4. Surround yourself with reminders.
5. Be consistent.
6. Keep learning about healthy living.
7. Share your goals with others.
8. Allow for setbacks.
9. Trust your plan.
10. Have fun!

- "When you hit a plateau, don't give up. Losing weight can be a lot of trial and error. Try eating fewer calories, exercising more, changing your workout days, or just try a completely new exercise. This is a lifestyle change, not a temporary fix. Challenge yourself, make goals, and find non-food-related rewards for goals you have reached. Have fun with it, and enjoy the changes that you are making towards being a happier and healthier you." —Amanda, 137 pounds lost

- "Take the focus off of everything you're not. You may not be perfect and super skinny. Focus instead on what you are. You are a strong person who wants to make a change. Challenge yourself to become better. Stop comparing yourself to others and start comparing yourself to yourself, and continually seek improvement." —Lisa, 83 pounds lost

- "If you've been stuck at a certain weight for a period of time, take a look at your food journal for the last few weeks or months. Have you been 'treating' yourself more than usual? Are your exercise minutes where they should be? Use the data from when you were losing weight to compare with what you're currently doing to see if [and] how you've gone off track. And then tweak as needed to start losing weight again." —Penny, 20 pounds lost

- "Typically a plateau for me happens when life gets so busy I quit paying attention, neglect counting calories, and don't exercise intentionally. During this time, I often don't eat enough for my body to burn additional calories and so it holds tight to the calories I already have. This is when I do what I can to survive the stress and then hop back on the wagon, counting my calories and working out intentionally. As I begin to pay attention and shake it up a bit, the pounds start coming off." —Rachel, 30 pounds lost

- "Make changes to your workout routine every few weeks. Little changes will matter: three sets of ten rather than two sets of twelve. Speed it up. Slow it down. Circuit train. Lighter weight for fifteen sets of five. The list is endless. Try each new routine for two to four weeks and switch it up. Your body won't get used to it and will be less likely to plateau." —Anonymous, 56 pounds lost

- "Make up your mind that you are going to be successful. Refuse to give up even when results are slow or nonexistent. You are getting stronger and the results will come. Be patient with yourself; the weight didn't appear overnight and it won't disappear overnight, but you can become a healthier you if you stay focused and don't give up. You are so worth the effort!" —Debbie, 92 pounds lost

Because every individual is unique, there's no way to actually predict when a plateau might happen, but we can look at nutrition, rest, and variation and how these jump-start your body, mind, and metabolism.

Eat the Right Nutrients at the Right Times

Make sure you're following your Spark Solution meal and fitness plan correctly. Are you eating 1,500 calories a day? Are you doing all your workouts? Are you eating all your meals and snacks, and drinking your milk? This is very important, so you don't eat too little for your body's needs, which can actually hinder your weight loss. In addition, track everything you eat, including the tastes taken while you cook and the nibbles from others' plates.

After a workout, remember to refuel with a balanced snack or meal within thirty minutes to two hours. Don't "save" your calories or wait to eat a snack. Your body needs those calories—a combo of carbs and protein—after you exercise.

And don't overlook your huge need for water. Hydration is very important for stable energy levels. You store three times as much water as energy (in the form of glycogen). Plus, hydration promotes muscle building, which powers your metabolism, while dehydration promotes muscle breakdown. So, drink up—before, during, and after your workout sessions. If you're exercising regularly or in a hot, humid climate, you might need more than eight 8-ounce glasses a day. Don't wait until you're thirsty to drink water.

Rest Is Important

Alternate your cardio and strength-training sessions, to allow for muscle repair. During a strength-training session, tiny tears occur in your muscle

fibers, which cause the soreness that lasts for a couple of days. (It's called delayed-onset muscle soreness, or DOMS.) For those tiny tears to repair themselves and rebuild your muscles stronger than before, your muscles need rest. Skip your rest days and you'll get weaker, leading to a plateau. (The "Fit to Live" chapter, page 327, further explains all you need to know about fitness.)

Active recovery is another way to rest your muscles. Research shows that engaging in lower intensity exercise after a strenuous workout session may be more beneficial than resting completely. There are two types of active recovery. The first is the typical cool down phase you perform at the end of your workout. Properly cooling down has been shown to help your muscles recover faster. The second type involves fitting in your NEAT minutes. In addition to helping your muscles rebound, active recovery also enhances relaxation and psychological recovery.

Make sure to get plenty of sleep too. A significant amount of muscle repair occurs during sleep. Skimp on shut-eye and you'll hinder your ability to recover from exercise, making plateaus more likely. We recommend getting seven to eight hours per night, both during the week and on weekends. If you're exercising intensely, with long workouts most days of the week, or training for an event such as a marathon, you might need more sleep.

Add Variety to Your Workouts

Incorporate variation into each workout. This concept should be applied to both cardio and strength training. Variety is critical because your muscles become very efficient at the exercises they are accustomed to doing. Switching things up or doing something radically different during each workout session is more challenging to your muscles.

Someone who does the same exercises will usually plateau sooner than someone who continually makes changes. If you don't feel comfortable doing a different workout each time you hit the gym, try to change your exercise routine at least every six to eight weeks. Changing your routine, as we discussed, is crucial to keeping your body's muscles surprised. They'll have to work harder, you'll be challenged, and you'll burn more calories and build more lean muscle in the process.

Skimp on Salt

Diets that rely heavily on frozen meals and canned or boxed foods are often quite high in sodium. And while sodium really has very little to do with actual weight loss, it is closely tied to overall health and well-being. Keeping salt in check is imperative to lowering blood pressure and risk of heart disease. Eating too much can cause puffy, swollen hands and feet, water retention, and bloating, which can artificially inflate the number you see on the scale and prevent you from fitting into your favorite jeans. Because our meal plan avoids highly processed foods, which we've already told you don't boost your metabolism the way whole foods do, you will have no trouble consuming less than 2,300 milligrams of sodium daily, which is the upper limit for healthy adults, according to USDA recommendations.

> "I don't use a salt shaker anymore. I keep salt in a container and use a measuring spoon when I do add salt. It keeps me aware of how much salt I am consuming."
> —*Barbara, 41 pounds lost*

For some of us (especially women), having a higher salt or sodium intake can lead to weight gain, water retention, and puffiness in the face, hands, ankles, and feet. Don't panic. Your body will return to normal in about three to four days. In the meantime:

- *Don't take any diuretics without a doctor's order.*
- *Remember there are no special foods or supplements to help remove the extra fluid from your body.*
- *Don't drink more water with the notion that it will "flush" the excess sodium from your body more quickly, but continue to drink at least eight 8-ounce glasses daily.*

If after three to four days the swelling does not decrease or continues to worsen, seek immediate medical attention if any of the following applies to you: you are continuing to gain weight daily, are on a doctor's prescribed diuretic, or have a history of heart disease, diabetes, congestive heart failure, or kidney disease.

Nutrition, rest, and variation all work closely together. When not followed properly, they can have a snowball effect: Repeating the same exercises can cause overtraining, which leads to plateaus and an inability to sleep. Lack of rest then impedes your progress, making recovery take much longer, especially if you're not well nourished and hydrated.

The human body is amazingly adaptable. By making a few changes in these areas, you can jump-start your routine and see those positive results in no time.

Tips from Successful SparkPeople Members to Help You Stay Strong

When your motivation starts to wane, read one of these tips from people who've been in your shoes—and walked many a mile to drop the weight and keep it off.

- "I switched to whole grains, switched from whole to skim milk, eliminated soda from my diet, planned all my meals and tracked my food, and quit eating out at restaurants. Making these changes to my lifestyle helped me to feel much more in control of my life." —Amber, 42 pounds lost

- "I chose for myself not to have weight-loss surgery because it is stomach surgery, not brain surgery. I am an emotional eater. When I went to the classes to prepare for possible surgery, I realized that everyone there still had the same mind-set: they were hungry. They complained about wanting to continue to eat after being full, craving things they knew were unhealthy choices, and not wanting to exercise. I was already there. That's when I told myself that having my stomach cut open wouldn't fix my problem." —Beth, 235 pounds lost

- "My hunger factor was huge in the beginning, and it was tough not to just give up and start eating more. The encouraging thing was that it did get easier every day and seeing big losses in the beginning was very motivating." —Kristina, 92 pounds lost

- "I feel better when I eat a balanced, clean diet. I educated myself on the difference between simple carbs and complex (smart) carbs, good fats versus bad fats, etc. I think ignorance is bliss. If you don't know exactly what is in the things you are eating, then you can make excuses for yourself, but you won't see the same results." —Marissa, 90 pounds lost

- "Initially I wanted to lose weight because I didn't want my grandson to remember me as a fat old lady who couldn't do anything. Losing the weight has given me a whole new life. I have gone from being morbidly obese and sedentary to a fit, active person. It's been a complete lifestyle change and transformation, inside and out." —Denise, 57 pounds lost

- "I started running nine months into my weight-loss journey. I could barely run a third of a mile without becoming totally exhausted and walking the rest of the way. I decided to work on increasing my distance. My number one fitness milestone is the first time I ran a mile without stopping. I felt so accomplished and excited! I cried with joy and pride right there on the trail." —Elicia, 92 pounds lost

- "Being a night owl, but working an early shift, makes it hard. But I do put a big focus on getting to bed early enough to get at least seven hours of sleep each night. I can tell a big difference in how I feel when I get enough sleep, so that is motivation enough to keep working at it." —Emily, 30 pounds lost

- "No secrets. What they've always said is true. It's all about hard work, exercise, healthy food choices, a support system, and your drive to succeed. Be sure to measure everything you put in your mouth. If you track your intake (food in) and output (exercise), you will lose much more weight." —Marie, 30 pounds lost

- "You are stronger than you think you are. When I first realized how heavy I had become, I sat down and sobbed. Once I dried my tears, I had an epiphany: I am not a victim. If I don't like how I look in pictures or what the scale says, I can change it. I am strong and have the power to change myself. This was extremely motivating to me." —Michelle, 103 pounds lost

- "Don't set impossible weight-loss goals. It will lead to frustration and certain failure. Make your goal a reasonable one, and once you reach it, then set another." —Tammy, 100 pounds lost

- "Exercise often and eat smaller food portions. I hated exercise before I started to exercise. I discovered that it can be so much fun. Exercise isn't boring and it isn't difficult. You just have to start slow and keep going. Eating smaller portions is also important. I didn't exactly change what I ate at first. I just ate less of everything. That helped more than anything." —Crystal, 71 pounds lost

- "When I have a craving, I stop and think about what I *really* want. Usually I'm thirsty, so I start with a glass of water. What else do I need? Salt? Tomato sprinkled with salt does the trick. Chocolate? Heat up skim milk and put unsweetened cocoa in it with some no-calorie sweetener." —Kristina, 92 pounds lost

- "I have so much more confidence now than I used to. It shows in the way I deal with everything else in my life. I am confident in the changes I've made. I credit SparkPeople for a lot of what I have accomplished. The resources they placed at my fingers are just wonderful. I stay active on the site." —Lisa, 83 pounds lost

- "Take small steps. We did not become overweight overnight. We are not going to become healthy overnight either. Have patience and keep moving forward. If you slip, pick yourself back up." —Amy, 62 pounds lost

- "I hated being fat. I feel better thin, and I feel better about myself. When I think about eating like I used to, I remember how I hated the way I looked and felt. That always brings me back to my healthy-living plan." —Joyce, 59 pounds lost

- "Always challenge yourself and believe you can rise to the challenge . . . because you can! When you hit your number, you're not done. This is a lifelong journey. Keep challenging yourself. Don't be defined by the numbers, particularly the scale. That's only part of your overall health." —Shelly, 20 pounds lost

- "Living a healthy lifestyle is important to me because I know it can do nothing but help my future. I can see my health has improved by a

few little things. I used to get sick with a cold at least once every month. Now I get sick maybe once or twice a year. I used to get heartburn a few times a day. Now I can't even remember the last time I had heartburn. Things like this show me that I've made real changes. When my fiancé and I start a family, I know I'll be able to pass this healthy lifestyle on to them, and have a happy, active, and healthy family." —Erin, 117 pounds lost

- "Don't set unrealistic or impossible short-term goals. It's much better to set attainable intermediate goals that you can celebrate on your way to your big overall goal." —Mikie, 41 pounds lost

- "Don't give up. If you get a ticket for going through a red light, you wouldn't then drive through red lights the rest of the day since you'd already done it once. So just because you eat something you shouldn't, or you skip a workout, doesn't mean your day is ruined or that you can't do this. You can! Always get back up and move forward." —Heidi, 79 pounds lost

- "The biggest thing for me was drinking water. It was easy, and I realized that it wasn't food my body craved but fluid. So not only did the weight come off and stay off, but my hair and skin improved tremendously with all the flushing of the toxic junk I was putting in my body. So not only was the weight coming [off,] making me feel younger and healthier, but I looked younger and healthier too. Start small and add something new every week. In no time you realize how far you have come and how much more you can do." —Ann, 50 pounds lost

- "Don't wait until everything is perfect because it will never be perfect and you will never start. Start today. There is no reason not to." —Christina, 30 pounds lost

- "Start with one or two things that you will commit to doing consistently, then add more as those become easier and more of a habit. Trying to change your whole lifestyle all at once is difficult, but changing one or two things is not as intimidating. Building positive momentum is essential to success." —Denise, 57 pounds lost

- "Really take the time to think about why you want to lose weight and write it down. You have to be doing this for the right reasons;

otherwise, it won't happen. Whenever I'm losing motivation, I return to my list to remind myself why I want to lose weight. I also add to my list over time as new things come up." —Layla, 31 pounds lost

- "Getting fit comes from changing the way you live. It's not a temporary behavior. Start small and build your foundation. Figure out what works for you. It may not be what works for someone else. Don't go it alone. Get support from friends, family, coworkers, and Spark-People members." —Diana, 68 pounds lost

- "Realize that making time for yourself is not the same as being a selfish person." —Una, 31 pounds lost

- "Don't think about the past or the future. Just think about *now*. Do what is good for you in this moment and remember that every good thing you do for yourself, whether it is eating well or moving more, is a step in the right direction, a step towards good health." —Lisa-Marie, 94 pounds lost

- "Everyone's bodies are different. What works for someone else may not work for you. And what worked for you before may not work for you now. The key is to find what your body needs and then start slow and steady with a sustainable plan. Also, find ways to overcome discouragement. There will be setbacks and plateaus. If you find a way to keep motivated through those times, the reward is worth it!" —Heidi, 58 pounds lost

- "Plan ahead as much as you can. Before I go to bed, I know when I'll be exercising the next day, what my three meals will be, with a few hundred calories of snacking leeway, and what my calories consumed [versus] burned will be. Having that knowledge makes me feel so accountable to myself and empowered, because I never have to scramble to meet my daily health goals." —Madeleine, 46 pounds lost

- "Never think you can lose weight quickly and keep it off. Start slow and find out what worked for others. Always reward yourself for your accomplishments, whether it is eating right, or getting five minutes more of exercise than you did before. It is important to remember that you can have things you enjoy occasionally, or you will not stick with it if you feel deprived. Always remember when you feel

discouraged that we all slip up. Just go forward and leave the past behind. We all hit plateaus. It is your body adjusting to the new you." —Bonnie, 50 pounds lost

- "Remind yourself from the beginning that it will not happen overnight, but imagine what you will look like and how you will feel in two weeks, a month, three months, six months, a year, if you are consistent. Then compare that new version of yourself to the image you have if you change nothing. The 'me' I saw if I made no changes was not a happy person. It was scary. That kept me focused on being consistent." —Kristi, 30 pounds lost

Monitor Your Medication

As you well know, weight can affect your health in all sorts of ways. Each time you shed a few pounds, if you take regular medication, you'll need to speak with your doctor about adjusting your dosage, which is determined by body weight. Losing even five pounds can affect how your body metabolizes medication and can lead to serious side effects. However, it is important that you don't make changes to your medication on your own. Let your doctor know that you are beginning a weight-loss program. Ask the doctor how often to check in during your weight-loss journey, and keep those appointments even if you feel better than ever.

Your doctor should know about your weight-loss goals even if you are not on medication, but if you are on medication for any of the following ailments, you will need closer monitoring:

- Depression or anxiety
- Diabetes
- GERD (gastroesophageal reflux disease) or other digestive issues
- Hyperlipidemia (high cholesterol)
- Hypertension (high blood pressure)
- Hypothyroidism

Motivation and Momentum

At age twenty-three, Julia was fed up. She weighed 282 pounds. She didn't like herself very much and, frankly, she didn't like others very much either. Though she was a talented photographer with a B.F.A. degree, she worked as a receptionist and sat all day long. She yearned for a life that fulfilled her, but her weight held her back.

"I am not happy with myself," she wrote in her blog in 2007. "I am tired of comparing myself to other people, and I am always the biggest girl in the room. So I am going to make a change."

She set a New Year's resolution to lose weight. Five days in, she was working out every day and hating it, but sticking with it and staying motivated. She was eating right, drinking water, and reading everything she could on SparkPeople. "Having support from others really seems to help," she wrote. "This website has been helping big time!"

Two weeks in, something major happened: Julia stopped avoiding the mirror, which had been her "biggest hardship" and decided to start loving herself again. *You're worth taking care of,* she told herself. *I really need to learn to love myself and stop treating myself like the enemy.*

Fast-forward to the present. She has lost 125 pounds, married her boyfriend of four years, and kept her promise to herself. "Now, thanks to my confidence, I am so friendly," she says, "and I have so many amazing friends in my life." She quit her receptionist gig and now balances two jobs, at a health food store and at an online book business, which requires her to lift heavy boxes all day long. She loves it! She also bike commutes, runs marathons, and works out for fun. Plus, she built the confidence to start taking photos again.

Recently a new doctor, unaware of her weight loss, confirmed that she's in stellar shape. "You must work out a lot," the doctor said as she listened to Julia's heart. "Your resting heart rate is super low." Julia beamed.

After four years, numbers no longer motivate Julia. Nor do inches, though she is maintaining her weight loss while continuing to gain strength and challenge herself. "What matters is that I feel good about myself. That I feel good—period."

Stacey noticed the same side effects of weight loss after dropping 97 pounds. "What started out as a goal to just 'get skinny' has turned into a desire to be the best and healthiest, happiest, fittest version of me possible," she says. Now thirty, she's been known to dance in the grocery store, and she's no longer afraid to head outside and enjoy the beauty of the Arizona desert where she lives. "Being healthy matters to me because I've seen the other side of life, and what being unhealthy is like," she says. "Any day of the week, I choose healthy. Healthy to me means happiness, longevity, confidence, and satisfaction. The option of being unhealthy is no longer on the table."

For those who lose weight and keep it off, weight loss becomes less about aesthetics and more about health. In our 2010 survey, 87 percent of our active members said they set out to get healthier, not skinnier, and 78 percent wanted to feel better about themselves.

Losing weight has a trickle-down effect, changing other areas of your life as well. You become more confident, which gives you the strength to make other changes. You have the energy to start conquering other areas of your life. Wendy (45 pounds lost) earned an M.B.A. Paula (125 pounds lost) says her dating life has "never been better." Denise (57 pounds lost) joined a co-ed softball team for the first time, at age fifty-seven.

As we said in the introduction, you make one healthy decision, which leads to another healthy decision and another and . . . you get the picture. Gone is the vicious cycle of dieting and guilt. In its place is a virtuous cycle of healthy living.

As the weight starts to come off, amazing changes happen. You start to trust yourself again. Sure, your pants might feel looser and you notice muscles you haven't seen in years, but there's more. Losing even 10 percent of your body weight (for a 200-pound person, that's 20 pounds) can have remarkable benefits, and that's another secret of super successful dieters:

they started with a goal of losing 10 percent or less, then upped their goal as the weight came off.

What will losing 10 percent of your body weight do for you?

- Improve your blood pressure

- Improve your heart health and lower your cholesterol levels

- Decrease your risk of developing diabetes

- Enhance your sex life

- Help you get a better night's sleep, for those with obstructive sleep apnea

- Reduce the pain associated with arthritis or joint disease

- Reduce lower back pain

- Improve your breathing

- Decrease your risk of developing colon and breast cancer

- Improve the health of your gallbladder

- Give you more energy

Let's learn more about how losing just 10 percent can impact your health from another of SparkPeople's experts, Dr. Birdie Varnedore, a neurologist, a mother of five, and one of SparkPeople's greatest success stories. Dr. Birdie lost 140 pounds, and her husband, Nick, lost 120. She appeared on the cover of a national magazine in a bikini and on a national morning show. She attributes much of her success to SparkPeople and uses it as a tool for her patients who have been affected by the potentially life-threatening consequences of obesity. She has written for SparkPeople's expert blog, DailySpark.com. Here's her best advice, as someone who knows firsthand how daunting it can be to set weight-loss goals:

> Many of you are just two weeks into a new lifestyle. Welcome! I'm sure you have an abundance of motivation and willpower, and I hope you use this powerful force to learn and integrate the Spark Solution principles early and successfully. Many of you are recommitting to your goals. You might be struggling to find your way back to consistency

and balance. Kudos to you for never giving up and for accepting that we are in it to win it!

Whether you're new to SparkPeople or a veteran, some of you may be feeling burned out and thinking about giving up. We are here to look for a "spark" that will start a fire. I hope you will decide not to take a break and will keep working until you find success.

Let's back up a bit and ask ourselves this question: Why lose weight? While your reasons for losing weight and maintaining that weight loss are as unique as you are, there are a few reasons many of us share, among them to improve one's health. I know it was on my reasons-to-lose-weight list. If you already carry the diagnosis of an obesity-related medical condition, such as high cholesterol, hypertension, or diabetes, that knowledge alone can be a great source of motivation and willpower. But what about the relatively healthy overweight person who wants to lose weight for health reasons, but doesn't really know yet what better health means? Losing weight for the sake of your health (as compared with an aesthetic motivation) is a socially acceptable reason to lose weight, but other than doing the right thing, do you know why you added it to the list? Do you know how your health will improve when you lose weight? Do you know how much weight you need to lose to start to improve your health?

When I was 140 pounds heavier, I was faced with the health consequences of uncontrolled yet modifiable risk factors—like obesity—on an almost daily basis. What did I say to myself then? Did I fully understand that I was putting myself at risk? I absolutely did know that I was risking my life by being obese, but like many, I willfully chose to ignore the risks and continued my unhealthy relationship with food.

The same relationship that caused my morbid obesity caused me to remain obese for more than a decade. Occasionally a young obese female who reflected my demographics would come to see me after a stroke or other obesity-related health crisis. I would get shaken up pretty badly for a few days, and I would make promises to myself that I was going to change, but I would slip right back into my carb-induced coma and continue to try to bury my thoughts. I knew I was killing

myself by carrying around more than 100 pounds of excess fat. Even though I was aware of this internal conflict at that time, I used it consistently as fuel for overeating and not changing my lifestyle.

Eventually, being surrounded by so much obesity-related illness, disability, and death, and in conjunction with the burning desire to become a better role model for my children (much less be there for them), I finally used my experience as a physician as fuel to change. I was no longer willing to live a life that was so incongruent in thought and in action. As I think back to the earlier stages of my weight-loss journey, this realization was perhaps one of the most important changes that enabled me to finally lose the weight.

This is just a little insight into how the concept of losing weight for my health shaped my journey. But how do you incorporate wanting to be healthier into your journey? Learning some of the known health benefits of weight loss is a start. The benefits are many, and the good news is that significant benefits can be achieved with only a 10 percent weight loss. For a 200-pound person, that's only 20 pounds! (I'm trying to be positive here—I know that losing 20 pounds is no small feat.)

What can a 10 percent weight loss do for you? A lot, especially if you suffer from lifestyle diseases, such as type 2 diabetes or hypertension.

1. *Are you diabetic? You could see some stabilization and improvement of your blood glucose levels.*

2. *Do you have hypertension? You could see a reduction in your blood pressure.*

3. *Is your cholesterol abnormal? You could see an improvement in your blood lipid levels.*

4. *Regardless of your other health conditions, losing 10 percent of your body weight puts you at a decreased risk of developing heart disease.*

Statistics prove that losing weight and maintaining weight loss are not easy pursuits, so if you lose 10 percent of your body weight, you should be proud of your achievement. You have improved your health. As you

continue to lose, you should continue to see improvement in your health and more. But if you eat and exercise like you did before losing weight, you will gain every pound back and probably more. Maintaining that 10 percent weight loss is only achieved by a permanent lifestyle change.

Congratulations on your continued pursuit of weight loss and your soon-to-be permanent lifestyle change. Even if you have not yet achieved a normal body weight, know that you are improving your health and that your efforts are worth it. If you achieved your weight loss by working on the fundamentals of a true lifestyle modification, and not through fad diets, you are well on your way to breaking free from the negative behaviors that lead to poor health.

Beyond the proven medical benefits, getting to a normal body weight should be your goal—and you can do it. Trusting that you can do it is another side effect of losing weight and building healthy habits. It starts small: you pass by a box of doughnuts without grabbing one, or maybe you have a doughnut, but you feel satisfied with one, not two. Or you find you've lost your taste for doughnuts altogether. All are side effects of healthy living. There might still be times when you have two doughnuts, an extra slice of pizza, or the whole bag of chips, but a single session of overeating won't undo all the healthy decisions you've made.

Beth, one of our most remarkable weight-loss stories, was bedridden at 460 pounds. Having lost 250 pounds, and counting, the Indiana native (known as "Indygirl" on SparkPeople.com) has gained quite a following on the site for her weight loss aphorisms. She overcame binge eating, started to exercise regularly, and almost completely abandoned the wheelchair and walker she relied on for years. She tells herself and others struggling with emotional eating, "One slice of pizza is always going to have less calories than two." And, "If you're going to think 'I may as well,' then you should think 'I may as well *not.*'" Plus, "Having a bad day is like getting a flat tire. You fix it and get back on the road. You don't throw a tantrum and pop the other three tires."

Makes perfect sense, right? These three mantras help her through the tough times, when her motivation wanes despite having the experience and know-how to transform her life.

Motivation is the trickiest part of weight loss. Our emphasis on it is what sets us apart. SparkPeople.com maintains a can-do attitude, and you'll notice that the tone on the site is overwhelmingly positive and encouraging—a marked difference from the rest of the Internet where, cloaked in online anonymity, people type mean things they'd never dare say in real life.

Among the experts SparkPeople works with is behavioral psychology expert Dean Anderson, whose interest in healthy living began more than a decade ago, when he confronted his own morbid obesity and health issues. He joined SparkPeople first as a member, losing 150 pounds and regaining his health. He now writes about motivation for the site. The remainder of this chapter is told from his point of view, from the unique perspective of an expert who has also been in the trenches of obesity and lived to tell the tale:

> Do you often find yourself wondering where your motivation went? Do you suddenly revert back to your "old ways" without really understanding why? If this sounds familiar, you may have some basic misconceptions about motivation—what it is, where it comes from, and what you can do to hang on to it.

> **What Is Motivation?**

> Being motivated doesn't mean that the struggle with opposing desires suddenly ends. It's human nature to pursue both the gratification of our senses (eating what and when we like) and the psychological gratification of achieving meaningful but more abstract goals (being healthy, fit, or attractive). Both of these pursuits are necessary for our survival, as individuals and within groups, and both are worthy of our understanding. Judging one of these pursuits as superior to the other is to deny half of what and who we are, and to set ourselves up for endless inner conflict and turmoil.

> At the same time, we cannot be blind or unthinking about our pursuits. In the realm of eating and food choices, the modern world (and often your own kitchen) is full of well-marketed, tasty foods that appeal to our innate desires (a sweet tooth and a fondness for rich foods) but are also nutritional nightmares. As long as we remain less than perfect, we

will struggle with this conflict between immediate and long-term grati-fication. No amount of motivation will make it go away.

Viewing motivation as the ability to resist the lure of "bad" foods or overcome the appeal of lying on the couch will only lead to frustration and self-blame. Instead, think of motivation as the ability to give your-self the chance to make conscious decisions and take responsibility for these choices. The main enemy of motivation is the tendency to see yourself as a helpless victim.

Your motivation will be as strong as the amount of consciously aware effort you put into making your own decisions, regardless of what those decisions might be. Your motivation will be weak when you con-sider yourself to be helpless against your own urges, feelings, and de-sires, or a victim of circumstances beyond your control.

So, what causes you to lose motivation in the first place? You may start a new nutrition or exercise program with excitement and full force, ready to succeed and reach new goals. What causes enthusiasm to die?

Unrealistic Expectations

When you have your hopes set on one thing (like seeing the number on the scale go down) but something else happens instead (the number doesn't change, or it goes up), of course it's difficult to keep doing what doesn't seem to be working. That's normal, and it's exactly how you're supposed to feel. These feelings help you avoid doing the same thing over and over again, expecting to get different results. But this natural reaction becomes problematic when the result you're hoping for isn't likely to happen, like seeing predictable and consistent changes in your weight every week, or expecting to go from confirmed couch potato to exercise maven by sheer force of will, without paying your dues.

So, if your motivation is lagging because you're not getting the results you expect, check to see whether your expectations are realistic or not. Here is what you should expect when it comes to weight loss:

Weight loss is not orderly or predictable. Shedding pounds is only one of many healthy changes your body undergoes when you de-

crease your caloric intake and/or increase your activity level. A lower number on the scale may be the least important of these changes, even though it may seem to be the most important. Everybody will respond differently. You may lose weight easily and quickly at first while your friend will have to wait weeks or months to lose that first couple of pounds. For others, weight loss may come in waves. All of this is perfectly normal.

Weight loss is not a simple calculation. Your body is a complex, living organism with many needs and priorities to juggle and difficulties to overcome (poor habits and thought patterns). A classic example of this complexity is how the stress you experience when your body doesn't meet your weight-loss expectations actually increases fat storage. There is a connection between your mind and your body. Instead of focusing on the number on your scale, you need to take a comprehensive view of this process of change and work hard to keep your mind from getting in the way.

Focus on what you can control. You will lose weight if you do your part to control what you eat and how much you exercise, and weight loss will probably occur at the expected rate. That's what happened for me, during the eighteen months it took me to lose 150 pounds, a rate of a little more than two pounds a week—the same as we lay out in this book. Those weeks where nothing changed, or I actually went backwards, drove me crazy and sapped my motivation until I finally realized I was focusing on the wrong things. When I started focusing on the small, positive changes I was making in my diet and in my capacity to exercise, life became easier and more rewarding. That, I believe, is our role in this process. The rest is not up to you, and trying to control what you can't control is a prescription for failure.

"You need to tell yourself you can do this. From the start, have realistic expectations. You will not lose 10 pounds in a week. Decide that you will be consistent with tracking and getting in some exercise. When you start to see results—scale moving, feeling better, and clothes getting looser—that will motivate you to keep going."
—Elizabeth, 144 pounds lost

Perfectionism

The idea that anyone can, or should, never overeat or never skip a workout is a form of false pride. Why would anyone think that he or she will be the first human being in history to pull this off, or that if you don't, you must be a miserable failure? The emotional upset of failed perfectionism can make it virtually impossible to stay motivated.

If you're holding yourself to a standard of perfection, or verbally abusing yourself for those bad days, give yourself a break. You must accept the fact that, along with the rest of us, sometimes your human appetites or feelings are going to win out over your good intentions—and it's not that big of a deal. Allow these occasions to teach you more about yourself, so that you can learn to do things differently.

But this learning won't happen if you spend your time and energy obsessing about your slip-ups or getting down on yourself. That kind of useless self-abuse is just a smoke screen you use to avoid your real responsibilities and opportunities. It's the polar opposite of honest self-appraisal, no matter how true or real it might feel to you. These may seem like harsh words, but getting past this problem is critical to success. Trust me, I had to learn this the hard way, and that cost me a lot of painful years and wasted effort. So, save yourself a lot of grief by learning how to keep things in perspective and avoiding unnecessary drama.

"My life is so much better now, and I never want to go back to where I was. That alone is very motivating for me. Of course I slip up. But life happens. There are days when exercising or eating as healthy as you would like to just isn't possible or you just don't feel like it. That is okay. I have changed my life so much, and maintained this lifestyle for over four years, that it would take a conscious effort for me to go back to my old ways. I don't want my old body back." —Erin, 104 pounds lost

Become Your Own Best Motivator

You've learned what motivation really is—taking responsibility for conscious actions—and how to prevent it from waning. To become your own best motivator, you must consistently do two things:

1. *Consciously choose to eat well and exercise as often as you can.* This isn't something you do once or at the beginning of your diet. It's something you have to do at every meal and snack, whenever you're thinking about eating or figuring out what to do with your time. It's a matter of trying to be mindful about what you're doing, instead of mindlessly reacting to your emotions, your circumstances, or your habits and natural predispositions. This can be as simple as taking a second to ask yourself, Is this what I want to do?

2. *When you do something different than what you think you should do, understand that this was also your choice.* This is where things can get a little tricky. Your natural inclination may be to figure out why this happened or, even worse, what's wrong with you that "makes" you do what you don't want to do. This is just the opposite of what you need to do. Simply accept the decision you made as a valid decision made by you. It doesn't matter whether it was right or wrong. Just think of it as a valid decision made under less than ideal circumstances. This will free you to look at the situation as a powerful and capable person. This way, you have the ability to modify the circumstances (in large or small ways), making it easier the next time around to make decisions in line with your intentions. That is the whole point.

Change Your Story, Change Your Results

Motivation is not something you find or lose, have or don't have. It's the product of how you see yourself in the world: active or passive, effective or ineffective, powerful or victimized, normal or pathological. If you want to be able to motivate yourself, you need to begin seeing yourself as active, effective, powerful, and normal.

Many situations can push you strongly in one direction or the other. If you tend to see yourself as a helpless victim, this is probably because at some formative point you were victimized and helpless to prevent it. If you feel powerless to manage your own feelings and soothe yourself, you probably didn't have much help learning how to do that when you were young.

But history is not destiny. From a psychological point of view, emotional "reality" is the product of whatever story you tell yourself about how things are and why you are the way you are. If you want or need to change your reality, then change the story you're telling yourself. This does not mean denying or ignoring your past or present circumstances, or inventing a nice fairy tale to take their places. If you're a single parent with a full-time job, a person with major medical or emotional issues to contend with, or someone who is so large that physical activity is very difficult, this will be harder for you than for some others. You need to acknowledge that and be realistic about the changes you can hope to make and how easily you can make them. But you can rewrite your story so these circumstances are not the determining factor in your success or failure. Your new story can be about how your creativity, ingenuity, and perseverance enable you to find full or partial solutions to these challenges, and how to do the best you can with what you have to work with.

The story you're telling yourself at any moment is the foundation of your motivation, or lack of it. Make sure you're telling yourself the story you need to hear. And the best way to really come to believe your story is to see it come true in the small, well-chosen steps you take every day.

Even in the those first few days, you'll notice a change, thanks to the Spark Solution, just like Rochelle, who's been on the program just a few days:

"SparkPeople has been really helpful with keeping my morale up. I can see myself slowly transitioning toward a better person. I know what my boundaries are, and I know what I need to do to push those boundaries and break down the barriers. All my barriers right now are self-imposed. I am my worst enemy and that's something that must change. Some days I feel like I haven't accomplished anything, but SparkPeople allows me to look back and see all that I have done to get where I am today, and that is definitely something to be proud of. It has only been a few days, but SparkPeople is definitely changing me for the better."

Consistency Equals Success: How to Stay Motivated

To change your life, you have to be consistent, which is easier said than done some days. Follow these three simple rules faithfully to make it

easier for you to be consistent with your healthy lifestyle habits—even on the toughest days.

Being motivated is your choice to make. Motivation is not a tangible object you possess or lack. Not having motivation is not the real problem, unless you really don't want to lose weight or live a healthy lifestyle. As long as you want these things, you have all the motivation you need.

Not wanting to eat your broccoli or work out when you're tired is understandable, but it doesn't mean you're not motivated. It just means you want two different and opposing things, and you have to make a decision. Telling yourself that you lack motivation is just a way of denying you really do have a choice. It makes the problem seem out of your control, and it makes you feel less powerful than you really are.

Acknowledge that the choice is yours to make. You can choose either option, without making excuses or inventing a theory like "lack of motivation" to justify it. Then, pay attention to how you feel about the choice you made and decide whether that is how you want to feel most of the time. Being consistent does not mean being perfect. There are going to be days when you decide to do something other than stick to your exercise and diet routine, and that's fine. But becoming consistent means giving yourself the power to choose.

Build momentum one step at a time. It's never easy to change old habits or start new routines. During those first two weeks—and beyond— you have to work at it pretty diligently, even when you don't feel like it.

Building momentum is the key to consistency in the long term, but getting started is the hardest part. Once you're moving, staying in motion and picking up speed becomes a lot easier. Continue to build on your healthy habits, adding new ones when you're ready and congratulating yourself every step of the way.

If you're stuck and need a push, find someone who knows about your plan and is willing to give you a push when you feel like slacking off. Each time you find yourself thinking about skipping an exercise session or blowing your meal plan, write down the reason for your choice. Share this reason with your cheerleader and get his or her

honest opinion about whether the reason for your choice is reasonable or just an excuse. You'll probably find that this makes it a lot harder for you to believe your own rationalizations.

Always have a plan B. Life is not scripted, so we always need to have a plan B ready, just in case. This will keep you on track when life doesn't go as planned. While you can't foresee every single problem that might come up, most of the time the things that get in your way are things that happen fairly often, like kids getting sick, extra hours at work, or days when you just don't feel very energetic. Those surprises won't throw you off track if you plan ahead. For example, have a friend or family member lined up to stay with your kids so you can make it to the gym, stock your freezer with some healthy meals for when you're short on time, and stash your exercise clothes at the office for a quick workout when you can't get away.

Don't Feed Negative Thoughts

Scientific evidence shows that the life span of any one emotion is only about ninety seconds. After that, we have to reboot that emotion or it goes away. Stepfanie, SparkPeople's editorial director and the coauthor of this book, uses that fact to help her deal with emotions that arise in any area of life:

I've taken that ninety-second life-span fact and combined it with another lesson gleaned from one of my favorite philosophy books to help myself move past rough patches of anxiety, fear, and self-doubt:

1. I acknowledge that I'm having a feeling, such as anxiety, when my to-do list is growing ever longer.

2. I take three deep, long, slow breaths, sometimes closing my eyes. Rather than putting life on hold, I allow myself to "loosen" that feeling, and feel its effect on my body. I don't react; I just feel.

3. I relax and move on.

Usually this works. Sometimes it doesn't. If three breaths aren't enough, I try more. I visualize the stress leaving my body. I imagine it coming out of

You'll get to know Stacey better in the next two chapters, but we wanted to share her thoughts on motivation, written in her own words. We think they perfectly capture what the Spark Solution is all about, what sets it apart, and what makes it so successful:

There is no right or wrong way to do this. Everyone's journey is unique. I've learned a lot about myself on this journey. Now I have a complete understanding of what the term "healthy lifestyle" really means for me, and I have a new lease on life.

For me, the concept of weight loss has always been a no-brainer: eat healthy and move more. It's really that simple. It's all the other stuff that's been my struggle. The emotional eating, bingeing, undereating, obsession, depression, etc. It was facing all that other stuff that was the hardest part of this journey. But working through it all little

my body as I exhale, never to return. Using the breath in tandem with the mind is a powerful practice.

Recently, a friend who struggles with an eating disorder wrote that she couldn't stop thinking about bingeing. It was consuming her thoughts and was stressing her out. The more she fought the thoughts, the stronger they became. I offered her this advice, telling her to remember that ninety-second rule with emotions. It helped. The tightness loosened, she resisted the binge, and eventually the urge dwindled away.

I used the same tactic when panic reared up in me during a stressful day of air travel. I closed my eyes, breathed, and felt the tentacles that had wrapped around my body and soul loosen. I chose to focus on breathing, on loosening panic's grip on me, on cutting off its food supply, and on calming my negative thoughts. Soon, the feelings dissipated.

Emotions are strong and powerful, and they can make us feel helpless. This simple exercise is just one way that I assert control when I'm feeling something that shakes my core. I hope it helps you too and allows you to find a moment of peace amid a chaotic life.

—Stepfanie Romine

by little is what made the biggest difference for me. I had to take a step back, evaluate my life, and acknowledge where I could do better. Then I worked at it one step at a time. That's a process I still practice today, and one I think is vital to success in anything we set out to achieve. It is true what they say: lots of little changes amount to big changes over time. It just takes time.

I'm in a place now where I never thought I'd find myself. I am living, breathing, day by day just doing my best, and trying to make the healthiest choices I can—setting a better example for my kids, enjoying being active with my family, and achieving things I never imagined I could do. And all this was possible while still having the kind of fun that doesn't always revolve around bad food or other bad habits.

After four years on this journey I certainly don't have all the answers. I am still (and always will be to some degree) a work in progress. But that's the important part: as long as we work on it, we are never failing. Giving up isn't an option.

Food for Life

Unlucky number thirteen. That's how many fast-food and take-out places were located within a mile of Stacey's house. She and her husband lived near the local mall, which meant they were in the middle of "fast-food heaven." Her meals came in boxes and were either handed to her through her car window or delivered to her front door. The kitchen was the place she went to fetch more soda, an after-dinner pint of ice cream, or a bag of chips for a snack.

A typical breakfast was a fast-food biscuit sandwich or burrito (or two) and potatoes, plus a large soda. Lunch was two roast beef sandwiches, a large order of fries, and a "bucket" of soda. Dinner sometimes came in two parts: a burrito the size of her head along with a bag of chips and guacamole earlier in the night, and sometimes after their sons went to bed the couple ordered pizza. Stacey could easily put away four slices of a large pizza and half a dozen buffalo wings, all dunked in ranch dressing, plus dessert. Regardless of what she ate, it had a sauce—sometimes one carton of sauce per nugget or a dozen packets of ketchup per order of fries.

After working long hours, she and her husband were tired. Restaurant food was convenient and, they believed, cheaper than cooking real meals. It tasted good, came in plentiful portions, and made them feel good—only so long as they kept eating. "I knew we were eating garbage," Stacey said. In one blog entry from 2008, she likened her eating habits to a garbage disposal and said she was desperately trying to change her ways.

To her, food served two purposes: pleasure and pain. This fast-food addiction was a vicious cycle, and Stacey's story is all too familiar. The food that gave her pleasure as she ate it was only masking the pain. As soon as she stopped, the pain she was fighting returned, so she ate more.

After tipping the scales at 225 and 265 pounds, respectively, Stacey and her husband decided together that enough was enough. "We did it for our sons," she said. "They deserved to have parents who did more than sit on the couch all the time." They were both eating their feelings and eating out of boredom. "It was something we shared when we couldn't share other parts of our lives," she said. Together, they committed to change.

So they dove right in, with Stacey activating her SparkPeople account and voraciously reading all she could about eating right and nutrition. "Once I realized the root of the problem and made significant changes to my diet (no more brown bags and pizza boxes), I discovered how much I actually enjoyed colorful foods and cooking. Now, the sight of the brown bags makes my stomach turn. Adding more nutritious sources of protein into my diet, and fruits and veggies, has been vital to my success in weight loss. Maintaining a diet rich in nutrients and clean foods makes me feel like a million bucks. Limiting the amounts of processed foods in my diet has played a vital role in my overall health. It just feels better."

They reached their goal weights: she reached 128 pounds and he, 215. Their relationship with each other and with their sons improved. Despite some financial hardships and other trying times as a family, they're committed to this healthy lifestyle.

Today, Stacey cooks big batches of healthy food on weekends, packs leftovers for lunches to avoid takeout temptations, and makes over their family favorites, like enchilada casserole and barbecue sauce. As a family, they shop together and cook healthy versions of their favorites, with room left over for a healthy treat each night.

This self-proclaimed sauce-and-dip addict has reformed her palate and found that she needs much less these days. Despite cutting her calories basically in half—to 1,500—Stacey was surprised to find that she wasn't overly hungry between meals, then or now. "Make your plate colorful. If you do that at every meal, you're going to be full," she says. "Healthy foods are providing you with the right stuff, not empty calories." Nutrition, she's learned, isn't some boring, esoteric branch of study. It affects our daily lives, and knowing the basics can mean the difference between a lifelong cycle of unhealthy habits or a life full of energy and vigor.

Before joining SparkPeople in 2001, Becky worked exclusively in private practice and at a community hospital in her small hometown in Indiana.

She has spent her career teaching people how to not only select and cook nutritious food that suits their tastes both on the tongue and in the wallet, but to also have fun while doing it. No two days are the same: teaching third-shift workers at an auto plant about limiting caffeine, and how to eat on an unconventional schedule; researching farm-to-table programs for the hospital cafeteria; and answering message board posts about managing cravings on SparkPeople. Everyone has to eat, and most of us enjoy doing it. Getting people excited about eating foods that fuel them is one of the best parts of her job.

Food is fuel, but it's so much more. Learning the basics of how to fuel your body properly is crucial to a healthy lifestyle, but it doesn't have to be dull or tedious. In this chapter, you'll learn more about what your body needs to burn calories and keep the weight off for life. Learning more about nutrition doesn't limit your food choices; it sets you free.

You already know that losing weight is about calories in versus calories out. Although the calorie is king, weight loss isn't based on calories alone; other calorie-providing macronutrients come into play as well: namely protein, carbohydrates, and fats. These three macronutrients provide the calories your body needs and perform other, unique functions in the body as well.

Entire books and diet plans aim to restrict certain macronutrients, eliminate them entirely, or hype one over another. For years the diet industry has tried to create a hierarchy in the nutrition kingdom. "Protein is all you need to lose weight." "Carbs are the enemy." "Fat is evil and should be avoided." Any of those fallacies sound familiar? Whom should you trust, and what should you eat, or not eat?

Your body needs all three macronutrients, and none is more important than the other, despite what you might hear on TV or read on the cover of a magazine. Any diet plan that asks you to severely restrict or eliminate any of these macronutrients should be avoided, as it can lead to issues in the long term, such as heart disease, kidney disease, or diabetes. The Spark Solution takes a middle-of-the-road approach using general recommendations from the Food and Nutrition Board of the Institute of Medicine of the National Academies. This ensures that you meet your nutritional needs while losing weight and allows more flexibility in your meals to suit your preferences.

Here is how the 1,500-calorie Spark Solution diet is broken down:

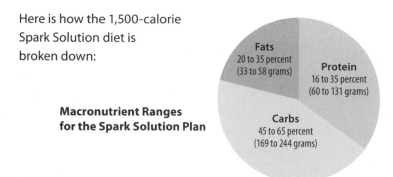

Macronutrient Ranges for the Spark Solution Plan

Why are these macronutrients important, and what role do they play in weight loss?

Protein

Protein, which provides the body with 4 calories per gram, plays some major roles in the body. It maintains and repairs body tissue, including muscle, makes the hemoglobin that transports oxygen, forms antibodies to fight infection, and produces enzymes and hormones to keep the body in balance and working properly.

Protein takes longer to digest than carbs, so it helps you feel fuller longer. Adding protein to your meals and snacks adds satiety, or that feeling of fullness; it gives your meals staying power. Protein also helps you maintain muscle mass during weight loss and assists in repairing your muscles after your workouts. For these reasons, we recommend at least 60 grams of protein daily.

Carbs

Like protein, carbs provide the body with 4 calories per gram, but their responsibilities are quite different. Carbs are energy food. They break down into glucose, which is the primary fuel for body cells and brain cells. They also play the martyr, allowing themselves to be used as energy so that protein can be used for other, more important functions.

We recommend that 45 to 65 percent of all calories come from carbs, to help balance blood-sugar levels and decrease cravings.

Fats

Fats provide the body with 9 calories per gram, which is more than twice as many as protein and carbs. For that reason, energy-dense fats are something you should limit but *never* eliminate or avoid. Fats supply the body with essential fatty acids, protect and insulate the body, and are a component of all cell walls. In addition, vitamins A, D, E, and K all require fat in order to be properly utilized by the body. Our plan provides a moderate amount of fat to keep you satisfied and your body working properly.

Fiber

Fiber is your friend when you're losing weight. Found only in plant food, it's a type of carbohydrate that is neither digested nor absorbed. It passes through the body; therefore, it contains no calories. It promotes regular bowel movements, by adding bulk to your stools, and softens them.

Bathroom habits aside, fiber has numerous other benefits. It boosts heart health, helps balance blood-sugar levels, and can decrease the risk of certain cancers. It fills you up, takes longer to chew, and helps ward off hunger because your body takes longer to process it. That's why our plan calls for at least 25 grams daily.

Fiber comes in two forms, each beneficial to the body. Soluble fiber, such as pectin, combines with water and forms a gummy substance, which coats the insides of the digestive tract. There, soluble fiber binds to cholesterol and reduces its absorption. This helps to lower blood cholesterol levels, delays the absorption of glucose, and helps with diabetes control.

Fat Versus Fats

When it comes to weight gain, a calorie is a calorie. Any food—pizza, steak, mashed potatoes, even broccoli—when eaten in excess of what the body needs, is converted and stored as body fat. That's why we shouldn't vilify healthy sources of fats. It's important to keep all foods in check, whether they're packed with nutrition or empty calories.

Soluble fiber is found in oats, seeds, beans, barley, blueberries, strawberries, peas, lentils, apples, citrus fruit, carrots, plums, and squash.

Insoluble fiber absorbs water, which bulks and softens stools. It keeps the digestive system running smoothly, reducing constipation, hemorrhoids, and other digestive problems, and it decreases risks of certain types of cancer. Insoluble fiber is found in oat or wheat bran, whole-grain products, skins of fruits and vegetables, and leafy greens.

Too much fiber too quickly may cause constipation or stomach discomfort. Increase fiber in your diet slowly, and be sure to drink eight 8-ounce glasses of water daily to allow your body to adjust comfortably.

Sodium

If fiber is your friend, sodium is your frenemy. Women especially know how salty foods at certain times of the month can cause your waistline to balloon temporarily and lead to dreaded water weight gain. In addition to making our favorite jeans feel too tight, excess sodium in the diet can lead to high blood pressure, heart disease, and kidney problems. We recommend no more than 2,300 milligrams daily, consistent with the most recent USDA guidelines.

However, sodium *is* important to the body. It regulates the movement of body fluids and blood pressure, helps your muscles and heart relax, and assists in transmitting nerve impulses. So you want to make sure you're getting at least 500 milligrams daily.

Shake Off Salt

1. *Take the salt shaker off the table.*
2. *Eat at home more, and when dining out, ask for foods to be prepared without added salt, when possible.*
3. *Choose low-sodium or no-salt-added versions of canned, boxed, and frozen foods.*
4. *Rinse canned vegetables and beans to remove up to 40 percent of the sodium.*
5. *Use acids like lemon juice and vinegar plus herbs and spices to add flavor to foods, rather than salt.*

Servings and Food Groups

We've just learned about food from a science perspective. Now let's talk about it from a real-world perspective. No one sits down to a home-cooked meal and thinks, *Mmm, carbs, fats, and protein!* Rather, you build a meal, and a diet plan, around the various food groups, which thankfully is much more enjoyable.

Just as you should be wary of any plan that asks you to eliminate a crucial macronutrient, you should be equally skeptical of one that forces you to cut out entire food groups. With the Spark Solution, there are no forbidden food groups and no need to knock out entire sections of the old food pyramid. Our 1,500-calorie-a-day plan brings all food groups to the plate to ensure you're getting not only the right balance of macronutrients but also the necessary vitamins and minerals.

Speaking of the food pyramid, it's gone. In its place is a plate, which is much easier to envision and translate into a real meal:

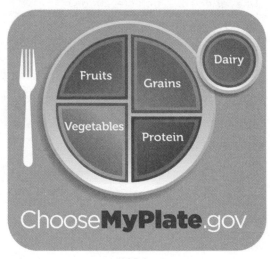

U.S.D.A.

Daily Servings for the Spark Solution Plan	
Vegetables	3 to 4
Fruit	2 to 3
Grains and Starchy Vegetables	5 to 6
Proteins	2 to 3 (to equal 60 grams)
Dairy	2, as part of a meal or snack
Fats	2, as part of a meal or snack

Vegetables

What to Eat

All non-starchy vegetables, both cooked and raw, and 100 percent vegetable juices.

Fresh, frozen, and canned are all acceptable.

Choose an assortment of veggies in various colors daily.

What to Limit

Vegetables cooked with heavy cream or full-fat cheese sauces, deep-fried, or breaded.

One Serving of Vegetables Equals:
½ cup cooked vegetables
½ cup raw vegetables, diced, chopped, sliced, or in sticks
1 cup raw leafy greens, such as lettuce, spinach, or kale
½ cup (4 ounces) 100 percent vegetable juice

Fruit

What to Eat

All fresh, frozen, and dried fruits, and canned fruit packed in water or its own juice.

What to Limit

Fruit canned in heavy syrup, or dried or frozen with added sugar.

One Serving of Fruit Equals:
½ cup fruit, whole, cubed, sliced, diced, puréed, or canned
1 small piece of fruit, such as an apple, orange, pear, peach, etc.
½ grapefruit
16 grapes
¼ cup dried fruit, such as raisins, prunes, apricots, etc.
½ cup (4 ounces) 100 percent fruit juice

Grains and Starchy Vegetables

What to Eat

Whole grains, such as 100 percent whole wheat, brown rice, oats, cornmeal, and barley, and starchy vegetables, like potatoes, sweet potatoes, corn, beans, lentils, and sweet peas.

Whole grains contain the entire grain kernel as well as all the beneficial fiber and nutrients. Cereals and bread products made with 100 percent whole-wheat flour, oatmeal, brown rice, popcorn, bulgur, quinoa (technically a seed), and corn tortillas are all whole grains. The fiber in whole grains means they take longer to digest and help keep blood-sugar levels stable.

Choose whole grains *at least* half the time.

What to Limit

Grains in the form of sugary baked goods, bread products that contain harmful trans fats, and refined grain products.

Refined grains have gone through a process that removes the outer layers, which creates a softer texture but also removes the fiber and key vitamins and minerals. White flour, white rice, corn flakes, white bread, and butter crackers are all refined grains. These grains are digested more quickly than whole grains.

A serving of fruit or veggies is easy to estimate, but grains can be tricky. For example, one large bagel or a tortilla the size of a dinner plate is four servings.

One Serving of Grains and Starchy Vegetables Equals:
1 slice bread
Half a hamburger or hotdog bun
1 mini bagel
1 small (2-inch diameter) biscuit
1 small (4-inch diameter) pancake
1 small (6- to 7-inch diameter) tortilla
5 saltine crackers

| 3 cups low-fat or fat-free popcorn |
| 1 cup no-sugar-added, ready-to-eat breakfast cereal |
| ½ cup cooked rice, pasta, potatoes, grain, or hot breakfast cereal |
| ½ cup cooked beans, peas, corn, or lentils |

Proteins

What to Eat

Formerly known as the meat group, in recent years this food group has been expanded to reflect today's more diverse diets. Meat (beef, pork, lamb), poultry, seafood, legumes and peas, eggs, cheese, cottage cheese, soy products, nuts, and seeds all fall into this food group.

Choose lean, low-fat animal *and* plant-based proteins.

You'll notice some overlap. Legumes (beans and lentils) and peas count as both proteins and starchy vegetables. If you're relying on them as the protein in your meal, count them in this group; if you use them as a side dish, count them as a starchy vegetable.

What to Limit

Processed meat (such as deli meat, hot dogs, and sausages), fatty cuts of meat, breaded or fried meat, and seafood packed in oil should all be eaten rarely. Cut off any visible fat, and use salty meats, such as bacon, Canadian bacon, and ham, in small quantities to add flavor rather than relying on them as a primary protein source.

Use full-fat cheese and processed cheese products sparingly.

The foods in this group vary greatly in the amount of protein they provide; therefore, portion size depends on the type of food. Choose a variety of proteins to total at least 60 grams daily. Your two servings of dairy also will contribute about 16 grams of protein each day.

Protein in One Serving:	
3 ounces cooked lean meat with no bones or skin: beef, pork, chicken, turkey, fish, seafood	20 grams

Protein in Partial Servings:	
1 large egg	6 grams
¼ cup egg whites	7 grams
1 ounce nuts or seeds:	5 to 6 grams
40 peanuts	
20 almonds	
15 cashews or walnut halves	
¼ cup sunflower seeds	
1 tablespoon nut butter	4 grams
½ cup cooked lentils, peas, or beans	7 grams
1 ounce low-fat hard cheese	7 grams
¼ cup grated low-fat cheese	
¼ cup low-fat cottage or ricotta cheese	7 grams

Dairy

What to Eat

Milk products are not created equal. Only fluid milk and yogurt count as a serving of dairy due to their high calcium content. Most cheese counts as a protein. Butter, cream cheese, and sour cream do not contain significant amounts of calcium or protein, so they count as fat sources and should be used sparingly.

Choose skim or 1 percent milk.

Opt for fat-free or low-fat yogurt in either Greek or traditional varieties. Artificially sweetened or "light" yogurts are good choices.

If you opt for nondairy milk and yogurt (made from soy, almond, or rice, for example), choose varieties fortified with calcium and vitamin D.

If you prefer chocolate milk, you can add 1 tablespoon light chocolate syrup to your milk.

What to Limit

Full-fat yogurt or yogurt with added sugar.

2 percent or whole milk.

Nondairy milks and yogurts that are not fortified with calcium and vitamin D.

One Serving of Dairy Equals:
8 ounces milk, skim or 1 percent
8 ounces yogurt, low-fat or fat-free
8 ounces soy milk or milk alternatives, fortified with calcium and vitamin D

Fats

What to Eat

While the body requires essential fatty acids, the amount required is quite small. It's important to include fats that benefit your health and limit fats that are damaging. For overall health, choose polyunsaturated fat or mono-unsaturated fat. These fats include canola, corn, cottonseed, olive, safflower, soybean, and sunflower oils. Other foods that contain healthy fats include fatty fish, nuts, seeds, and avocados.

What to Limit

Saturated fats have been linked with heart disease and include the fats found in meat, dairy, shortening, butter, coconut oil, palm oil, palm kernel oil, stick margarine, and partially hydrogenated oils.

Trans fats are made in a process that changes vegetable oils into semi-solid fats. These fats can raise blood cholesterol levels and should be avoided in the diet. Look for ZERO TRANS FAT on the nutrition label.

One Serving of Fat Equals:
1 teaspoon oil, zero trans-fat margarine, butter
1 tablespoon low-fat spreadable margarine
2 tablespoons low-fat salad dressing
1 tablespoon regular salad dressing
2 tablespoons avocado (about ¼ fruit)

What About Drinks?

These days, 1 in 5 calories we consume comes from beverages. Sure, we need to stay hydrated, but drinking your calories can be a major cause of packing on the pounds. Liquid calories go down quickly with no chewing, which allows little time for the brain to respond with its typical "full" message to stop eating. Start counting what's in that glass, cup, can, or mug, and take inventory of your daily gulping habits.

Beverage	Serving Size	Calories	Added Sugar	How Often?
Water	1 cup (8 ounces)	0	0	Drink when thirsty, at least 8 glasses (64 ounces) a day
Skim or 1 percent milk, or nondairy milks fortified with calcium and vitamin D	1 cup (8 ounces)	90 to 100	0	Up to 2 servings daily to provide protein, calcium, and vitamin D
100 percent fruit juice	½ cup (4 ounces)	60 to 80	0	No more than 8 ounces daily
Regular soda	12 ounces	150	10 teaspoons	Avoid
Diet soda	12 ounces	0	0	No more than 32 ounces daily
Fruit drinks	20 ounces	250 to 300	At least ⅓ cup	Avoid
Sports drinks	20 ounces	120 to 150	Almost 3 tablespoons	Consume only during hard exercise lasting more than 90 minutes; otherwise, avoid
Tea and coffee (unsweetened)	8 ounces	0	0	Limit intake to less than 400 milligrams caffeine daily (about 24 ounces)
Flavored teas and coffee drinks	12 ounces	Varies	Varies	Avoid or choose low-calorie, diet versions, since these drinks can contain 300 to 600 calories
Alcohol	12 ounces beer 5 ounces wine 1.5 ounces distilled spirits	100 to 200	Not applicable	Though men can drink two alcoholic beverages daily and women can drink one, during weight loss it's best to limit alcohol to no more than two servings a week, as a snack, or avoid it.

The Golden Rule of Healthy Eating: Always Measure Portions

FD was trying to shed a few pounds, so he started tracking his food on SparkPeople and measuring his portions. After a few days, he was hooked and already feeling better about his weight-loss chances. He learned that the oversize bowls he used for pasta held more than 2 cups of noodles. A serving size is half a cup, so he was often eating four times what he thought he was! That's an extra 250 calories, or 3.7 added pounds a year, with a weekly pasta dinner.

He also discovered that the "splash" of half-and-half he used in his coffee was more like 3 tablespoons (60 calories and 6 grams of fat). Multiply that times two 8-ounce cups of coffee seven days a week and that's an extra 840 calories and 84 grams of fat (almost 12.5 pounds).

Measuring portions helped keep FD on track, and he dropped 10 pounds within a couple of months. Measuring portions keeps you from convincing yourself you only had "a few" chips when you know the bag was full when you opened it. Luckily, it's easy to recover from portion distortion.

Use Measuring Cups

It's just as easy and quick to serve yourself using a measuring cup as it is a spoon or a ladle, but you'll be exact every time. Stock your kitchen with measuring spoons, dry measuring cups, and a liquid measuring cup. You can choose stylish ones to match your décor or pick up a cheap set at the dollar store—both will get the job done. Consider having a spare set so you always have them clean and ready. You might also want to buy a small, inexpensive food scale.

Shrink Your Dishes

A single serving of pasta would look skimpy in the large, deep bowls FD was using. Once he used smaller bowls, the 1 cup combination of pasta and broccoli topped with ½ cup of marinara sauce seemed like much more food.

Take Advantage of Generous Portions of Vegetables

A serving of leafy greens is 1 cup, the size of a baseball. Once you've got a serving of dairy, fruit, protein, and whole grains, fill up on vegetables. You can trick your eyes and brain into thinking you're eating more calories than you really are.

Liquid Calories Count

Unless you're drinking water, use the tallest, skinniest glass possible. Studies have shown that people pour more liquid into short, squat tumblers. Use a liquid measuring cup for your milk, juice, and even wine, then pour it into a glass, to make sure you're drinking what you think you're drinking.

Raw or Cooked?

When possible, weigh and measure the ready-to-eat version of your food. Measure the roasted meat, the cooked pasta, and the sautéed green beans.

Record It All

Whether you are using a journal or SparkPeople.com to record your food, look up and enter everything you eat and drink. You will quickly see which food choices are costing you too many calories and where adjustments need to be made.

Laura, who lost more than 100 pounds, said that buying a food scale and an extra set of measuring cups and spoons to take to work was the most important thing she did. She lost 5 pounds in the first two weeks!

What do you do when you are dining away from home at a restaurant, a friend's party, or a business meeting? Use your hands. Here's how: Look at the food on your plate. Then look at your hand, comparing the size of the serving on your plate to the size of your hand, using the following table for reference. While this technique isn't quite as accurate as measuring and weighing your food, it does provide a good estimate, and you can avoid the awkwardness of pulling out a measuring cup during a business lunch. Also, if the food is already on your plate, create a dividing line, separating out one portion and subtly pushing the rest aside.

About the Size of My . . .	Serving Size	Best for . . .
Clenched fist	8 ounces (1 cup)	Beverages Soups Cereal Fresh fruit Casseroles Salads
Cupped hand	4 ounces (½ cup)	Grains and pasta Beans Cooked potatoes Pudding and ice cream Cooked vegetables
Open palm (the portion should be as thick as your hand)	3 ounces	Meat and fish
Thumb	1 tablespoon	Condiments Nut butters
Tip of your thumb	1 teaspoon	Fats and oils

The Spark Solution Plate

Pick Out Your Plate

Have you noticed the trend of restaurants serving food in large bowls? Once upon a time, only soups, stews, and other liquids were served in bowls, but now it seems that at home and when dining out we're reaching for bowls.

Buck the trend and use a plate. With a bowl, it's much easier to eat with one hand, shovel food into your mouth, and dine away from the kitchen table. Eating with a knife, fork, and plate requires more attention and time, which can allow your body to realize when it's full and prevent overeating.

Pitch the platters and oversize plates too. Choose one with a 9-inch diameter eating space.

Divide and Conquer

Visualize that your plate has four equal sections. For breakfast, you'll fill three-quarters of the plate with three of the four food groups. At lunch and dinner, you'll fill the entire plate. Add two total servings of dairy to any meal or snack.

Don't worry about eating exactly 1,500 calories once you start designing your own meal plan. If you're over or under by 50 calories or less a few times a week, you'll be fine, as long as you stay in the recommended ranges for macronutrients and keep up with your fitness plan.

Getting Comfortable in the Kitchen

With our Spark Swaps meals, you'll see how you can continue to eat familiar, comforting foods while still losing weight. You'll learn how to adjust portions and feel satisfied with fewer calories. And you'll understand how to fuel your body properly to maintain energy levels and take on all the challenges life brings you.

Now that you know what to eat and why you should eat it, let's talk about *where* to eat. To regain control over your weight and your health, you need to know what's going into your body. That means cutting back on packaged and processed foods, eating fewer restaurant meals, and spending more time in the kitchen. You don't have to love to cook, you

don't have to spend hours creating fancy meals, and you don't have to blow your budget on fancy ingredients and equipment. But you do need to get more comfortable in the kitchen. That's why we're here.

Stress-Free Meal Planning

Keep an Updated List on the Fridge
When you run out of something, write it down. Make this a habit for everyone in your house. This will avoid those mad dashes to the supermarket halfway through a recipe. Before recycling or throwing away the empty container of an item, write it on the list.

Plan Before You Shop
At least once a week, plan your meals for the days ahead, keeping your schedule in mind. Do you have a busy week coming up? Do you have company coming or a weekend trip planned? How much time do you have to cook each night this week? Plan meals based on how much time you have available. One night you may have only thirty minutes to cook and eat, so you need something fast. The next day you may have more time to try out that new recipe you've been eyeing.

Be Ready for Anything
Choose a variety of quick recipes, dishes that yield leftovers, and meals that require more time so cooking always fits into your schedule. Lean on your slow cooker for really busy nights, and be flexible. Life can change without notice, so keep quick, healthy staples on hand to avoid fast-food runs.

Write Your List, Check It Twice
Take the list off your fridge, along with your weekly meal plan, and create one master grocery list that includes everything you'll need for meals and snacks. Divide your list into sections to make your shopping trip more efficient (unless pushing a heavy cart around the supermarket is your idea of cardio!). If you clip coupons, don't forget them, and if something is on sale, make a note on your list. We have a shopping list template in the appendix of this book, along with detailed lists of everything you'll need for Week 1 and Week 2.

Shop Smart

Avoid shopping with kids (it makes it easier to skip the snacks and sweets aisle), shopping on an empty stomach, and shopping when you're in a bad mood, if possible. This will help minimize impulse purchases. Stick to the perimeter of the store, which is where the healthier food items are located, and if something isn't on your list, don't buy it. But be flexible. If broccoli is on sale but asparagus is on the list, make the swap.

Unpack with Purpose

When you get home, spend a few minutes putting away the groceries in logical places, keeping similar items together and setting full packages behind any that are half empty. This will make cooking more efficient. Another idea is to put all the ingredients you'll need for a recipe in one place, so you can easily grab them when you're ready to cook.

Don't Leave Out the Leftovers

According to *The Wall Street Journal,* Americans waste 25 percent or more of the food they buy. You can help cut down on your food waste (and save money) by buying only the amount of food you know you can eat in a week or so—sticking to your shopping list and limiting impulse purchases—and using your leftovers. Maybe you save your leftovers, but do you ever eat them? Rather than look at leftovers with disdain ("This, again?") think of them as an insurance policy. By cooking a bit extra and saving what's left over, you can guarantee a healthy meal tomorrow or the next day, even if you're busy. Your future self will thank you later.

A note about leftovers: For some people, leftovers are a binge waiting to happen. For others, they're a time saver. If having leftover food around is a positive weight-loss technique you're using to keep your calorie intake in control, continue to make extra portions and store them for later. If leftovers are a source of temptation, then stick to just the amount of food you need for one meal.

Clean and Organize the Kitchen

You don't have to tackle the entire kitchen all at once. Break it down into different sections on different days or different weeks. Perhaps begin with your pantry, then move to your cupboards. Next, hit the refrigerator and freezer. Throw out all outdated food items. Group similar items together.

Put healthy snacks in your line of sight. If you have a designated space for your pantry staples, you can easily spot when you need to purchase more. Don't forget to clean out the spice cabinet (if you can't remember when you bought it, throw it out), the appliance jungle (donate any single-use appliance you don't use regularly), and the utensil drawers.

The Spark Swaps Assembly Line

Reaching for a frozen meal is tempting, but its convenience is trumped by its sky-high sodium level and lack of staying power. It's fine in a pinch, but even if you hate cooking or just don't have time, you can still put a homemade meal on the table. With some help from the supermarket, you can assemble a healthy meal in fifteen minutes or less. Plus, preparing your own food—whether by the assembly-line method or by actually cooking—has been proven to increase fruit and veggie consumption.

The following no-cook ideas assume you have a decently stocked kitchen and some leftovers.

Build Your Own Burrito

Choose your wrap: whole-grain or corn tortillas, or iceberg or Romaine lettuce leaves. Add protein: 3 ounces leftover ground beef or turkey, rotisserie chicken, or canned beans (½ cup). Top with at least two veggies: lettuce, onions, peppers, tomatoes, corn, radishes, or carrots. And finish with flavor: salsa, olives, avocado, low-fat sour cream, or shredded cheese.

A few possible combinations:

- Pinto beans, chipotle salsa, mixed greens, chopped red pepper, and guacamole in iceberg lettuce wraps
- Shredded chicken, salsa verde, pepper jack cheese, onions, and green bell peppers in two corn tortillas
- Leftover ground beef, lettuce, onions, chopped black olives, and low-fat sour cream in a whole-wheat tortilla

Kitchen-Sink Salad

Add whatever you have in the fridge to turn a salad into a satisfying and filling meal. Start with dark, leafy greens: don't skimp—at least 2 to 3 cups. Add a handful (½ cup) each of two or three different vegetables, a serving of leftover or precooked protein, something tasty to sauce it up, and a fun topping. Serve it with a slice of toast or toss it on precooked whole grains.
   A few possible combinations:

- Mixed greens, tuna packed in water, sliced red onion, sliced fennel, and grated carrots, topped with low-fat balsamic vinaigrette and chopped olives
- Romaine lettuce, thawed frozen (and cooked) shrimp, shredded Parmesan cheese, sliced tomato, and sliced fennel, tossed with low-fat Caesar dressing
- Arugula, sliced almonds, chopped cooked chicken, grapes, and chopped celery, tossed with low-fat honey-mustard dressing

Egg Scramble

Eggs are among the simplest proteins to cook. Coat a skillet with cooking spray. Sauté chopped raw veggies or heat leftover ones. Add one whole egg plus one egg white per person, plus cheese, or another protein source if desired, and cook, stirring often, until the eggs are set. It's less fuss than an omelet and just as much flavor. Serve with toast or roasted potatoes.
   A few possible combinations:

- Spinach, onions, and chicken with feta cheese
- Bacon, cheddar cheese, tomato, and onion
- Tomatoes, kale, and roasted peppers with basil

Super Spaghetti

Start with whole-wheat pasta and a jar of no-salt-added sauce that's loaded with vegetables. Brown extra-lean ground beef or turkey in a skillet, stir in a can of tuna packed in water, or add cooked lentils or white

beans. Mix the pasta, sauce, and protein together, top it with a bit of grated cheese, if desired, and serve it with cooked (from frozen) veggies or sneak some veggies into the sauce.

A few possible combinations:

- Penne and spicy tomato sauce with tuna and capers or olives
- Rigatoni and mushroom sauce with ground beef
- Fettuccine and marinara with chicken, topped with goat cheese (sneak grated zucchini into the sauce)

Burgers and Fries

Use a countertop grill or your oven's broiler for quick burgers any time of year. Choose extra-lean chicken, beef, or turkey burgers that are preformed to save time, or reach for a box of frozen veggie burgers. Skip the bun and serve the burger over greens alongside potatoes (from frozen), which have come a long way in terms of quality, or microwave "baked" potatoes. Get creative with your toppings.

A few possible combinations:

- Turkey burger over mixed baby greens with chopped red onion, sweet potato wedges, and chipotle salsa
- Beef burger over spinach with blue cheese and onions, plus a baked potato
- Indian-spiced veggie burger over microwave-steamed kale with roast potatoes and curry sauce or chutney

Beans, Greens, and Grains

Canned beans, frozen green veggies, and heat-and-eat grains make meals a snap. Microwave the veggies until almost hot, and drain and rinse the beans. Microwave a serving of each, or heat together in a skillet over medium. Top with cheese or sauce. Serve with instant brown rice, quinoa, or couscous.

A few possible combinations:

- Black-eyed peas, collard greens, and barley, topped with smoked paprika and hot sauce

- Black beans, kale, and quinoa, topped with salsa and chopped avocado
- White beans, broccoli, and farro, topped with sun-dried tomatoes and capers

Loaded Baked Potato

Consider these starchy sides a blank canvas. Choose either white or sweet potatoes, microwave until tender, then top with a leftover protein, some veggies, and a sauce. Return to the microwave to warm your toppings.
    A few possible combinations:

- Sweet potato with pork tenderloin, peppers, and spinach, plus pineapple salsa
- White potato with chicken, arugula, and tomatoes, plus pesto and a sprinkle of Parmesan cheese
- Sweet potato with lean beef, broccoli, and peppers, plus red curry sauce

Stir-Fry

Open the fridge. Grab anything that's fresh, and toss it into a pan. You'll need a protein, a grain, and at least two veggies. Season to please, and think beyond typically Asian flavors.
    A few possible combinations:

- Tofu with broccoli slaw and peanut sauce over cooked brown rice
- Chicken with carrots, peppers, broccoli, and curry sauce over quinoa
- Pork with peppers, onions, cabbage, and barbecue sauce over couscous

Tasting Plate

On the nights you're too tired to cook, when you're tempted to just stand in front of the fridge or in the pantry eating whatever strikes your fancy, make a tasting plate instead.
    Fill a plate with a portion of several of these: vegetables (two to three), nuts, cheese, fruit, and whole-grain crackers, bread, or a rice cake. Serve

with a little bowl of low-fat dip. You're snacking, but it takes two minutes to prepare, if your veggies are already cut, and you won't dive face-first into a bag of potato chips.

A few possible combinations:

- Celery, carrots, and cucumbers with white bean hummus, sprouted-grain crackers, cheddar cheese, grapes, and almonds
- Bell peppers, cherry tomatoes, and jicama with guacamole, a segmented orange, baked tortilla chips, and chicken
- Radishes, cucumbers, and cauliflower with low-fat ranch dip, apple slices, rye crackers, and a single-serving cup of plain yogurt

Quick Quesadillas

Fold a tortilla in half, add beans or meat, a bit of cheese, and finely chopped fresh veggies. Spritz it with cooking spray, then heat it in a skillet until golden brown on both sides. Slice it into wedges and serve with salsa.

A few other combinations:

- Beef and cheddar cheese with green onions and peppers
- Fat-free refried black beans and pepper jack cheese with cilantro and tomatoes
- Chicken and Mexican cheese blended with spinach and mushrooms

Making Convenience Foods Healthier

In a perfect world, we would all cook healthful, balanced meals from scratch seven nights a week. But who's perfect? When you're trying to eat right, work out, and live your life, there's no harm in getting some help from the supermarket. According to one survey of SparkPeople members, more than 60 percent of them rely on a microwave, a can opener, and a toaster oven for dinner from time to time.

However, we all know a can of soup or a frozen cheese pizza doesn't constitute a well-balanced meal. The trick to eating right with these short-cut foods is to use them as a basis for your meal, not as your entire meal.

You can boost the nutrition of any convenience food. Here's how:

- Frozen meals have come a long way in recent years. Choose a low-sodium one that has lean protein, veggies, and whole grains.

- Add canned tuna, black beans, or chicken breast packed in water to any meal that lacks protein.

- Add frozen or canned vegetables to either a boxed preparation of macaroni and cheese or a jar of spaghetti sauce. (Choose whole-wheat or whole-grain pasta when possible.)

- Add an extra serving of vegetables to frozen meals.

- Make a green salad to serve alongside a frozen pizza.

- Add extra vegetables to frozen pizzas.

- Skip extra cheese, deluxe, or pepperoni frozen pizzas and choose vegetable-heavy varieties instead. Top with cooked chicken breast chunks or small amounts of low-fat pepperoni before baking.

- Use spice packets sparingly, to reduce sodium in boxed rice or noodle dishes.

- Serve a piece of whole-wheat toast topped with a slice of low-fat cheese or a poached egg, to make a soup meal more filling.

- Choose broth-based rather than cream-based soups.

- Add a cup of frozen vegetables and half a cup of canned beans to any soup to bulk it up.

- Add a serving of fruit and a glass of milk to round out any meal.

Convenience foods are often high in sodium, so it's best to choose low-sodium varieties and eat them only on occasion.

Fit to Live

In the last chapter, you met Stacey, the thirty-year-old woman who was addicted to fast food and had little energy for life before losing 97 pounds. We've also quoted her several times throughout the book.

Stacey lives with her husband and two sons in Phoenix, where it's over 110 degrees five months of the year. Despite the heat, she could usually be found in layers of clothing, disguising her body. The heat also kept Stacey and her husband indoors as much as possible; they spent more time on the couch than anyplace else. As recently as 2008, Stacey couldn't climb a flight of stairs without wanting to collapse. She didn't have the energy to get off the couch and play with her two sons. She didn't run, and she hated exercise.

When we interviewed her for this book, Stacey was just arriving at her gym. She's a regular now, and several people greeted her as she made her way to the cardio machines. Stacey knew that diet alone would only take her so far, so she started moving and hasn't stopped.

"You'll rarely find me doing nothing," she said. Stacey's workouts began in her surroundings: the beautiful Arizona desert. She started walking the hills near her home and graduated to hiking. Now her weekends, when not spent challenging her kids to races across the park or taking them to the lake to swim, are devoted to hiking.

Just one year after she took her first step toward healthy living, the woman whose life once revolved around the couch hiked thirty-two miles through the Grand Canyon in two and a half days. "The feeling of accomplishment I had when I reached the top of the canyon at the end of our journey was incredible," Stacey said. "I cried like a baby, because I never

in a million years thought I would ever be able to achieve such an unfathomable feat." Not only is she looking forward to doing that hike again, but also the rim-to-rim Grand Canyon hike is on her fitness bucket list. "I love that no vacation is off-limits because we aren't in good enough shape," she said. "I feel like a healthier lifestyle means life has more options now, and I also have more time to explore those options."

Stacey's evolution from couch potato to super mom didn't happen because she forced herself to spend hours doing activities she hated. She didn't exercise every day, and she didn't push herself to the max each time she hit the gym or went for a hike. She found activities she loved so that exercise felt like playtime and not work.

Fitness isn't about punishment, and it isn't just about looking good in a bikini (though that's a fine goal if it suits you). It's about being strong enough to take on whatever life brings. Whether your fitness goal is to run a 5K or hike the Grand Canyon, exercise starts with a single step and a single thought. But beyond that, what do you do? How do you get from not being able to climb stairs without cursing and gasping for breath to running (or walking) a mile without stopping?

It's normal to be confused about fitness when you get started. What exactly should you be doing anyway? How do you know which exercises to do? How long should you exercise? How often? Which types of exercises offer the best results? For many people, not knowing what to do is a huge hurdle, so they end up doing nothing at all.

The four categories of exercise we've talked about before should be a weekly part of any fitness program for optimal health and weight-loss results: NEAT plus cardio, strength training, and flexibility.

Cardio Exercise

Cardio strengthens your heart and lungs, helps you maintain a healthy weight, lowers your risk of countless diseases, and makes you feel good. Cardiovascular exercise includes any type of continuous movement that uses the largest muscles of the body in a "rhythmic" way to elevate the heart rate for at least ten continuous minutes. The ideal workout plan will include a variety of cardio exercises for best results.

- *How Hard to Work.* Each cardio workout should increase your heart rate to a somewhat challenging level for you. Monitoring your heart rate is a good way to measure exactly how hard you're working, but you can also use the "talk test" or the rate of perceived exertion (estimate how hard you're working on a scale of 1 to 10). The talk test is easy: exercise at a rate where having a conversation becomes slightly challenging. When you're new, aim for low-intensity cardio. As you get fit, try to increase the intensity every few weeks.

- *How Often.* Aim for three to six cardio sessions each week, with beginners starting at the lower end of that range and gradually doing more over the course of several weeks or months as they get accustomed to it. We don't recommend daily cardio, so take at least one day off from training each week.

- *How Long.* Each cardio session should range from ten to sixty total minutes, but be sure to start at a length you can handle, then gradually progress. These sessions can be broken up into multiple, shorter sessions. Beginners should aim for ten to twenty minutes per session, the thirty- to forty-five-minute range is for intermediates, and forty-five minutes or more is for people who have been exercising for a while.

- *What Counts.* The key to an activity counting as cardio is that it uses your major muscles repeatedly, elevates your heart rate, and lasts for at least ten minutes. When you move fast enough and long enough, almost any type of movement can become a cardio workout. But some general examples include walking, running, bicycling, skating, swimming, dancing, hiking, kickboxing, step aerobics, elliptical training, rowing, stair climbing, and jumping rope. The most important thing is to find a form of cardio you enjoy. That will ensure you'll stick with it.

Sample Cardio Schedule

How do you fit three to six days of cardio into a weekly plan? Start with three days a week, but work up to five to six days per week, gradually adding time and sessions as you get fitter. Never take more than two days

off between sessions, as you'll start to lose your fitness level quickly there-after.

Here are some ideas for how to structure your schedule, depending on how many sessions you're doing each week:

	Day 1	Day 2	Day 3	Day 4	Day 5	Day 6	Day 7
3 workouts	Cardio		Cardio		Cardio		
4 workouts	Cardio	Cardio		Cardio	Cardio		
4 workouts	Cardio		Cardio		Cardio		Cardio
5 workouts	Cardio	Cardio		Cardio	Cardio		Cardio
5 workouts	Cardio	Cardio	Cardio	Cardio	Cardio		

Four Cardio Crimes

Cardio Crime #1: You use little or no resistance on machines.

If you can move extremely fast, the machine is probably on such a low resistance level that momentum is helping you move, instead of your mus-cles. Therefore, you're not burning as many calories or gaining the strength and endurance that comes with added resistance.

Spark Solution: Pump up the resistance on the bike, elliptical, or stair climber to a challenging level for a much more effective workout.

Cardio Crime #2: You use the treadmill (or elliptical) at a zero percent incline.

Treadmills help propel your body. You don't have to do as much work when the belt is doing some of that movement for you. Walking on a flat road outside is more challenging and burns more calories than walking on a flat (zero percent incline) treadmill at the same speed.

Spark Solution: Increase the incline. If you like to get outside when the weather is nice, varying the incline will more likely mimic an outdoor route. Plus, you'll burn about twice the calories at a 5 percent incline in the same amount of time.

Cardio Crime #3: You don't change up your speed.

Repeating your workouts day after day can result in a plateau, since your body quickly gets used to doing the same thing all the time. Changing your

Strength Training

Whether you call it resistance training, weight lifting, toning, or body sculpting, all these terms refer to strengthening your muscles by performing exercises against resistance. Strength training also strengthens your bones, tendons, and ligaments, which improves your fitness, appearance, and metabolism so that you can manage your weight. Each strength-training workout should include at least one exercise for each of your major muscle groups (arms, chest, back, core, and legs).

- *How Hard to Work.* Aim for one to three sets of eight to fifteen reps (e.g., three sets of ten pushups) of each exercise. How many reps you

---

speed and intensity level can help prevent a plateau and offer a greater challenge.

Spark Solution: Try interval training. Most treadmills offer programs you can follow, so take advantage of them. Changing speed is also a great way to improve your fitness level and increase your calorie burn.

Cardio Crime #4: You skimp on or skip warming up, cooling down, or stretching. *Your body can't go from a state of rest to an aerobic level (or vice versa) in a matter of seconds. It takes a few minutes to prepare for exercise and recover from it. Without warming up, cooling down, and stretching, you're not making the most of your workouts. Plus, you could be increasing your chances of injury or other complications.*

Spark Solution: Designate a few minutes per session for these tasks. If you're short on time, jog from the parking lot to the gym as part of your warm-up, and walk slowly to your car as you continue to cool down, for example. Warming up helps lower your risk of injury and prevents aches and pains. A proper cooling down slowly decreases the heart rate to prevent dizziness, fainting, and that post-workout muscle soreness. Stretching can help prevent injury by promoting recovery, decreasing soreness, and ensuring that your muscles and tendons are in good working order.

do will probably be dictated by the amount of resistance you're using. Here is some guidance on choosing weights:

Choose a weight that's moderately challenging for you, one that's not so heavy you can't lift it with proper form and control, but not so light that you could lift it forever.

The resistance should fatigue your muscles within eight to fifteen reps, which means you couldn't possibly lift another repetition in good form beyond that.

Weights will vary for each type of exercise and muscle group you're working, since some muscle groups are stronger than others, just as certain exercises are inherently more complex or challenging than others.

Which weights you use will continue to change as you get stronger, and this continual progression is what improves your strength and boosts your fitness level over time.

- *How Often.* Target every major muscle group at least two times per week, making sure to rest from resistance training for at least one to two days between strength-training sessions. You can do cardio on your "off" days from strength training, if you'd like.

- *Which Exercises.* You could follow a workout DVD or take a class at your fitness center for varied workout ideas. SparkPeople.com offers hundreds of structured workouts and videos that you can follow with little or no equipment, but you'll also find a sample plan on the following page.

- *What Counts.* Resistance comes in many forms. During pushups, squats, and planks your own body weight provides resistance, which strengthens muscles. Other forms of resistance include dumbbells, weight machines, kettlebells, resistance bands or tubes, medicine balls, Pilates reformer machines, and more. There are endless options for strengthening your body. The key is to use resistance, perform exercises that target each muscle group, and work at a challenging level until you reach fatigue in your muscles, which is the inability to complete another rep in good form.

Sample Strength-Training Schedule

Start with at least one session per week that targets every major muscle group, but work up to at least two (or possibly three for advanced exercisers) strength-training sessions each week. Always rest at least one to two days before training the same muscle group again. Although there are many ways to structure your workout week, for simplicity's sake we're showing only a couple variations for breaking up your strength training (full-body routines or upper, lower, or core routines):

	Day 1	Day 2	Day 3	Day 4	Day 5	Day 6	Day 7
1 workout				full body			
2 workouts	full body				full body		
6 workouts total, 2 per muscle group	upper body	lower body	core		upper body	lower body	core
3 workouts	full body			full body		full body	

The Truth About Spot Toning

You cannot take weight off specific body areas by doing exercises that target those areas. This concept is called spot training, and unfortunately it doesn't burn fat. When you lose weight, you're unable to choose the area in which the reduction will occur. Your body determines which fat stores it will use. For example, doing sit-ups will strengthen your abs but will not take the fat off your stomach. Similarly, an activity like running burns fat all over your body, not just your legs. You can, however, compliment a balanced exercise program with a selection of weight-training exercises to gradually lose weight and tone the body.

That goes for your abs too. The fact is, the only way to get a flat stomach is to strip away the fat around the midsection. This is accomplished by doing cardio exercise (to burn calories) and strength training (to increase metabolism), and following a proper diet. Abdominal exercises will help build muscle in your midsection, but you will never see the muscle definition unless the fat in this area is stripped away.

Three Strength-Training Mistakes

Strength-Training Mistake #1: Your weights are too light.
The point of strength training is to overload your muscles so they can become stronger. Without the challenge of this overload, you're wasting your time with strength training, because light, unchallenging weights don't offer the same benefits.

Spark Solution: You want a weight that's challenging, but not so heavy that you risk injury. Here's a good rule of thumb to follow. If you can easily perform more than twelve repetitions of an exercise, then your weight is too light—time to take it up to the next level. On the other hand, if you can only perform four reps in good form, your weight might be too heavy. The proper weight for you is one that you can lift in good form for about twelve reps.

Strength-Training Mistake #2: You only use weight machines.
For the most part, strength-training machines have a two-dimensional movement pattern, so they don't offer the variety or range of motion that other exercises (such as those using free weights) provide. In fact, the machines are doing a lot of the work for you. Because they support you so much, you don't have to balance, control, or stabilize your body on your own; therefore, you use your muscles less.

Flexibility Exercise

Stretching is another name for flexibility exercise, which can help lengthen your muscles and develop an appropriate range of motion for specific sports and daily activities. Flexibility exercises increase joint mobility, improve coordination, enhance your posture, and may help reduce injuries. People often think of stretching as nonessential, or they speed through it, but it warrants attention and priority in any workout plan.

- *What to Do.* You should stretch all of your major muscle groups (arms, chest, back, core, and legs) at least three to six times per week. The

Spark Solution: Add free weights to your routine, plus your own body's weight, as in our plan. Free weights require you to do all the work, which engages more muscle fibers. You'll get a better workout in the same amount of time. You can also do a larger variety of exercises instead of being limited to the machines your gym has available, helping prevent plateaus. There are pros and cons to both machines and free weights, so a combination of the two is ideal for achieving maximum results.

Strength-Training Mistake #3: You rest a long time between sets.

Long rests can decrease the overall intensity of your workout. Some studies show that long resting periods will decrease levels of hormones that help you build strength and reduce your overall calorie burn, making your workouts less effective.

Spark Solution: For most people, a thirty- to ninety-second rest period in between sets is sufficient. Watch the clock or even set a timer on your watch to go off when it's time to resume your next set. Another option for maximizing your workout time and calorie-burning potential is to do a circuit, where you move quickly from one exercise to the next, with very little rest, or do cardio activity in between strength-training sets.

best and probably easiest way to do this in conjunction with your workouts is to simply stretch after you do your strength and cardio exercises.

- *How Much.* Hold each stretch in a slow and controlled manner for fifteen to thirty seconds. Don't push, bob, or bounce.

- *How Far to Stretch.* On a scale of 1 to 10 where 10 is "ouch" and 1 is "rest," stretch to a 5 or 7. Over time, you'll become more flexible and should be able to stretch further while still maintaining a stretching intensity of 5 to 7 on that scale. But even if you swear you're not and never will be flexible, you should still stretch to the best of your ability on that scale. But never to the point of pain.

- *What Counts.* Besides basic stretches that you might do after a workout, class, or run, many mind–body exercises, such as yoga and Pilates, incorporate flexibility training as well. For stretching ideas, check out SparkPeople.com's exercise demos and videos.

We've given you the basic rundown of how much exercise you need to reach your goals during the first two weeks. Next comes the hard part: How do you fit it all into your schedule for the rest of your life? And maybe more important, how can you do all that exercise and still have a life?

That, readers, is the million-dollar question. Like many things in weight loss, and in life, most of us know what to do, but that doesn't mean we know how to put that knowledge into practice. Lack of time is the biggest hurdle we face when trying to fit in exercise.

That's where our Spark Swaps workout plan comes in. With this approach, you'll get in the workouts you need for fitness and weight loss, while also maximizing your calorie burn during your sessions, and all day long. Our plan includes the exact exercises you need, along with the best possible tips for squeezing all the NEAT lifestyle activity into your day, so you can crank up your calorie burn and drop weight more easily than you ever thought possible.

Spark Swaps Secrets of Being Fit to Live

The Spark Swaps plan is built on three concepts, which aim to make fitness simple and approachable.

Maximize Your Time

Although cardio, strength training, and flexibility training are each separate and distinct types of exercise, you can maximize your results—and spend less time exercising—by grouping these exercises together in a single workout. Rather than running for an hour (cardio), only to have to hit the gym and pump out another thirty minutes of weights (strength training) followed by stretching (flexibility), there are plenty of ways you can elevate your heart rate and burn extra calories in a single workout that counts for *all* types of exercise. Plus, you can accomplish it in less time.

While there is absolutely nothing wrong with keeping these workouts separate and distinct, if time isn't on your side, then we have the plan for you. We're getting rid of isolated exercises that only work a single, small muscle at a time. Besides not training your body functionally, these moves burn very few calories, don't add up to an aerobic benefit, and force you to spend more time in the gym. Instead, we combine full-body and multi-joint moves into a functional workout that gives you everything you need.

Forget All-or-Nothing Exercise

While you may have the best intentions to exercise consistently and really put that solid hour in at the gym each day, many of us fail to do so when we get busy or stressed. Too often we can't fit our usual routine into our extra-busy days, so we choose to do nothing instead. Now how does that make any sense?

It's like Beth's mantras about overeating. Just like she tells us not to toss the whole day over a slice of pizza, the same goes for your exercise plan. If you can't fit in your full session, why does it make sense to do nothing instead? Wouldn't you want to burn 50 or 100 calories instead of zero? Lose half a pound instead of none? Get the benefit of just ten or fifteen minutes of exercise instead of none?

We know that short workouts still count. Ten-minute bouts of fitness are the foundation of the SparkPeople program, and research has shown that they still help people improve their fitness levels. Ten minutes may seem insignificant when you're used to doing more, but it really does add up. Not only does it keep you consistent (many of us know just how motivating an exercise streak can be), but it also helps you maintain your fitness level, burn calories, and work toward your goal. If your all-or-nothing mentality leads you to not exercise at all during a month, you'll burn zero calories and lose a lot of momentum. But if you do what you can, even if it's not a full workout, you'll burn thousands of calories, which could prevent you from regaining weight and may even help you lose a few extra pounds.

Next time life gets in the way, don't get caught up in the all-or-nothing mentality when it comes to fitness (or food). Every small step you can take toward your goals is still going to get you closer than standing still. With this workout plan, doing anything at all trumps doing nothing. Your goal is to get moving, and to do something even if you can't fit in the full workout prescribed. Trust us. It makes a real difference.

Smart Exercise Swaps

Without knowing it, a lot of people waste their workout time by doing activities that don't offer much benefit. When it comes to fitness, all movement counts. But we should maximize our results for the least amount of time possible. Sometimes that's as simple as choosing a more effective strength-training move over one that doesn't offer such great results. Other times, it's a small tweak you can add to your program to ramp up your results. We're all about efficiency—we want to get you well exercised and on your way—and that's what you've been doing the last two weeks.

Here are some of our favorite ways to maximize results and burn calories during common cardio and strength exercises.

Cardio Spark Swaps

Instead of: Treadmill with zero incline
Try: Treadmill with 5 percent incline

Calories Burned in 30 Minutes (2 miles):	
Treadmill walking 4 miles per hour (15-minute-mile pace)	168
Treadmill walking 4 miles per hour (15-minute-mile pace) with a 5 percent incline	277
Bonus: 109 extra calories burned, or 65 percent more calories	

The Benefit: You'll engage more muscles in your glutes, thanks to the incline, and burn more than 50 additional calories per mile.

Instead of: Steady-state cardio
Try: Interval training

Calories Burned in 30 Minutes:	
Treadmill walking (4 miles per hour; 15-minute-mile pace)	168
Intervals of walking and running	224
Bonus: 56 extra calories burned, or 33 percent more calories	

The Benefit: In one Australian study, volunteers rode a stationary bike for either 40 minutes at a steady pace or 20 minutes of intervals, alternating 8 seconds of sprints with 12 seconds of easy pedaling. After fifteen weeks, those using interval training had lost three times more body fat, despite working out less time. Intervals are proven to burn more fat and calories and keep your metabolism elevated longer, even after your workout ends.

Instead of: Stationary cycling
Try: Spinning class

Calories Burned in 30 Minutes:	
Exercise bike (6-minute-mile pace)	148
Spinning class	262
Bonus: 114 extra calories burned, or 77 percent more calories	

The Benefit: Let's face it. Sitting on that lone stationary bike can be boring. You're more likely to get a better workout and push yourself harder (which means more calories and fat burned) in an indoor cycling class led by a qualified instructor with a kick-butt workout and a motivating soundtrack. Just hop on the bike and enjoy the ride!

Instead of: Resting between sets
Try: Circuit training

Calories Burned in 20 Minutes:	
Strength training	72
Circuit training	200
Bonus: 128 extra calories burned, or 178 percent more calories	

The Benefit: You'll get the heart-pumping benefits of cardio along with your strength training and torch on average 178 percent more calories per 20-minute session.

Instead of: Exercising on an empty stomach, which can lead to a shorter or less intense workout

Try: Eating something before you work out, to maintain pace and intensity

Calories Burned in 30 Minutes:	
Running (12-minute-mile pace; pace slowed due to lack of energy)	299
Running (10-minute-mile pace)	374
Bonus: 75 extra calories burned, or 25 percent more calories	

The Benefit: It's a myth that you'll burn more fat if you exercise on an empty stomach. Here's why: you need energy (which comes from food) to make the most of your workouts. Studies show that when you have energy readily available, you feel better and are able to work harder during your workout sessions. So stop skipping breakfast or starving yourself before a run. Eat a small snack first and you'll probably lose more weight.

Instead of: Exercising in the fat-burning zone

Try: Exercise at a higher intensity

Calories Burned in 30 Minutes:	
Cardio in the fat-burning zone	175
Cardio at a higher intensity	300
Bonus: 125 extra calories burned, or 71 percent more calories	

The Benefit: Many gym machines have "fat burning" workout zones marked on them, which involve exercising at a low intensity. It's physiologically true that your body will use more body fat as fuel when you work out at a lower intensity compared to a higher intensity. But sitting burns even more fat as fuel than walking leisurely does and you don't hear anyone telling us to not exercise in order to burn fat, right? The truth is that weight loss depends on the total calories burned, not the sources of those calories. You burn far more calories working harder for less time than working less hard for longer.

For example, in high-intensity exercise (performed at about 70 percent maximum heart rate), 33 percent of the energy you use comes from fat

and 66 percent comes from glucose. You're burning about 600 calories per hour (200 calories from fat). In low-intensity exercise (the fat burning zone, which is working at roughly 50 to 60 percent maximum heart rate), your fat-to-glucose usage is almost fifty-fifty. You're burning 350 calories per hour (175 calories from fat).

Instead of: Stationary bike
Try: Elliptical machine

Calories Burned in 30 Minutes:	
Stationary bike (6-minute-mile pace)	148
Elliptical machine (moderate pace)	337
Bonus: 189 extra calories burned, or 128 percent more calories	

The Benefit: Both are great forms of low-impact cardio and are easy on the joints. But you'll get more calorie burn for your time by choosing the elliptical. Why? You're standing, bearing your own weight, which uses more muscles, even your core muscles. And ellipticals with handles you can push or pull also engage your upper body, helping you burn more calories than pedaling with your legs alone.

Instead of: Other cardio machines
Try: Rowing machine

Calories Burned in 30 Minutes:	
Stair-stepping machine	224
Rowing machine (moderate to vigorous pace)	318
Bonus: 94 extra calories burned, or 42 percent more calories	

The Benefit: Rowing is one of the most effective forms of cardio because it engages 80 percent of your muscles. Almost nothing can top its calorie-burning potential.

Instead of: Walking or running on a treadmill
Try: Walking or running outdoors

Calories Burned in 30 Minutes:	
Running on a treadmill (10-minute-mile pace)	355
Running outdoors (10-minute-mile pace)	374
Bonus: 19 extra calories burned, or 5 percent more calories	

The Benefit: The treadmill actually propels your body, so you do less work on your own. That means you're not burning as many calories as you would if you did the same workout outside. Run outdoors to burn about 5 percent more calories.

Instead of: Any other swimming stroke
Try: Freestyle swimming

Calories Burned:	
Breaststroke (15 minutes)	187
Freestyle swimming (30 minutes)	224
Bonus: 37 extra calories burned, or 20 percent more calories	

The Benefit: Most recreational swimmers don't have the skill or technique needed to perform other swimming strokes at high enough levels—and for long enough—to get a good workout. Most people, however, can execute a freestyle stroke longer and with greater intensity, which translates into a better workout. Freestyle swimming also recruits more muscle fibers than any other stroke.

Even though 30 minutes of the breaststroke would burn more calories, most people can't sustain that kind of a workout, so 30 minutes of the less intense freestyle stroke is a better workout.

Instead of: Doing strength training before cardio
Try: Doing cardio before lifting weights
The Benefit: Which order is better? When it comes to fat burning, do cardio first. Published in the *Journal of Strength and Conditioning Research,* one study examined how many calories exercisers burned doing one of

four workout combinations: running only, strength training only, running followed by strength training, and strength training followed by running. Researchers found that while all exercisers experienced a strong after-burn (a higher rate of calories burned when at rest after exercise) for the two hours after working out, the strength-training-only and the running-then-strength-training groups had the highest exercise after-burn of all. So what does this mean? Although it's just one study, the conclusion is that we might burn more calories after working out if we do our cardio first.

Strength-Training Spark Swaps

Instead of: Crunches
Try: Planks
The Benefit: Basic crunches only engage one of the muscles in your core. Plus, they're not that functional and can lead to back problems (especially if you already suffer from back pain). The plank is the hero of core exercises. It engages every muscle in the core and abs, plus the back and shoulders, and even the legs.

Instead of: Low weights with high reps
Try: Heavier weights with fewer reps
The Benefit: The heavier weight you lift, the bigger the calorie burn. Not to mention, the less time you spend in the gym. In one study, weight lifters torched nearly twice as many calories in the two hours after their workouts when they lifted 85 percent of their maximum load for eight reps than they did when lifting only 45 percent of their maximum load for fifteen reps. For strength training to really be effective, pick a weight that challenges you within eight to fifteen reps. If you can do more reps than that, the weight is too light.

Instead of: Upright rows
Try: Bent-over rows
The Benefit: Upright rows are controversial because the movement can compress the nerves in the shoulder area, impinging the shoulder. Instead,

try bent-over rows, bending forward from the hip and pulling the weights up to your shoulder. This move is safer and also engages more muscles in the back.

Instead of: Biceps curls
Try: Pull-ups
The Benefit: Biceps curls are yet another isolating exercise that recruit just a tiny bit of muscle. Pull-ups are a multitasking move that works tons of muscle groups at once—including your biceps—in a completely functional way. Not strong enough to do full pull-ups? Try the assisted pull-up machine at the gym, or a lat pull-down machine, which works similar muscles.

Instead of: Seated leg-extension machine
Try: Squats
The Benefit: Leg extensions are a very popular exercise for targeting the muscles along the front of your thighs, the quadriceps. The problem is this exercise poses major risks to the knees. Lifting heavy weights in this position, with all the resistance focused at your ankles, is not what the knee was designed to do. If you have any kind of knee problem or use too much resistance during this exercise, you can easily run into big trouble. On top of that, it's an isolating movement that targets a single muscle group, which isn't functional (or a good use of time). Instead, try squats with or without added weight to work your thigh muscles naturally, safely, and effectively. This movement also uses more muscle groups and burns more calories.

Instead of: Donkey kicks
Try: Lunges
The Benefit: Want to reshape your butt? Get off your hands and knees and get on your feet. When the American Council on Exercise compared specific gluteal exercises to a traditional lunge, to see which exercises targeted the butt muscles most effectively, lunges came out on top.

Instead of: Chest presses
Try: Pushups

The Benefit: The chest press is a great move for the chest, shoulders, and triceps, but you'll get more results from pushups. Pushups use the same movement but engage even more muscles, including your core and legs. That means a higher calorie burn and a more functional body, plus a tighter belly. If you're not yet strong enough to do pushups on your toes, modify by placing your knees on the floor.

Instead of: Gym machines
Try: Free weights
The Benefit: You'll be standing, balancing, and using more coordination when using free weights, which means you'll recruit more muscle fibers for better results and a higher calorie burn.

Instead of: Exercising every day
Try: Resting one to two days each week
The Benefit: Your muscles rebuild and your body gets stronger not just during workouts, but also during the recovery period between your exercise sessions. Always allow your body to rest from intense exercise at least one to two times a week. We promise you'll see better gains in strength and endurance, plus avoid burnout.

Simple Ways to Boost Calorie Burn

- *Don't hold on.* Leaning on the handles or console of a cardio machine feels easier for a reason: it takes weight off your lower body so you're not working as hard. Resist the urge to relax or hold on by focusing on good posture.
- *Don't fear the weights.* Strength training can help improve your appearance and boost your metabolism so you burn more calories, even at rest.
- *Use more muscle.* Compound exercises, which work multiple muscle groups at once, save you time. Whenever you can, try to combine exercises, working the upper and lower body at the same time.

- *Lower slower.* Use a two-four count during strength training: take two seconds to lift but four seconds to return the weight. Research shows that exercisers who lower the weight in this slow, controlled manner gain nearly twice the strength as those who take less time.

What Counts as Exercise?

We know how important it is to be active, and so we try to count every activity we do as exercise or cardio. Big mistake, and one of the most common ones. While any activity is better than no activity, only those activities that meet the requirements for cardio activity give your body the health and fitness benefits we exercise in order to reap. Plus, tracking calories burned from every little thing you do is misleading. You're only really burning "extra" calories when you're working pretty darn hard, not when you're simply walking leisurely through the mall or doing some light cleaning.

You may think that since you work out regularly you don't need to worry about doing additional active things each day. You hit the gym before work in the morning, so when your spouse brings up the idea of an evening walk with the family after dinner, you think, *I better not overdo it after today's tough workout*. Or when you're rushing through your weekend errands, you park in the closest spot to the door, brushing off the usual advice to park further away because you already worked out today.

Unfortunately, a lot of us fall into the trap of thinking we don't need to be active because we already exercise. But when experts and fitness professionals talk about the benefits of living an active lifestyle, they're talking about one that includes planned workouts and additional daily activity that gets you on your feet. If you think about it, you only spend a few hours in the gym each week. Even if you're there six days a week for an hour at a time, there are still more than a hundred waking hours in your week when you're not exercising. And for those of us with desk jobs, at least forty of those hours are spent sitting. Several more hours involve driving (sitting), watching TV (sitting), playing on the computer (sitting), and other passive activities, like letting the dishwasher wash your dishes for you.

Years ago, there was no such thing as obesity or the health problems associated with it. People were on their feet all day long, simply moving

because they had to in order to survive. We didn't drive long distances, spend hours watching TV, or sit at computers all day. We farmed, weeded, built, tended, carried, walked, harvested, hauled, cooked, and cleaned—everything. On top of that, we didn't have remote controls (or TVs for that matter), dishwashers, washing machines, or automatic lawnmowers. And we think modern life is hard! Just think of the calorie burn and the muscle-building potential of all that activity each day.

Building a More Active Lifestyle

Even though fitness is Nicole's job and her passion, even she tries to squeeze in activity whenever she can. After teaching a Pilates class during lunch (her planned workout for the day), she also bikes to and from the library. On Wednesdays, after an hour-long Spinning class, which always kicks her butt, she also walks for an hour after dinner. At the grocery store, she skips the cart and hauls groceries in a basket. On weekends, she rarely sits down. She visits the farmers' market or pick-your-own farm, washes dishes by hand, cooks big batches of food for the week ahead, hang-dries her laundry on the line outside, cleans the house, and mows the lawn, on top of the hour or so she spends in the gym.

These activities aren't workouts, but they burn far more calories than napping or sitting at the computer would. All of it adds up to what experts call an active lifestyle, one that includes planned workouts but also light activities, some of which are work—like gardening—and others of which are more enjoyable—like dancing or a game of bowling.

Here are a few ways you can bring more activity into your fit lifestyle, no matter how much time you have on your hands:

- For a dinner out, choose a place within walking distance of your house (up to two miles away) and walk to and from the restaurant.
- At work, opt for the restroom farthest away from your workstation. (With all that water you're drinking, those steps will surely add up!)
- Take the stairs any chance you get: at work, the mall, and even in your home.
- Shun some labor-saving devices, like remotes and the dishwasher, a few nights a week.

- When watching TV, try a few simple exercises, like the plank, pushups, squats, or lunges.

- Play with your kids (or your pet). Don't be an onlooker. Get involved. I only have a dog, but she loves a game where I chase her around the house. It's intense enough to get my heart rate up.

- Choose active dates and outings with friends: bowling, Ping-Pong, and miniature golf will keep you on your toes and off your tush.

- Sit on an exercise ball at your computer to help strengthen your core and posture muscles.

- Wear a pedometer. It'll encourage you to walk more often, and you'll be surprised at the number of creative ways you'll find to get on your feet.

Remember, there's more to fitness than just working out. You'll feel stronger, fitter, and more energetic when you incorporate little bursts of activity into your days on top of working out. Plus, you'll burn more calories, which can help you manage your weight.

51 Ways to Burn 100 Extra Calories*

Exercises

Bicycling: 23 minutes at a casual pace
Cardio dance class: 15 minutes
Elliptical machine: 8 minutes
Jumping rope: 9 minutes at a moderate intensity
Lifting weights: 15 minutes at a vigorous intensity
Pilates: 24 minutes
Rowing machine: 13 minutes
Running: 9 minutes at a 10-minute-mile pace
Running stairs: 6 minutes
Swimming: 15 minutes at a moderate intensity
Walking: 20 minutes at a 20-minute-mile pace
Walking stairs: 11 minutes
Water aerobics: 23 minutes
Yoga: 20 minutes
Zumba: 11 minutes

Sports and Leisure Activities

Basketball, shooting hoops: 20 minutes
Bowling: 30 minutes
Dancing around your living room: 20 minutes
Darts: 35 minutes
Football, playing catch: 35 minutes
Frisbee: 30 minutes
Golfing, carrying your own clubs: 15 minutes
Miniature golf or a driving range: 30 minutes
Ice skating: 18 minutes at a moderate pace
Kickball: 13 minutes
Skiing, downhill: 10 minutes
Soccer: 13 minutes at a casual pace
Softball or baseball: 18 minutes

CONTINUED ON PAGE 350

Tennis, doubles: 21 minutes
Tennis, singles: 15 minutes
Treading water: 23 minutes at a moderate intensity
Volleyball, recreational: 26 minutes
Waterskiing: 15 minutes

Yard Work

Mowing the lawn: 20 minutes
Painting the house: 18 minutes
Raking leaves: 23 minutes
Shoveling snow: 15 minutes
Washing the car: 20 minutes
Weeding the garden: 18 minutes

Everyday Activities

Carrying an infant: 24 minutes
Cleaning: 26 minutes at a moderate intensity
Cooking: 34 minutes
Getting frisky: 15 minutes
Mopping the floor: 20 minutes
Playing with the kids: 23 minutes
Pushing a stroller: 35 minutes
Rearranging furniture: 14 minutes
Shopping: 38 minutes
Sweeping: 23 minutes
Walking the dog: 26 minutes
Washing dishes: 40 minutes

*Calories are approximate

NEAT Sheet

Date			
Time of Day	**Activity**	**Minutes Sitting**	**Minutes Standing or Moving**
Woke up:			
Total Minutes Awake:		**Total Minutes Sitting:**	**Total Minutes Standing or Moving:**
To calculate the percent of your day spent sitting, divide your total minutes sitting by your total minutes awake:			

Total Sitting _____ ÷ **Total Awake** _____ = _____ **percent**

Menu of Workouts

Changing up your cardio while meeting your goals can be tricky for new exercisers, so we took the guesswork out of it. We selected ten common workouts for several calorie ranges so you can choose a cardio activity based on the amount you want to burn on any given day. You can also see how your favorite workouts stack up in terms of efficiency. (For more ideas or specific activities, visit SparkPeople.com.)

How long will it take to burn . . .

200 Calories?

- Bicycling: 46 minutes at a casual pace cycling around town
- Bicycling on a stationary machine: 24 minutes
- Cardio dance class: 30 minutes
- Elliptical machine: 16 minutes
- Intervals of walking and running: 26 minutes at a 10-minute-mile pace or slower
- Jumping rope: 18 minutes at a moderate intensity
- Running: 18 minutes at a 10-minute-mile pace
- Walking: 40 minutes at a 20-minute-mile pace
- Water aerobics: 46 minutes
- Yoga, power, or vinyasa style: 42 minutes

300 Calories?

- Bicycling on a stationary machine: 36 minutes
- Cardio dance class: 45 minutes
- Elliptical machine: 24 minutes
- Intervals of walking and running: 39 minutes at a 10-minute-mile pace or slower
- Jumping rope: 27 minutes at a moderate intensity
- Running: 27 minutes at a 10-minute-mile pace
- Swimming: 45 minutes at a moderate intensity
- Walking: 32 minutes at a 15-minute-mile pace
- Walking: 60 minutes at a 20-minute-mile pace
- Yoga, power, or vinyasa style: 63 minutes

400 Calories?

- Bicycling on a stationary machine: 48 minutes
- Cardio dance class: 60 minutes
- Elliptical machine: 32 minutes
- Intervals of walking and running: 52 minutes at a 10-minute-mile pace or slower
- Running: 36 minutes at a 10-minute-mile pace
- Spinning: 44 minutes
- Stair-stepping machine: 52 minutes
- Walking: 54 minutes at a 15-minute-mile pace
- Walking: 44 minutes at a 15-minute-mile pace with a 5 percent incline
- Zumba: 44 minutes

500 Calories or More?

- Elliptical machine: 40 minutes
- Intervals of walking and running: 65 minutes at a 10-minute-mile pace or slower
- Running: 35 minutes at a 9-minute-mile pace
- Running: 45 minutes at a 10-minute-mile pace
- Spinning: 55 minutes
- Stair-stepping machine: 65 minutes
- Swimming: 75 minutes at a moderate intensity
- Tennis: 55 minutes
- Walking: 55 minutes at a 15-minute-mile pace with a 5 percent incline
- Zumba: 55 minutes

Shopping Lists

Week 1

Protein

8 to 10 ounces raw, unsalted almonds (amount for both weeks)

½ pound reduced-sodium bacon (amount for both weeks)

3 ounces Canadian bacon (amount for both weeks)

2 15-ounce cans low-sodium black beans

1 15-ounce can cannellini (white kidney) beans (if you can't find, use Great Northern or navy beans)

2½ pounds boneless, skinless chicken breasts

1 pound bone-in chicken breasts

1 dozen large eggs

1 pound white-fleshed fish (such as cod or tilapia)

1½ pounds 96 percent lean ground beef

1 12- or 16-ounce jar natural unsalted peanut butter (amount for both weeks)

0.5 ounces (1 tablespoon) shelled, unsalted pistachios (or another type of nut, if preferred)

1 pound pork tenderloin

1 ounce reduced-fat breakfast-style sausage

4 ounces fresh or frozen shrimp (about 4 medium)

1 2.6-ounce can or pouch chunk tuna, packed in water

3 ounces low-sodium deli-sliced turkey

Dairy

4 ounces (1 stick) unsalted butter (amount for both weeks)

1 pound (16 ounces) low-fat cheddar cheese (amount for both weeks)

4 ounces 2 percent cottage cheese

2 ounces (or small container) low-fat feta cheese

½ pound (8 ounces) Monterey jack cheese

½ pound (8 ounces) Parmesan cheese (amount for both weeks)

2 to 3 ounces low-fat Swiss cheese (amount for both weeks)

1 pint slow-churned vanilla frozen yogurt (amount for both weeks and more)

1 pint slow-churned ice cream (amount for both weeks)

1¼ gallons skim milk

1 ounce (1 tablespoon) light whipped topping

1 quart plain, fat-free plain Greek yogurt (may use low-fat sour cream for ¼ cup of this, if preferred)

4 ounces light Key lime pie yogurt (swap another flavor or plain Greek yogurt, if preferred)

4 ounces light strawberry yogurt (swap for plain Greek yogurt, if preferred)

Veggies

FRESH

1 avocado

2 bell peppers (1 red, 1 green)

1 pound carrots

1 head of celery (amount for both weeks)

1 small bunch cilantro

3 cucumbers (1 English variety, if possible)

1 head garlic

2 small knobs gingerroot, or 1 small jar minced ginger, no sugar added (amount for both weeks)

¾ pound green beans (or 2 cups frozen)

1 small bunch green onions

2 to 3 ounces red leaf lettuce (or buy 1 head; one leaf to be used next week)

2 heads Romaine lettuce or 4 to 8 ounces bagged Romaine or mixed greens

¼ to ½ ounce mint

3 to 4 ounces mushrooms

1 large red onion

2 white or yellow onions

1 bunch parsley

2 small parsnips

1 pound fingerling potatoes (about 12)

3 medium red potatoes

6 radishes (or 1 small bunch)

6 ounces packaged rainbow slaw

¼ to ½ ounce rosemary

15 to 20 ounces bagged spinach

½ to ¾ ounce thyme

3 slicing tomatoes

1½ pints grape or cherry tomatoes

2 small zucchini

CANNED

24 ounces jarred low-sodium salsa

FROZEN

12 to 14 ounces corn kernels

8 ounces stir-fry vegetables

Fruit

FRESH

3 apples

2 bananas

4 to 6 ounces blackberries or other choice of berries (can opt for frozen)

1 pint blueberries (or 8 to 10 ounces frozen)

⅛ or less cantaloupe (about ½ cup chopped)

2 to 3 ounces cherries (can opt for frozen)

1 medium bunch grapes (amount for both weeks)

⅛ or less honeydew melon (about ½ cup chopped)

1 kiwi

2 lemons

1 lime

2 oranges

1 peach

1 small pineapple (about 1 cup chopped, plus save 2 slices for next week, or buy canned)

1 pint strawberries

1 small watermelon (1 cup chopped)

CANNED OR DRIED

4 ounces jarred unsweetened applesauce

4 to 6 ounces dried cranberries (about 4 tablespoons) (amount for both weeks)

4 ounces fruit cocktail in water or juice (or other canned or fresh fruit)

4 ounces mandarin oranges packed in water or juice

Grains

*Note: You will have extra bread products
for next week*

1 loaf whole-wheat bread

1 10-ounce box whole-wheat couscous

1 pound whole-wheat flour

6 ounces whole-wheat elbow macaroni

1 32- to 48-ounce canister old-fashioned oats

1 8-ounce box panko (Japanese-style
breadcrumbs) or whole-wheat
breadcrumbs, if you can't find panko

1 6-count package whole-wheat pitas

1 approximately 1-ounce single-serving bag
unsalted pretzels

8 to 16 ounces brown rice (heat-and-eat is fine)

1 14-ounce box instant brown rice

1 8-count package whole-wheat Sandwich
Thins

1 10- or 12-count package 6-inch corn tortillas

1 10- or 12-count package 7-inch whole-
wheat tortillas

1 approximately 1-ounce single-serving bag
baked tortilla chips

Drinks

1 12-ounce can light beer (optional)

flavored water (optional)

Pantry Items

baking powder

baking soda

balsamic vinaigrette

balsamic vinegar

black pepper

brown sugar

capers (optional)

chili powder

dark chocolate or dark chocolate chips,
plus 2 dark chocolate kisses

light chocolate syrup (optional)

cinnamon

cooking spray (olive oil or vegetable oil)

cornstarch

ground cumin

curry powder (yellow and dark varieties)

Dijon mustard

flaxseeds (ground, if you don't have a grinder)

graham crackers (low-fat honey or cinnamon)

honey

hot sauce

hummus

ice cream cone (sugar or plain, as you prefer)

all-fruit or reduced-sugar jam

real maple syrup

olive-oil mayonnaise

microwave popcorn

miso paste

olive oil

onion powder

whole-wheat pancake mix

smoked paprika

sweet paprika

light ranch dressing

red pepper flakes

red wine vinegar

salt

toasted sesame oil

low-sodium soy sauce

sugar

tartar sauce

dried thyme

vanilla extract

white wine vinegar

Week 2

Protein

2 15-ounce cans low-sodium black beans

1 15-ounce can cannellini (white kidney) beans (if you can't find, use Great Northern or navy beans)

¾ pound 96 percent lean ground beef

1¾ pounds boneless, skinless chicken breasts

20 ounces homemade or low-sodium chicken stock

8 boneless, skinless chicken thighs (about 1½ pounds)

1 pound cod or other white-fleshed fish

1 dozen large eggs

2 slices lean deli-sliced ham (or another type of meat, if preferred)

2 to 3 ounces dry-roasted unsalted peanuts (or another type of nut, if preferred)

3 ounces extra-lean roast beef

1 pound salmon fillets

½ pound extra-lean ground turkey breast

Dairy

2 to 3 ounces crumbled blue cheese (optional)

4 ounces 2 percent cottage cheese

1 to 2 ounces low-fat cream cheese

1 ounce provolone cheese (or use Monterey jack left over from last week)

2 ounces part-skim ricotta cheese

1 ounce string cheese (or use Monterey jack left over from last week)

8 ounces fat-free evaporated milk

1 gallon skim milk

16 ounces fat-free plain Greek yogurt (may use low-fat sour cream for a few tablespoons of this, if preferred)

8 ounces fat-free vanilla Greek yogurt

Veggies

FRESH

1 pound asparagus

4 avocados

¾ ounce basil

4 green bell peppers

1 head bok choy

1 pound broccoli (or 10 ounces frozen florets)

7 medium carrots

1 small head cauliflower

1 small bunch chives

1 bunch cilantro

1 head garlic

1 small bunch green onions

2 heads or 8 to 10 ounces bagged Romaine lettuce

4 to 5 ounces mushrooms

1 small, 1 medium, and 3 large yellow or white onions

1 large red onion

1 banana pepper

3 hot peppers: 1 red Anaheim, 1 serrano, and 1 of your own heat preference

2 small russet potatoes

3 ounces bagged spinach

1 sun-dried tomato or 1 tablespoon roasted red pepper (fresh, dried, packed in water, or substitute sun-dried tomato paste)

1 sweet potato

2¼ pounds slicing tomatoes

1 pint grape or cherry tomatoes

1 Roma tomato

1 small zucchini

CANNED

1 small jar low-sodium salsa verde

1 15-ounce lentil-vegetable canned soup (or other variety of your choice)

2 15-ounce cans unsalted diced tomatoes

Fruit

FRESH

1 apple

4 bananas

1 pint berries (any kind)

⅛ or less cantaloupe (about ½ cup chopped)

2 lemons

9 limes

2 mangoes

1 orange

1 peach

1 pear

1 pint strawberries

CANNED OR DRIED

1 small can pineapple stored in natural juice (if no fresh is left over from last week)

2 to 3 ounces raisins (about 2 tablespoons)

Grains

1 slice cinnamon-raisin bread (or whole-wheat bread, if preferred)

1 approximately 1-ounce single-serving bag baked potato chips

1 small box low-fat whole-wheat crackers (will use only 4)

1 small package whole-wheat English muffins (will use only 2)

1 pound whole-wheat spaghetti (½ pound could be angel-hair instead)

2 10- or 12-count packages 6-inch corn tortillas

Drinks

1 12-ounce can diet root beer soda

Pantry Items

semisweet chocolate chips (unless you purchased them last week)

unsweetened grated coconut

unsweetened coconut flakes

light coconut milk

whole cumin seed

fig bars

graham crackers (chocolate)

all-fruit orange marmalade

prepared yellow mustard

powdered sugar

light ranch dressing

lemon sorbet

ice cream sprinkles (optional)

Sriracha (Thai hot sauce)

vegetable oil

red wine

Worcestershire sauce

Chances are, you already have plenty of the items we included in our weekly shopping list. If your kitchen is already well stocked, use the following template to create a shopping list that suits your needs and your budget:

Protein	Fruit (fresh or frozen)
Dairy	**Fruit (canned or dried)**
Vegetables (fresh or frozen)	**Grains**
Vegetables (canned or dried)	**Drinks**
Pantry	

About the Authors

Becky Hand, R.D., M.Ed.

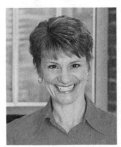

Becky Hand's teenage son and friends bolted in the back door and headed straight for the brownies cooling on the counter. "May we have some, Mrs. Hand?" they asked as they poured themselves glasses of milk. "Of course," she answered, cutting the brownies and plating them with a scheming smile on her face. The boys sang praises about those brownies, so Becky just had to let them in on the secret ingredient: puréed black beans. "What?" they screamed, mouths dropping wide open.

As a registered dietitian for more than twenty-five years, Becky knows that a sense of humor goes a long way when introducing unfamiliar foods and developing new eating habits. She is passionate about improving the health and wellness of people in her rural community as well as the lives of people throughout the world via SparkPeople. Whether it be during her weekly radio talk show, planting seeds at a school's veggie garden, bringing farm-fresh produce to the local hospital's cafeteria, coaching adults and children during their weight-loss adventures, or tackling a tricky question on the message boards at SparkPeople, Becky is deeply dedicated to the mission of health improvement and disease prevention.

Becky enjoys the slower pace of her life on the family farm in southern Indiana, where she lives with her husband and son, and she connects weekly with her daughter, who is attending college, also in Indiana. Becky unwinds by digging in the soil of her small vegetable and herb garden, preparing new recipes, sewing, and walking in the woods with her canine companions. She is committed to having her family eat meals together at the kitchen table—it is often the only time to connect and catch up—and eagerly encourages other families to do the same.

Stepfanie Romine

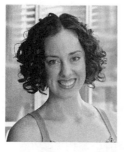

Stepfanie Romine is editorial director at SparkPeople.com. She manages *DailySpark,* the healthy living blog written by the site's experts, and *SparkRecipes,* where she develops and curates healthy recipes. A certified yoga teacher since 2009, she earned degrees in French and journalism from Ohio University. Romine began her career as a newspaper copy editor, business reporter, and columnist.

After more than a decade of disordered eating habits and an unhealthy obsession with dieting, Romine steadily gained weight in her early twenties. In 2005, while teaching essay writing in Seoul, South Korea, she joined a gym and committed to losing the excess weight. She shed almost fifty pounds and learned to love healthy living.

Until joining the SparkPeople team in 2008, Romine still saw exercise as an obligation. Since then, she has found her passion for fitness: She learned to ride a bike, started running, and took up hiking. She has a daily Ashtanga yoga practice and is training for her third half marathon. Exercise changed her life, freeing her from anxiety and providing stress relief.

Romine and her boyfriend, Sam, along with their two cats, recently moved to the North Carolina mountains in search of a simpler life with healthy living at the forefront. This is her second book.

Meg Galvin

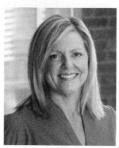

At SparkPeople.com, Chef Meg Galvin develops healthy recipes, tests some of our best member-submitted dishes, and teaches the fundamentals of cooking through informative and entertaining videos, blogs, and articles. A World Master Chef since 2005 (one of only twenty women in the world with that title), Chef Meg hosted the regional television show *The Dish* and a series of cooking videos on a local station. She has appeared on TV and radio, and in print, both locally and nationally as a SparkPeople expert. A faculty member at the Midwest Culinary Institute at Cincinnati State Technical and Community College, she trained at Le Cordon Bleu in London and uses clas-

sical French cooking methods and farm-fresh foods to create flavorful and satisfying healthy dishes.

Raised in a large farm family in central Kentucky, Chef Meg now lives in northern Kentucky with her husband and three teenage sons. On any given day, this world-class chef can be found hitting the pavement on long runs or cheering on her boys at their numerous sporting events. She balances her busy schedule by incorporating her home life and career, bringing her kids into the kitchen, and testing recipes on—and with—her family. This is her second book.

Nicole Nichols

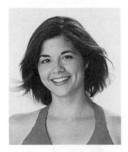

Nicole is a fitness trainer and health educator who helps people of all skill levels integrate simple but powerful fitness techniques into their daily lives. She's known for her approachable style, which makes working out fun and accessible. Coach Nicole contributes regularly to magazines, websites, television programs, and radio, helping to motivate people to live healthier lives. In 2011, Nicole received national recognition as America's Top Personal Trainer to Watch by the American Council on Exercise and Life Fitness.

Nicole has designed and taught health programs on the topics of eating disorders, body image, and self-acceptance; strength training for women; exercise for seniors; and prenatal exercise. She has created two major fitness DVDs along with more than fifty free workout videos, making her one of the most-watched exercise instructors on the Internet.

Nicole has a bachelor's degree in health promotion and education, specializing in exercise and fitness, from the University of Cincinnati. She currently holds a chair on the dean's advisory council for the College of Human Services at the University of Cincinnati, where she was the youngest graduate to ever receive their Distinguished Alumni honor. Nicole maintains several fitness certifications, including ACE Personal Training, AFAA Group Exercise, efi Sports Medicine Group and Personal Training, Spinning, PiYo, and prenatal and postpartum exercise design, and is comprehensively trained in mat and reformer Pilates through Balanced Body University. She is the editor-in-chief of SparkPeople.com.

Chris "SparkGuy" Downie

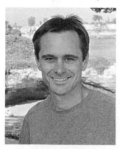 Chris "SparkGuy" Downie is the founder and CEO of SparkPeople, where he and his team "spark" millions of people to reach their goals and lead healthier lives. After earning a business administration degree from the University of Cincinnati, Downie worked for Procter & Gamble, where he used proven health, goal-setting, and motivation techniques to get fit, manage stress, and create the fuel he needed to reach his goals. Inspired by his success, Downie left Procter & Gamble to cofound an Internet company that became eBay's first acquisition. With the freedom and capital to do whatever he wanted, Downie founded SparkPeople in 2001. Today, SparkPeople has nearly forty employees, has more than fourteen million members around the world, and operates eight websites. His innovations include SparkCoach, a personalized virtual coaching program that helps people reach their goals, and SparkAmerica, a national campaign to help people get more exercise, eat healthier foods, and enjoy active, healthy lives. As SparkPeople's resident motivation expert, Downie corresponds directly with members daily. A hands-on CEO, Downie has written more than ten thousand personal messages to members, offering encouragement and congratulations alike. Downie frequently "spreads the spark" via motivational speeches and events and in the national media. Downie is the author of the *New York Times* bestseller *The Spark*. He lives in California with his wife, Karina, and two sons.

About SparkPeople.com

SparkPeople.com is one of the leading diet, fitness, and healthy-living destinations on the web, with more than fourteen million members; free weight-loss, nutrition, and fitness-tracking tools; and a positive community of people committed to reaching their goals and supporting one another along the way. SparkPeople combines the science of nutrition and fitness with the science of motivation and the power of social networking. The company has eight websites, including SparkRecipes.com, with more than 444,000 healthy and delicious recipes. Join us online. Use special code SPARKSOLUTION to get your SparkPoints.

Acknowledgments

SparkPeople Would Like to Thank

The SparkPeople experts and coaches who contributed to this book, including Dean Anderson, Chris "SparkGuy" Downie, Jen Mueller, Nicole Nichols, and Dr. Birdie Varnedore.

Erin Aiello, Tina Sweep, Stacey, Julia, Beth Donovan, and all the other members who contributed to the book. Thank you for sharing your success with us!

Catherine Murray (Photo Kitchen), our incredible food photographer, who brought our Spark Solution meals to life on these pages along with her assistants, Beth and Missy.

Our agent, Stephanie Tade, for her contagious enthusiasm and sage advice. Thank you for believing in us—again!

Our editor, Gideon Weil, for his incredible insight, guidance, and vision. You get us. Welcome to the SparkPeople family.

Our assistant editor, Babette Dunkelgrun, for her invaluable assistance throughout the entire process and her keen eye for details.

Jessie Hoffman of Parlour and Diane Amon, for their hair and makeup skills at the photo shoots.

Peggy Neal, for testing every recipe in the book and sharing her remarkable talent as a food stylist.

Peggy Beebe, for her assistance in food prep and styling.

Elliott Giles for taking the fitness photos, and Fran Santangelo of Bene-FIT Studio for allowing us to use her space for those photos.

Julie Niesen Gosdin for the use of her lovely kitchen as the backdrop for our photos.

Malinda Hartong, for our author headshots.

Becky Would Like to Thank

My mom and dad, who exposed me to the ultimate labor of love: fresh foods from the family farm.

My husband, Eric, who encourages me daily to reach for the stars.

My children, Rachel and Nathan, who pitched in and assisted with all the household chores so that I could dedicate the time to writing this book.

Stepfanie Romine, for continued support and encouragement that "it would become a book."

My SparkPeople family for igniting the spark in "this old flame" by pushing me to new heights and awesome adventures. A big woohoo to all of you!

Stepfanie Would Like to Thank

Sam Klontz, for his constant support, for not letting me take anything too seriously, and for handling our big move to the mountains while I wrote this book. I love you.

Becky Hand, for taking this leap of faith with me. We wrote a book!

Meg Galvin, for her continued commitment to making our books the best they can be and for working, without complaint, on an incredibly short deadline. We did it again!

Tami Corwin, for yet another opportunity to help change lives, and for your invaluable guidance. Our eleventh-hour editing sessions make me a stronger writer.

Chris Downie, for creating SparkPeople and a life-changing culture that makes me excited to go to work each morning, and for helping me see life (and this book) through a different lens.

Kim Nietch, my Ashtanga yoga teacher and friend, for all those early-morning Mysore practices. Without yoga, so much would be impossible.

Gideon Weil, for your unwavering confidence and trust. Thank you for having faith in me as a writer.

Meg Would Like to Thank

My family, both those living in the house putting up with all the madness and the ones a telephone call away. My husband, Mark, and sons, Noah, Ian, and Josh, for stepping up to the plate (or should I say the sink?) and helping with dishes, groceries, and household chores. They have become certified tasters! My sister, Ann, Dad, and Betty for the phone calls of encouragement and support.

The SparkPeople team for all their faith in me and commitment to spreading the word that it's easy and fun to live a healthy lifestyle.

Index

INCREASE YOUR ODDS OF
WEIGHT-LOSS SUCCESS
WITH SPARKCOACH!

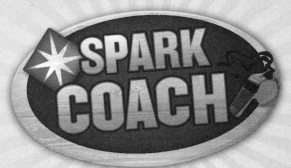

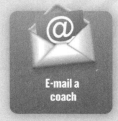 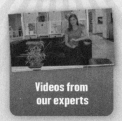 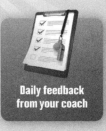

E-mail a coach | **Videos from our experts** | **Daily feedback from your coach**

Don't lose momentum! Stay motivated!
Get a FREE trial today at
www.SparkCoach.com

With SparkCoach you'll get:

- A personalized program with daily guidance and feedback

- Video-based virtual coaching and instruction from our experts

- Direct access to SparkPeople coaches via e-mail—including SparkGuy and the authors of *The Spark Solution*

Start your FREE TRIAL today
at www.SparkCoach.com

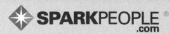

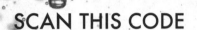

SCAN THIS CODE
WITH YOUR SMARTPHONE TO BE LINKED TO
THE BONUS MATERIALS FOR

THE SPARK SOLUTION

on the Elixir mobile website,
where you can also find information about other
healthy living books and related materials.

YOU CAN ALSO TEXT
SPARK to READIT (732348)

to be sent a link to the Elixir mobile website.

Facebook.com/elixirliving   Twitter.com/elixirliving   www.elixirliving.com

P9-DNX-318